NEUROSCIENCE RESEARCH PROGRESS

THE DENTATE GYRUS

STRUCTURE, FUNCTIONS AND HEALTH IMPLICATIONS

NEUROSCIENCE RESEARCH PROGRESS

Additional books and e-books in this series can be found on Nova's website under the Series tab.

NEUROSCIENCE RESEARCH PROGRESS

THE DENTATE GYRUS

STRUCTURE, FUNCTIONS AND HEALTH IMPLICATIONS

FENG-RU TANG
EDITOR

nova
Medicine & Health
New York

DOI: https://doi.org/10.52305/CGUL9251

Library of Congress Cataloging-in-Publication Data

ISBN: 978-1-68507-212-4

Published by Nova Science Publishers, Inc. † New York

CONTENTS

PREFACE

The dentate gyrus (DG) is one of the most sensitive regions to various brain insults due to the occurrence of neurogenesis in its subgranular zone. Thus, it may serve as a brain sensor to radiation exposure, chemical and biological toxins, alcohol abuse, smoking, drug treatments, hormone imbalances, stress, pain, hypoxia, brain trauma, malnutrition and aging. DG is also involved in the pathogenesis of multiple neurological and neuropsychological disorders including intractable temporal lobe epilepsy (TLE), Alzheimer's disease (AD), major depressive disorder (MDD), post-traumatic stress disorder (PTSD), and schizophrenia.

Over decades of research, our understanding regarding the function and physiology of the DG is ever-changing. While it is commonly believed that the dentate granule cells are primarily responsible for executing higher brain functions such as learning and memory, there is increasing evidence demonstrating that the glial cells, particularly microglia, astrocytes and oligodendrocytes, are also involved in memory formation. Therefore, a book that systematically reviews DG structure, function and health implications is needed to update clinicians and researchers with state-of-the-art knowledge.

In the first three chapters of this book, the recent progresses in the study of DG development with relevant molecular mechanisms, the cytoarchitectonics of DG with laminar and sublaminar distribution of different types of neurons and glial cells, as well as afferent and efferent of the DG and their neurophysiological roles will be described respectively. In Chapters 4 and 5, DG as a brain sensor to radiation exposure, and pre- and post-natal radiation-induced DG damage and cognitive impairment will be reviewed accordingly. The involvement of DG in pathogenesis of neurological disorders including TLE and AD will be discussed in Chapters 6 and 7. Finally, in the last two chapters, i.e., Chapters 8 and 9, the roles of DG in the development of neuropsychological disorders including MDD, PTSD and schizophrenia will be presented.

Neurologists, neuroscientists, neuropsychologists, radio-oncologists, paramedics and medical students will find this book informative and timely for the current understanding of the normal physiology of DG, and its role in the development of cognitive impairment after radiotherapy or accident ionizing radiation exposure and of other neurological and neuropsychological disorders.

Dr. Feng-Ru Tang
Singapore Nuclear Research and Safety Initiative,
National University of Singapore

In: The Dentate Gyrus
Editor: Feng-Ru Tang
ISBN: 978-1-68507-212-4

Chapter 1

THE DEVELOPMENT OF THE DENTATE GYRUS AND THE RELEVANT MOLECULAR MECHANISMS INVOLVED

Kimberly Ho Jen Ni*
Radiation Physiology Lab,
Singapore Nuclear Research and Safety Initiative,
National University of Singapore, Singapore

ABSTRACT

The dentate gyrus is the structure that governs continuing neurogenesis in adult mammals. As such, its development and the molecular mechanisms involved are of great scientific interest. Such an important function is of course regulated by a wide variety of molecular mechanisms and structures. There have therefore been many studies done on the subject; however, most studies have a narrow focus on a few select mechanisms. In this chapter, we hope to provide a thorough overview of the full process of dentate gyrus development, through examining both the histological process of development as well as a list of the molecular mechanisms involved.

* Corresponding Author's Email: snrkhjn@nus.edu.sg.

Keywords: dentate gyrus, development, neurogenesis, molecular mechanisms, precursor cells, radial glia, Cajal-Retzius cells, Reelin, Wnt, BMP, NeuroD, Sox2, SDF1/CXCR4

INTRODUCTION

As the site responsible for adult neurogenesis, it is essential for the dentate gyrus to sustain the relevant precursor cell niche in the subgranular zone. This process is likely reliant on the developmental mechanisms involved in the formation of the dentate gyrus. There have been several studies outlining the developmental process of the dentate gyrus [1, 2], as well as the molecular mechanisms underpinning such [3]; however, there are few studies which describe both in the context of each other. As such, in this chapter, we consolidate and synthesise the current body of knowledge on the formation of the dentate gyrus, to provide a comprehensive view of both the histological and molecular processes involved in the development of the dentate gyrus. This chapter will be split into three parts. Firstly, we will explore the histological development of the dentate gyrus. Secondly, we will focus on some of the more prominent molecular mechanisms involved. finally, we will summarise the first two sections and provide an overview of the roles of various molecular mechanisms in each stage of DG development, as well as provide some suggestions on future research directions.

HISTOLOGICAL DEVELOPMENT OF THE DENTATE GYRUS

We will first describe the histological development of the dentate gyrus. This section shall be split into two parts. In the first part, we outline the key structures involved in dentate gyrus development, followed by the outline of the process of DG development.

Key Structures in Development of the Dentate Gyrus

According to Hatami [3], there are four main key structures implicated in the development of the dentate gyrus. These are the cortical hem (CH) and anti-hem, the radial glia, Cajal-Retzius cells, and the meninges surrounding the developing dentate gyrus.

Cortical Hem (CH) and Anti-Hem

The cortical hem (CH) and anti-hem are long, narrow stripes which run rostro-caudally along the neuroepithelium, which is the precursor to the cerebral cortex. The neuroepithelium is flanked by the CH medially, and laterally by the anti-hem [4]. These two structures are patterning/signalling centres which secrete signal morphogens responsible for providing spatial cues and regulating the proliferation and structure of the developing cortex [3]. In particular, the CH is responsible for secreting important ligands involved in the formation of the DG, Wnt and BMP, and any deficiencies in this structure can cause abnormal development of the hippocampus [5].

Radial Glia

Radial glia are specialised cells present in the developing nervous system of all vertebrates, identifiable by their long radial processes. They are best known as support cells, facilitating the migration of newly matured neurons [6]. In the context of dentate gyrus development, they form a horseshoe-shaped scaffold, which is an early indicator of the eventual shape of the dentate gyrus [2]. This scaffold begins at the fimbrial region and runs to the pial side of the cortex and hippocampal fissure (HF) [3].

Cajal-Retzius Cells (CR)

Cajal Retzius cells are a unique class of neurons, possessed of an unusual morphology with characteristic horizontal dendrites [7]. They are found in the marginal zone/layer I of the developing and adult cortex, throughout all vertebrates except fish [8]. They mainly originate from the CH, close to the hippocampal primodium. Other sources include the pallial septum and the ventral pallium [7]. They produce Reelin, a protein required for the migration of neurons along the radial glial scaffold [3].

Surrounding Meninges

The meninges are three membranes that surround the brain and spinal cord. In mammals, they are the dura mater, the arachnoid mater, and the pia mater. Cerebrospinal fluid is found in the subarachnoid space between the arachnoid mater and the pia mater. The meninges surrounding the developing dentate gyrus secrete bone morphogenic protein 7 (BMP7), which is implicated in dentate gyrus granule cell differentiation [3].

Stages in the Development of the Dentate Gyrus

As a biological process, the development of the dentate gyrus is not strictly demarcated into clearly delineated stages. Various studies utilise their own methods of outlining the developmental stages of the dentate gyrus. In this chapter, we will be following Li's [9] division of the dentate gyrus into 6 distinct steps: 1) the definition of the dentate neuroepithelium, 2) the formation of the primary radial glial scaffolding, 3) the radial migration of granule neurons to form the primordial granule cell layer, 4) the establishment of the precursor pool in the hilus, 5) the radial transformation of the tertiary matrix, and finally 6) the differentiation of the dentate granule cells.

Defining the Dentate Neuroepithelium

The development of the dentate gyrus begins with the expansion of the undifferentiated neuroepithelium sheet of the early cortical primordium, of which the hippocampal formation comprises the most caudomedial portion [3]. At this point, the hippocampus and dentate gyrus are still indistinguishable from the cortex as a whole [9]. Signal morphogens are produced from the CH and anti-hem, which provide spatial cues and regulate the regional proliferation and architecture in the developing cortex [10]. Differentiation of the cortical neuroepithelium is thus initiated. The cortical neuropithelium generates a blueprint for the eventual structure of the cortex in response to the signal morphogens via region-specific neurogenesis and gliogenesis [3]. During this process, the dentate neuroepithelium is thus defined as part of the medial pallium ventricular zone (VZ).

Forming the Primary Radial Glial Scaffolding

Once the dentate neuroepithelium has been defined, the next distinctly identifiable morphological event is the generation of the primary radial glial scaffold utilised by early granule cells to migrate from the VZ towards the hippocampal fissure (HF). The scaffold is first apparent in mice at around E14.5 and can be identified using markers expressed in radial glial cells [11]. This scaffold is horseshoe-shaped, an indication of the eventual structre of the dentate gyrus. It originates from the fimbrial region and runs to the pial side of the cortex and the HF [9]. The formation of the scaffold is initiated by a chain of interactions involving reelin (Reln), Disabled1 (Dab), and integrin beta 1 (Itbg1) [12]. The early granule cells migrating along this scaffold constitute the secondary proliferative matrix of the DG. They are a unique phenomenon; they continue undergoing mitotic division at various differentiation stages while they migrate [3]. Cajal-Retzius cells (CR cells) are also involved in this step as they provide factors essential for

DG precusor migration. Alongside the DG precursor cells, they originate in the CH and migrate towards the HF, while producing reelin, encoding a protein required for the migration of neurons along the radial glial scaffold [13, 14].

Radial Migration of Granule Neurons to Form the Primordial Granule Cell Layer

Once the radial glial scaffold has been formed, the immature granule neurons commence their migration towards the hilus. Once there, they form the primodial granule cell layer, otherwise known as the tertiary proliferative matrix [2]. This process is regulated by the receptor CXCR4, which receives the chemokine SDF1, likely by way of functioning as a chemoattractant for granule neurons [15, 16]. This process will be elaborated upon later in the chapter, in the sections focusing on the molecular mechanisms of dentate gyrus development.

Establishing the Precursor Pool in the Hilus

When the DG precursor cells have migrated to the hilus, they continue proliferating in order to establish the pool of precursor neurons required to be maintained for adult neurogenesis. Radial glia also participate in this migration, and have recently been hypothesised to be the actual precursors. Molecules found to be involved in this step include Lef1 and LRP6, in whose absence the amount of actively proliferating precursor cells in the hilus was found to be greatly lessened [17]. The same phenomenon was also observed in the absence of CXCR4 [15, 16].

Radial Transformation of the Tertiary Matrix

At this point, the animal would be ready for birth, but the development of the dentate gyrus is by no means fully completed. This stage as well as the following one take place predominantly as postnatal occurrences. Once the pool of precursor neurons has been established, they start to become more structurally defined and more radially organised. At birth, the radial glial processes still retain their horseshoe formation as established in stage 2 [12], but by P4, they have been shifted to be directly next to the developing granule cell layer. This process is governed by the protein Reelin (Reln). Reln mutants fail to achieve this reorganisation, and the hilus continues to be bereft of radially oriented mature radial glial cells [12-18, 19]. During this stage, the radial glial cells, as well as the CR cells, interact with the pial basement membrane through beta-1 integrin and fak protein signalling in order to form the contours of the dentate gyrus and radial glial scaffolding [12-20]. After the restructuring of the hilus to produce the mature granule cell layer with its fully developed network of radially oriented radial glial processes, the tertiary matrix begins to form in the second week after birth.

Differentiation of Dentate Granule Cells

This final step is one that all neurons must eventually undergo, not just neurons of the dentate gyrus. Cells at this stage undergo a final differentiation into a mature neuron of the appropriate phenotype. This is a complex process which involves a tangled web of signalling networks made up of regulatory transcription factors which are themselves controlled by extracellular signalling cues. For DG cells in particular, the Wnt pathway seems to be essential for the correct development of mature granule neurons; however, the effects of Wnt mutants have been observed to be quite pleiotropic, hence, it is difficult to determine if the Wnt pathway affects later developmental stages directly or indirectly [2].

Molecular Mechanisms Involved in the Development of the Dentate Gyrus

We move on now to the molecular mechanisms involved in the development of the dentate gyrus. There are, of course, a wide variety of molecules and interactions involved in so lengthy a process, so we shall only be going through the most prominent ones. Some molecules will already have been mentioned in the previous subsection. At the end of this chapter, there will be a diagram to summarise which molecules and interactions are involved in which stage of dentate gyrus development.

Reelin Signalling

Reelin (Reln) is an extracellular matrix protein, produced by CR cells, and implicated in stages 3 and 5 of DG development. It affects the radial glial scaffold, granule cell migration, and granule cell orientation. In stage 3, CR cells encode Reln, which triggers the formation of the radial glial scaffold and the migration of the granule cells along the scaffold, via a chain of interactions involving Disabled1 (Dab1) and beta-1 integrin [12]. Mice lacking in the Reln protein, otherwise known as reeler mice, are thus unable to form the radial glial scaffold and direct the migration of granule cells. As a result, they exhibit an absence of the DG granule layer, and demonstrate aberrant placement of granule cells within the hilus. In stage 5, Reln governs the shifting of the radial glial processes to be next to the granule cell layers, and the orientation of the granule cells towards the hippocampal fissure. Reeler mice thus exhibit granule cells whose dendrites are not uniformly pointed towards the hippocampal fissure, and instead are haphazardly orientated in different directions [21].

Wnt

Wnt is a ligand secreted by the CH [22, 23] and is implicated in stages 1, 2, and 4 [2]. In particular, the ligands secreted by the CH are WNT2a, -2b, -3a, and -5a. They are prominently implicated in the proliferation and organisation of the DG precursor pool [24-27]. Most important is Wnt3a, which begins to be expressed quite early on in the development of the DG, and is confined to the CH [22-26]. Effects of mutations in Wnt3a include the absence of the DG at the medial border of the hippocampus, as well as the subiculum, CA1, and CA3 regions being significantly smaller at the caudal region, and totally absent at the rostral region. A lack of the Wnt receptor, low density lipoprotein receptor-related protein 6 (LRP 6), results in severe abnormalities observed in the hippocampus [5]. Furthermore, the presence of several Wnt modulators in the CH greatly supports the idea that strict regulation of Wnt/beta-catenin signalling is essential during hippocampal development.

Bone Morphogenic Proteins (BMPs)

BMPs are a class of proteins, variants of which (BMP4, -5, -6, and -7) are produced by the telencephalic roof plate in early stages of DG development, and later on by the CH [22-24]. Absence of BMP signalling can cause a lack of important structures in the telencephalic medio-dorsal region, such as the choroid plexus (ChP) and the CH, which then results in severe deficiencies in DG development [28, 29]. Once the CH is fully formed, BMPs do not appear to be essential in ascertaining the properties of DG precursor cells. As BMP receptors BMPR-1a and BMPR-1b differ in function, so too do the BMP ligands; BMPR-1a promotes the proliferation of the embryonic telencephalon, while cell cycle arrest and differentiation are governed by BMPR-1b [30]. BMP ligands have also been implicated in the differentiation of DG granule cells. [31] found that BMPs fulfil an important function in maintaining quiescence in neural stem cell (NSC) populations. Deficiency in the receptor BMPR-1a (achieved in vitro through the use of morphogen proteins NOGGIN and CHORDIN to antagonise the BMP population in the mature hippocampal proliferation niche [32, 33]) leads to an overproduction of neurons by adult NSCs, leaving them no resources and energy with which to proliferate and thereby reducing the population of NSCs [31]. BMPs have also been observed in vitro to have the ability to modulate astrocyte gene expression, which supports their capability to induce the expression of specific astroglial characteristics in adult NSCs [34, 35]. The differential expression of BMPR-1a receptors is responsible for the contrary observation that BMPs are required both for the quiescence of NSCs as well as for the differentiation and maturation of granule cells [36]. BMPR-1a is expressed by NSCs in the adult DG, and are promptly downregulated in intermediate precursor cells. In contrast, neurons express BMPR-1b [31- 37]. Lastly, BMP also operates via the activin receptor type 1 (ACVR1), which then induces the expression of Lef1 [38], an important transcription factor gene activated by both WNT and BMP ligands [39]. Lef1 will be later explored in further detail in its own subsection.

SDF1 and CXCR4

Stromal cell-derived factor 1 (SDF1) is a chemokine secreted by CR cells, which interacts with chemokine receptor type 4 (CXCR4). It is a chemoattractive protein that aids DG granule cell precursors in their migration from the neuroepithelium to the DG granule layer [15]. In mice deficient in CXCR4, a large number of granule precursor cells do not reach the DG, and remain as clumps within the hilus [2]. The DG and migration path thus end up with fewer actively dividing cells. Additionally, cell differentiation is irregular, and the DG is smaller and abnormally shaped [16]. This points to SDF1, aside from regulating the migration of granule cell precursors, possibly also being involved in the regulation of their proliferation in the hilus [2].

Lef1

Lef1, as mentioned earlier, is a transcription factor involved in Wnt signalling [40]. It is greatly expressed in the DG precursor cells, but less so in those located in the adjacent (CA) region [41]. It is implicated in stages 1, 2, and 4 of DG development. Mouse embryos lacking Lef1 have been found to be devoid of any DG granule cells [40]. In fact, the whole hippocampal region, including the CA areas, are missing in mouse embryos homozygous for a fusion Lef1-lacZ gene, which codes for a mutated protein which lacks a DNA binding domain as well as hinders transcriptional activation by other LEF/TCF proteins [3]. Thus we can conclude that the generation of DG granule cells is regulated by Lef1, which, in tandem with the other LEF/TCF proteins, also regulates the general development of the hippocampal area. Mutations in Lef1 and LRP6 can also result in grave oversimplification of the primary radial glial scaffolding, which results in the failure to generate a proper structure for the upper blade of the DG. Such mutations also result in the number of dividing precursors in the hilus to be significantly reduced [3-17].

NeuroD

NeuroD is a family of basic helix-loop-helix (bhlh) neuronal differentiation genes which are involved in stage 6 of DG development. Mice with mutations in one of these genes have specific abnormalities in the generation of DG neurons, but neurons in other parts of the hippocampal region are unaffected [42]. The reason that other hippocampal neurons are unaffected seems to be because of the redundant expression of other genes in the NeuroD family in other parts of the cortex [43]. However, strangely enough, even with this mutation, there are still the rare few abnormal cells that develop with some characteristics of granule neurons, such as the ability to extend axons to the correct targets, as well as some of the characteristic markers of granule neurons. This suggests that there are other genes that contribute to the development and differentiation of DG neurons that may or may not work in tandem with NeuroD [2]. Members of the NeuroD family which have been specifically studied include Neurog2, a gene encoding for a transcription factor which is expressed in the embryonic neuroepithelium; and Neurod1, another transcription factor gene, whose products are expressed in the cortical plate and tertiary matrix of the DG, along a dorsal-ventral gradient. Neurog2 encourages the development of multipotent stem cells into neurons, via the activation of several neuronal differentation genes, such as the NeuroF family [44, 45]. It is essential for the production of glutamatergic neurons [45-47]. All dividing precursor cells in the matrix express Neurog2 during DG formation [43-48]. Mutants lacking Neurog2 exhibit a grievously underdeveloped DG at birth because of deficiencies in the division and development of DG neurons. Specifically, such mutations cause the radial glial scaffold to exhibit an abnormal conformation, resulting in the disruption of precursor cell migration [48]. Since this phenomenon is also present in Wnt mutants, it suggests that Neurog2 is part of the downstream Wnt signalling process [17-48, 49]. As for Neurod1, it plays a critical role in the survival of DG neurons. Mutants lacking this gene exhibit the complete absence of both the DG and cerebellum [42-50, 51]. Conversely, the overexpression of Neurod1 results in premature maturation of DG granule cells [52, 53].

Beta1-Integrin

Beta1-integrin has been found to be expressed in radial glial cells [54] and bind Reln [55]. Mice without this protein exhibit a reduced ability of the neuronal and radial glial cell processes to communicate with the basement membrane. The formation of the glial scaffold and the positioning of DG granule cells is also negatively affected in such mice [12]. The defects observed were similar to those in reeler mice; however, they were less pronounced in Beta1-integrin deficient mice, thereby suggesting that Reln and Beta1-integrin work along the same pathway to organise the formation and structure of the radial glial scaffold and granule cell migration in stages 2 and 5 of DG development [12].

Sox2 Dependent Gene Expression

SOX2 is a pivotal transcription factor that regulates the expression of many other important genes in DG development, including some mentioned above, such as Wnt3a, CXCR4, and Reelin [56]. It is expressed primarily in the undifferentiated neuroepithelial cells within the primordial hippocampus and adjacent cortical hem, and ceases expression during cell differentiation [56]. The deformities present in SOX2 knockout mutants is dependent on the stage at which SOX2 is deleted. Early SOX2 mutants demonstrate much more severe defects in DG development than late SOX2 knockouts. Furthermore, the defects observed in SOX2 knockouts are similar to the ones observed in knockouts of other genes. For example, the lack of differentiated neurons and proliferating progenitor cells, as well as an abnormal radial glial scaffold, are characteristic of Reelin knockouts, and the abnormally shaped DG is similar to the effects observed in CXCR4 mutants. Reelin, CXCR4, Wnt3a, and several other genes were also found to be downregulated in SOX2 knockouts [56]. Hence, SOX2 can be said to be a "master regulator" of multiple gene pathways involved in the development of the dentate gyrus.

Conclusion

In this chapter, we have outlined the development of the dentate gyrus in terms of both the histological stages and the molecular mechanisms. Below is a table summarising the different molecules involved in each stage of dentate gyrus development.

Table 1. Signalling Molecules involved in each stage of dentate gyrus development

Developmental Stage	Reelin	Wnt	BMP	SDF1/ CXCR4	Lef1	NeuroD	Beta-1 Integrin	Sox2
Defining the Dentate Neuroepithelium		✓	✓		✓			✓
Forming the Primary Radial Glial Scaffolding		✓			✓			
Radial Migration of Granule Neurons to form the Primordial Granule Cell Layer	✓			✓				
Establishing the Precursor Pool in the Hilus		✓		✓	✓			
Radial Transformation of the Tertiary Matrix	✓						✓	
Differentiation of Dentate Granule Cells						✓		

The development of the dentate gyrus is essential to sustain the ability of the dentate gyrus to perform neurogenesis over the course of an organism's life. As this is a lengthy and complex process that extends beyond gestation into early postnatal development, many different proteins and molecular mechanisms are involved. The sheer number prevents us from outlining all of them in detail; hence, the list of molecular mechanisms explored above is non-exhaustive, including only the most prominent ones. Future research may hopefully be able to draw connections between the different molecular mechanisms involved and provide a more extensive overview of the development of the dentate gyrus. Additionally, while mice have been established to be a good model organism for the development of humans and mammals in general, it would also be beneficial to have human-specific studies on the development of the dentate gyrus. Although it is currently difficult to obtain human tissues for traditional research methods, it is hoped that the development of bioimaging technology will be able to provide more comprehensive insights into the development of the human dentate gyrus in the future.

REFERENCES

[1] Cowan, W., Stanfield, B., Kishi, K. *The development of the dentate gyrup Current topics in developmental biology*: Elsevier; 1980. pp. 103-157.

[2] Li, G., Pleasure, S. J. 2005. Morphogenesis of the dentate gyrus: What we are learning from mouse mutants. *Dev. Neurosci.* 27, 93-9.

[3] Hatami, M., Conrad, S., Naghsh, P., et al., 2018. Cell-biological requirements for the generation of dentate gyrus granule neurons. *Frontiers in cellular neuroscience.* 12, 402.

[4] Subramanian, L., Remedios, R., Shetty, A., et al. *Signals from the edges: The cortical hem and antihem in telencephalic development. Seminars in cell & developmental biology*. Elsevier. 2009. pp. 712-718.

[5] Yoshida, M., Assimacopoulos, S., Jones, K. R., et al., 2006. Massive loss of cajal-retzius cells does not disrupt neocortical layer order. *Development.* 133, 537-45.

[6] Campbell, K., Götz, M. 2002. Radial glia: Multi-purpose cells for vertebrate brain development. *Trends in neurosciences*. 25, 235-238.

[7] Villar-Cerviño, V., Marín, O. 2012. Cajal-retzius cells. *Current Biology*. 22, R179.

[8] Martínez-Cerdeño, V., Noctor, S. C. 2014. Cajal, retzius, and cajal–retzius cells. *Frontiers in neuroanatomy*. 8, 48.

[9] Li, G., Pleasure, S. J. 2005. Morphogenesis of the dentate gyrus: What we are learning from mouse mutants. *Developmental neuroscience*. 27, 93-99.

[10] Grove, E. A., Fukuchi-Shimogori, T. 2003. Generating the cerebral cortical area map. *Annual review of neuroscience*. 26, 355-380.

[11] Eckenhoff, M. F., Rakic, P. 1984. Radial organization of the hippocampal dentate gyrus: A golgi, ultrastructural, and immunocytochemical analysis in the developing rhesus monkey. *Journal of comparative neurology*. 223, 1-21.

[12] Förster, E., Tielsch, A., Saum, B., et al., 2002. Reelin, disabled 1, and β1 integrins are required for the formation of the radial glial scaffold in the hippocampus. *Proceedings of the National Academy of Sciences*. 99, 13178-13183.

[13] Rickmann, M., Amaral, D. G., Cowan, W. M. 1987. Organization of radial glial cells during the development of the rat dentate gyrus. *Journal of Comparative Neurology*. 264, 449-479.

[14] Del Río, J. A., Heimrich, B., Borrell, V., et al., 1997. A role for cajal–retzius cells and reelin in the development of hippocampal connections. *Nature*. 385, 70-74.

[15] Bagri, A., Gurney, T., He, X., et al., 2002. The chemokine sdf1 regulates migration of dentate granule cells. *Development*. 129, 4249-4260.

[16] Lu, M., Grove, E. A., Miller, R. J. 2002. Abnormal development of the hippocampal dentate gyrus in mice lacking the cxcr4 chemokine receptor. *Proc. Natl. Acad. Sci. U S A*. 99, 7090-5.

[17] Zhou, C. J., Zhao, C., Pleasure, S.J. 2004. Wnt signaling mutants have decreased dentate granule cell production and radial glial scaffolding abnormalities. *J. Neurosci*. 24, 121-6.

[18] Frotscher, M., Haas, C. A., Förster, E. 2003. Reelin controls granule cell migration in the dentate gyrus by acting on the radial glial scaffold. *Cereb. Cortex*. 13, 634-40.

[19] Weiss, K. H., Johanssen, C., Tielsch, A., et al., 2003. Malformation of the radial glial scaffold in the dentate gyrus of reeler mice, scrambler mice, and apoer2/vldlr-deficient mice. *J. Comp. Neurol*. 460, 56-65.

[20] Beggs, H. E., Schahin-Reed, D., Zang, K., et al., 2003. Fak deficiency in cells contributing to the basal lamina results in cortical abnormalities resembling congenital muscular dystrophies. *Neuron*. 40, 501-514.

[21] Stanfield, B. B., Cowan, W. M. 1979. The morphology of the hippocampus and dentate gyrus in normal and reeler mice. *Journal of Comparative Neurology.* 185, 393-422.

[22] Grove, E. A., Tole, S., Limon, J., et al., 1998. The hem of the embryonic cerebral cortex is defined by the expression of multiple wnt genes and is compromised in gli3-deficient mice. *Development.* 125, 2315-25.

[23] Mangale, V. S., Hirokawa, K. E., Satyaki, P. R., et al., 2008. Lhx2 selector activity specifies cortical identity and suppresses hippocampal organizer fate. *Science.* 319, 304-9.

[24] Furuta, Y., Piston, D. W., Hogan, B. L. 1997. Bone morphogenetic proteins (bmps) as regulators of dorsal forebrain development. *Development.* 124, 2203-12.

[25] Galceran, J., Fariñas, I., Depew, M. J., et al., 1999. Wnt3a-/--like phenotype and limb deficiency in lef1(-/-)tcf1(-/-) mice. *Genes Dev.* 13, 709-17.

[26] Lee, S. M., Tole, S., Grove, E., et al., 2000. A local wnt-3a signal is required for development of the mammalian hippocampus. *Development.* 127, 457-67.

[27] Caronia, G., Wilcoxon, J., Feldman, P., et al., 2010. Bone morphogenetic protein signaling in the developing telencephalon controls formation of the hippocampal dentate gyrus and modifies fear-related behavior. *J. Neurosci.* 30, 6291-301.

[28] Cheng, X., Hsu, C. M., Currle, D. S., et al., 2006. Central roles of the roof plate in telencephalic development and holoprosencephaly. *J. Neurosci.* 26, 7640-9.

[29] Fernandes, M., Gutin, G., Alcorn, H., et al., 2007. Mutations in the bmp pathway in mice support the existence of two molecular classes of holoprosencephaly. *Development.* 134, 3789-94.

[30] Panchision, D. M., Pickel, J. M., Studer, L., et al., 2001. Sequential actions of bmp receptors control neural precursor cell production and fate. *Genes Dev.* 15, 2094-110.

[31] Mira, H., Andreu, Z., Suh, H., et al., 2010. Signaling through bmpr-ia regulates quiescence and long-term activity of neural stem cells in the adult hippocampus. *Cell Stem Cell.* 7, 78-89.

[32] Scott, I. C., Steiglitz, B. M., Clark, T. G., et al., 2000. Spatiotemporal expression patterns of mammalian chordin during postgastrulation embryogenesis and in postnatal brain. *Dev. Dyn.* 217, 449-56.

[33] Fan, X., Xu, H., Cai, W., et al., 2003. Spatial and temporal patterns of expression of noggin and bmp4 in embryonic and postnatal rat hippocampus. *Brain Res. Dev. Brain Res.* 146, 51-8.

[34] Gross, R. E., Mehler, M. F., Mabie, P. C., et al., 1996. Bone morphogenetic proteins promote astroglial lineage commitment by mammalian subventricular zone progenitor cells. *Neuron.* 17, 595-606.

[35] Sun, Y., Hu, J., Zhou, L., et al., 2011. Interplay between fgf2 and bmp controls the self-renewal, dormancy and differentiation of rat neural stem cells. *J. Cell Sci.* 124, 1867-77.

[36] Bond, A. M., Peng, C. Y., Meyers, E. A., et al., 2014. Bmp signaling regulates the tempo of adult hippocampal progenitor maturation at multiple stages of the lineage. *Stem Cells.* 32, 2201-14.

[37] Lim, D. A., Tramontin, A. D., Trevejo, J. M., et al., 2000. Noggin antagonizes bmp signaling to create a niche for adult neurogenesis. *Neuron.* 28, 713-26.

[38] Choe, Y., Kozlova, A., Graf, D., et al., 2013. Bone morphogenic protein signaling is a major determinant of dentate development. *J. Neurosci.* 33, 6766-75.

[39] Armenteros, T., Andreu, Z., Hortigüela, R., et al., 2018. Bmp and wnt signalling cooperate through lef1 in the neuronal specification of adult hippocampal neural stem and progenitor cells. *Sci. Rep.* 8, 9241.

[40] Galceran, J., Miyashita-Lin, E. M., Devaney, E., et al., 2000. Hippocampus development and generation of dentate gyrus granule cells is regulated by lef1. *Development.* 127, 469-82.

[41] Lein, E. S., Hawrylycz, M. J., Ao, N., et al., 2007. Genome-wide atlas of gene expression in the adult mouse brain. *Nature*. 445, 168-76.

[42] Liu, M., Pleasure, S. J., Collins, A. E., et al., 2000. Loss of beta2/neurod leads to malformation of the dentate gyrus and epilepsy. *Proc. Natl. Acad. Sci. U S A*. 97, 865-70.

[43] Pleasure, S. J., Collins, A. E., Lowenstein, D. H. 2000. Unique expression patterns of cell fate molecules delineate sequential stages of dentate gyrus development. *J. Neurosci.* 20, 6095-105.

[44] Seo, S., Lim, J. W., Yellajoshyula, D., et al., 2007. Neurogenin and neurod direct transcriptional targets and their regulatory enhancers. *Embo j.* 26, 5093-108.

[45] Wilkinson, G., Dennis, D., Schuurmans, C. 2013. Proneural genes in neocortical development. *Neuroscience*. 253, 256-73.

[46] Schuurmans, C., Armant, O., Nieto, M., et al., 2004. Sequential phases of cortical specification involve neurogenin-dependent and -independent pathways. *Embo j.* 23, 2892-902.

[47] Berninger, B., Costa, M. R., Koch, U., et al., 2007. Functional properties of neurons derived from in vitro reprogrammed postnatal astroglia. *J. Neurosci*. 27, 8654-64.

[48] Galichet, C., Guillemot, F., Parras, C. M. 2008. Neurogenin 2 has an essential role in development of the dentate gyrus. *Development.* 135, 2031-41.

[49] Hirabayashi, Y., Itoh, Y., Tabata, H., et al., 2004. The wnt/beta-catenin pathway directs neuronal differentiation of cortical neural precursor cells. *Development.* 131, 2791-801.

[50] Miyata, T., Maeda, T., Lee, J. E. 1999. Neurod is required for differentiation of the granule cells in the cerebellum and hippocampus. *Genes Dev*. 13, 1647-52.

[51] Schwab, M. H., Bartholomae, A., Heimrich, B., et al., 2000. Neuronal basic helix-loop-helix proteins (nex and beta2/neuro d) regulate terminal granule cell differentiation in the hippocampus. *J. Neurosci.* 20, 3714-24.

[52] Roybon, L., Hjalt, T., Stott, S., et al., 2009. Neurogenin2 directs granule neuroblast production and amplification while neurod1 specifies neuronal fate during hippocampal neurogenesis. *PLoS One.* 4, e4779.

[53] Boutin, C., Hardt, O., de Chevigny, A., et al., 2010. Neurod1 induces terminal neuronal differentiation in olfactory neurogenesis. *Proc. Natl. Acad. Sci. U S A.* 107, 1201-6.

[54] Pinkstaff, J. K., Lynch, G., Gall, C. M. 1998. Localization and seizure-regulation of integrin β1 mrna in adult rat brain. *Molecular brain research.* 55, 265-276.

[55] Dulabon, L., Olson, E. C., Taglienti, M. G., et al., 2000. Reelin binds α3β1 integrin and inhibits neuronal migration. *Neuron.* 27, 33-44.

[56] Mercurio, S., Alberti, C., Serra, L., et al., 2021. An early sox2-dependent gene expression programme required for hippocampal dentate gyrus development. *Open Biology.* 11, 200339.

In: The Dentate Gyrus
Editor: Feng-Ru Tang
ISBN: 978-1-68507-212-4

Chapter 2

CYTOARCHITECTONICS OF THE DENTATE GYRUS

Feng-Ru Tang**, *PhD, MD
Radiation Physiology Lab,
Singapore Nuclear Research and Safety Initiative,
National University of Singapore, Singapore

ABSTRACT

Emerging evidence has suggested the involvement of glial cells, including microglia, astrocytes, and oligodendrocyte in memory formation either directly or indirectly. The traditional granule cell-dominated hypothesis of the involvement of the dentate gyrus (DG) in hippocampal memory formation and brain disorders may therefore need be supplemented with the participation of the laminarly and sublaminarly distributed different types and subtypes glial cells in DG. This is because the activity of glial cells in different sublayers may be affected by the local neural circuit, and meanwhile glial cells may also closely fine tune intra- and extra-DG inputs to granule cells to control their activity and therefore be involved in memory formation. The abnormal changes of any cell type may significantly affect the activity

* Corresponding Author's Email: tangfr@gmail.com.

of all the other cells leading to DG related disease genesis. In line with the rapid development of the research on glia in memory formation, an updated cytoarchitectonics of DG including both neuron and glia is provided in this chapter. The laminar and sublaminar distributions of respective glutamatergic granule and mossy cells, GABAergic interneurons with many different subtypes and their axon and dendritic branches, microglia, astrocytes oligodendrocyte and NG2 cells are described. The pre- and post-natal development of neurons and glial cells in DG, and the different type of cells at the various developmental stages in the subgranular zones (SGZ) are also reviewed. Finally, the functional roles of each type of cells in DG are mentioned briefly. It is hoped that neurologist, neuropsychologists, radio-oncologist, neuroscientists and toxicologist will have a better, comprehensive understanding of the structure of DG in order to design novel approaches to detect or diagnose brain insult-induced DG damage and treat DG related diseases targeting both neuronal and glial elements.

Keywords: dentate gyrus, granule cells, mossy cell, interneurons, microglia, astrocytes oligodendrocyte and NG2 cells

INTRODUCTION

The dentate gyrus (DG) is the first region where all sensory modalities from the entorhinal cortex flow in. It has three layers, i.e., the molecular layer (stratum moleculare), the granule cell layer (stratum granulosum) and the polymorphic cell layer (or hilus). The subgranular zone, where the hippocampal neurogenesis occurs, is located between the granule cell layer and the polymorphic cell layer. Comparative neuroanatomical study indicates that the basic trilaminar structure of DG is common across all species. Layers of DG are arranged in a "V" or "U"-shaped configuration in which the open portion is directed toward 'the fimbria in transverse sections. The granular layer is made up of densely packed spherical or oval bodied neurons with dendrites entering the molecular layer and axons passing through the polymorphic layer to synapse with the dendrites of pyramidal cells in CA3 area of the hippocampus.

DG along with many other fields of the hippocampal formation create a banana shaped structure that, in the rat, runs from the septal nuclei rostrally to the temporal cortex caudally. Its long axis is named as the septotemporal axis whereas the axis at the right angle to the long axis is named as the transverse axis. The granule cell layer between the CA3 area and the CA1 area is called the suprapyramidal (above CA3 area) blade whereas the portion opposite to the suprapyramidal is the infrapyramidal (below CA3 area) blade. The region connecting the suprapyramidal and infrapyramidal blades (at the apex of the "V" or "U") is called the crest [1].

The Granule Cell Layer

Granule Cells (GCs)

Pre- and Post-Natal Development of the Granule Cells

The granule cells are principal neurons in DG. In the human, the granule cell layer of DG first appears in the 13-14th gestational weeks [2], approximately at the time when pyramidal cell formation terminates in Ammon's horn. The granule cell continues to grow after birth [3]. All cytoarchitectonic layers of DG can be distinguished by the 24th week although the majority of granule cells are formed before the 34th gestational week [4]. At term, the granule cell layer includes ~70% of adult granule cells. The migration of immature cells from the hilus to the granule cell layer continues during the first eight postnatal months [3, 5]. The development of the infrapyramidal blade appears 4-5 weeks later than the suprapyramidal blade [2, 6]. In the suprapyramidal blade of DG of 28-week-old fetus, the outer two rows of granule cells displayed a thin lightly stained cytoplasmic rim. In the infrapyramidal blade, granule cells with stained cytoplasm appeared 4 weeks later (in a 32-week-old fetus). From the 24th gestational week to the postnatal 11.5^{th} month, the surface of the different subregions of DG has increased differently. The surface of the granule cell layer is doubled at 40th weeks, five times larger at the postnatal 11.5th month than at the 24th gestational week. The molecular layer becomes three times larger by term and increases approximately 20 times up till the 11.5th postnatal month, whereas the surface area of the hilar region increases 10 times between the 24th gestational week and the 11.5th postnatal month. It suggests that postnatally the most rapidly growing area is the molecular layer where dendrites of granule cells are located. Glial cells are formed continuously from the 24th week, but an increased proliferation of oligodendrocytes starts in both Ammon's horn and DG at 1 year of age that probably represents the onset of myelination.

In rodents (rat), the earliest forming regions of the granular layer lie at the two extremes where cells at the temporal levels originate earlier than the septal level. The granule cells lying between the septal and temporal levels originate latest. Neurogenesis in the suprapyramidal limb precedes that in the infrapyramidal limb during the prenatal period, when approximately 15-20% of the total population arises in both the septal and temporal levels. Approximately 85% of granule cells are formed postnatally from postnatal day 1(P1) to P20, and the adult cytoarchitectonic pattern of the rat DG is reached at P 20.

There is a decreasing growth rate during the first three postnatal weeks [7], but a 35-43% linear increase between 1 month and 1 year [8]. The total granular layer volume grows linearly with age, but the average volume of a single granule cell nucleus in the ventral DG decreases with age. The granule cell neurogenesis in the septal and temporal extremes is significantly lower than in the combined septal and temporal levels. The infrapyramidal limb (facing the thalamus) has more neurogenesis than the suprapyramidal limb at the septal extreme instead of at the temporal extreme, where granule cell neurogenesis is virtually non-existent. The cells in the hilus and molecular layer of the DG arise earlier than the granule cells and the hilus is formed mainly during E15-17 when the cells in the deep part of all other hippocampal regions are forming[8].

In monkeys, approximately 85% of granule cells are formed prenatally. Granule cell formation continues until the end of the first postnatal month with a small percent of granule cell proliferation in the adult animals [9, 10]. The formation rate in the adult monkeys is much lower than rodents, and is only one tenth of the latter [10]. In humans, granule cell genesis begins during gestation weeks 10.5 to 11, and it continues during the second and third trimesters, after birth and all the way into adulthood although at the latter stage, neurogenesis is reduced significantly [11, 12].

Morphology of the Granule Cells

The cell body of the granule cells is elliptical with a size of 10 μm x 18μm (width x height) [13] and their spiny apical dendrites and dendritic branches extend throughout the molecular layer. The granule cell bodies are tightly packed and form a "V"- or "U"- shaped structure with the thickness of the granule cell layer ranges from 4 to 8 neurons or ~60 μm. It is estimated that the total number of granule cells in one DG of the rat, monkey and human is approximately 1, 10 and 15 million respectively and this number does not vary in adult animals with neurogenesis [14, 15]. In 6-month-old male rats, the number of dendrites of the first, second and third order of granular cells increases in a ratio of 1: 2: 3, whereas the total length of the dendrites increases in a ratio of 1: 4: 5 respectively. The mean number of origin points of dendritic branches is 10, and the mean number of free dendritic endings is 12 [16]. Compared to the infrapyramidal blade, the total length of the dendritic trees of granule cells in the suprapyramidal blade is longer (3500 μm vs. 2800μm, respectively). More dendritic spines are found in the suprapyramidal blade (1.6 spines/μm) than those in the infrapyramidal blade (1.3 spines/μm) [17]. The average density of spines increased considerably with age in isolated dendritic segments as well as over the whole length of a dendrite. The density is 0.03, 0.04, 0.09, 0.1, 0.17, 0.23, 0.48, 0.62 spines/μm at P2, P5, P8, P10, P15, P20, P30, P180 respectively. Synaptogenesis starts in the perinatal period in form of immature axo-somatic and axo-dendritic contacts [18]. The mature principal neurons can be labelled with NeuN and calbindin, whereas immature granule cells are labelled by doublecortin (DCX) or NeuroD.

Functionally, granule cells are involved in sorting incoming information, preparing it for subsequent processing in CA3 area, to associate sensory information with the appropriate context, and functionally integrating newly generated neurons in adult. These cells have therefore, been considered as a pre-processor and make an important contribution to the hippocampal learning, memory, spatial orientation and navigation, and mood regulation. Abnormal changes of the granule cells may be involved in many neurological and neuropsychological disorders such as Alzheimer's disease, epilepsy, schizophrenia, and depression which will be discussed in details in other chapters in this book.

Pyramidal Basket Cells

In the granule cell layer, there are some inhibitory neurons called pyramidal basket cells which are located just within the granule cell layer at its border with the polymorphic layer. The cell body of these cells is pyramidal-shaped with a large diameter of 25–35 μm. Pyramidal basket cells have a single, principal aspiny apical dendrite that protrudes into the molecular layer and divides into several aspiny branches. These cells also have several basal dendrites that divide and extend into the polymorphic cell layer. Their axons form pericellular plexuses around the cell bodies of the granule cells to negatively regulate granule cell activity as their terminals are GABAergic and form symmetric, inhibitory axo-somatic synapses. A single pyramidal basket cell may influence as many as 10,000 of the granule cells [1, 19]. The ratio of pyramidal basket cells to granule cells are different between the two blades and between the blade at the septal and temporal levels of DG, i.e., it is 1:100 in the suprapyramidal blade and 1:180 in the infrapyramidal blade of the septal level. At the temporal level, the ratio is 1:150 and 1:300 for the suprapyramidal and infrapyramidal blade respectively [20]. It suggests that the granule cells in the suprapyramidal blade are more powerfully regulated by pyramidal basket cells than those in the infrapyramidal blade, and granule cells in the temporal level are less controlled by pyramidal basket cells than those at the septal level. Further functional comparison between the role of pyramidal basket cells on the granule cells in the suprapyramidal and infrapyramidal blades or in the temporal and septal levels is still needed.

Biochemically, pyramidal basket cells are parvalbumin-, cholesystokinin (CCK) - vasoactive intestinal polypeptide (VIP)-, type 3 neuropeptide Y- or nitric oxide synthase (nNOS)- immunopositive [21-25].

The Subgranular Zone (SGZ)

The subgranular zone is a narrow layer of cells located between the granule cell layer and the hilus of DG. Different type of cells at various developmental stages are located in the subgranular zones. Type-1 cells (also called B cells) are a group of radial-glia-like neural stem cells which express astrocytic marker glial fibrillary acidic protein (GFAP), brain lipid binding protein (BLBP), SRY-Box Transcription Factor 2 (SOX2), and nestin. Type 2 cells (also called D cells) are daughter cells generated by Type 1 cells by asymmetrical division, and are proliferating intermediate progenitor cells (IPCs) which are nestin and DCX positive, but GFAP negative. These type 2 cells can give rise to neuroblasts (Type 3) that subsequently differentiate into immature dentate granule neurons. Type 3 cells are DCX and polysialated form of neural cell adhesion molecule (PSA-NCAM) positive, but nestin negative [26-28]. The postmitotic immature neurons then migrate to the granule cell layer and become mature neurons which could be labelled by NeuN and calbindin (CB). The entire process of differentiation, maturation, and integration of the new granular cells occurs during 6 to 8 weeks after birth in mice [29, 30].

Other cells in the subgranular zone include postmitotic calretinin immunopositive neurons, different glial cells, the cells in the blood vessels such as endothelial cells and cannabinoid receptor type 1 (CB1 R) immunopositive cells or total molecular layer cells (TML-Cs). TML-Cs have high axonal density in the middle molecular layer and are positioned to mediate feedback inhibition of medial perforant path inputs [31, 32]. Neurophysiological study indicates that cannabinoid receptor type 1 (CB1 R) immunopositive TML-Cs can mediate cannabinoid sensitive feed-forward and feedback inhibition of dentate perforant path inputs [33].

THE POLYMORPHIC CELL LAYER

The polymorphic cell layer or the hilus of DG has more than 20 types of cells based on Golgi studies [34] and these hilar neurons play a critical role in the normal activity of DG and in brain disease genesis [35-39].

Based on the morphology and physiology of hilar cells, two groups of cells could be categorized, i.e., regular-spiking cells with characteristics of pyramidal cells and fast-spiking or moderately fast-spiking neurons that correspond to GABAergic interneurons [40, 41]. The former is spiny and has thorny excrescences, with dendrites mostly in the hilus [40], and is called spiny hilar cell or mossy cell [39, 42]. The faster-spiking cells have no thorny excrescences, usually few spines and dendrites in all DG cell layers. They are GABAergic interneurons and have been characterized into many different subtypes [22, 43-46].

Mossy Cells (MCs)

Mossy cell is named as such as it appears to be covered by moss at low power after Golgi staining which corresponds to large thorny excrescences at high power [34]. These cells are the most common types of cells in the polymorphic layer of DG comprising more than 30% of hilar cells in rodents. MC has large triangular or multipolar cell body with a diameter of 25–35 μm. Three or more thick dendrites originate from the cell body, extend for long distances within the polymorphic layer or pierce the granule cell layer and enter the molecular layer occasionally, but these dendrites never enter the adjacent CA3 area in the rat. Each principal dendrite bifurcates once or twice and generally gives rise to a few side branches with all of its proximal dendrites being covered by very large and complex spines, the so-called thorny excrescences which is the most distinctive feature of MC where the mossy fiber axon terminals synapse with MC. The distal dendrites of MC have typical pedunculate spines. Hilar mossy cells also distinguish the DG from other hippocampal subareas (CA1–3 areas) by using glutamate as the neurotransmitter which is also released by granule cells, whereas in CA1–3 areas, the only glutamatergic cell type is the pyramidal cell. Hilar mossy cells of the mouse are calretinin immunopositive [47, 48]. Axons arising from these cells form a strong calretinin immunopositive belt in the inner third of the dentate molecular layer (IML).

At the electron microscopic level, calretinin-immunopositive boutons make asymmetric synaptic contacts primarily on spines and, occasionally, on dendritic shafts of granule cells. It accounts for the majority of asymmetrical synapses in the inner molecular layer [49]. MCs projects to the distal ipsilateral and contralateral IML whereby they activate local circuit GABAergic neurons (interneurons), which in turn inhibit GCs [50]. Recent study suggests that dorsal and ventral mossy cells differ in their axonal projections throughout DG of the mouse hippocampus [51]. The major inputs to MCs are from local interneurons, GCs and CA3 back projection [52]. The cholinergic nuclei of the septum and diagonal band also innervate MCs [53].

Neurophysiological study indicates that the primary effect of MCs is not excitation but inhibition of GCs, as MCs activate interneurons that in turn silence GCs [54]. On the other hand, it has been reported that the net effect of MCs on GCs is excitatory as deletion of hilar MCs in slices does not induce disinhibition of GCs from a perforant path stimulus [55]. Functionally, MCs are active during behavior such as spatial navigation and may contribute to spatial coding. These cells have more plasticity in remapping than GCs and their spatial tuning differs from GCs. It suggests a central role of MCs in the processing of spatial information by the DG

[39, 56, 57]. Mossy cells may also be involved in epileptogenesis [58], novel object recognition [59] and anxiety [60].

Hilar-Perforant-Path-Associated Interneurons (HIPP)

This group of cells is located subjacent to the granule cells, has dendritic trees limited to the hilar region, covered with long thin spines, but no thorny excrescenses. The axon of HIPP cells crosses the granule cell layer, gives rise to an extensive axon arborization in the outer two-thirds of the molecular layer to innervate granule cell dendrites [44]. Several collaterals are also present in the inner one-third molecular layer [61]. The axon collaterals studded with a large number of small to medium-sized (0.2-1μm) axon terminals may cross the hippocampal fissure, where they form small local arbors in the stratum lacunosum moleculare of the CA1 area and in the subiculum [44, 61, 62]. Their axonal plexus can extend for as much as 3.5 mm along the septotemporal axis of DG (the entire length of DG in the rat is only ~10 mm) and may generate as many as 100,000 synaptic terminals [1].

The most postsynaptic targets of HIPP are GABA-negative dendritic shafts and spines of principal cells (76%), whereas other target elements contain GABA (8%). Synaptic inhibitory interactions exist between cholecystokinin (CCK) immunopositive hilar commissural associational path (HICAP) cells and among SOM immunopositive hilar perforant path-associated (HIPP) interneurons. Moreover, HICAP and HIPP cells inhibit parvalbumin (PV) immunopositive perisomatic inhibitory basket cells (BCs), whereas BCs and HICAPs rarely target HIPP cells. HICAP and HIPP cells produce slow, weak, and unreliable inhibition onto postsynaptic interneurons [63]. HIPP cell activity contributes to inhibitory effects of acetylcholine in DG and that M1 muscarinic receptors mediate the cholinergic activation of HIPP cells as well as the control of background context memory salience [64].

At the electron microscopic level, boutons of HIPP cells form symmetrical synapses, even at their nonvaricose segments, with spiny dendritic shafts and spines of presumed granule cells [40]. In the hilus, the dendrites of HIPP cells are covered by numerous asymmetrical synapses, most of which show characteristic features of mossy fiber terminals [44]. It therefore seems that the HIPP cells largely mediate feedback inhibition of granule cells by terminating on distal granule cell dendrites and spines in conjunction with entorhinal afferents [43, 44].

Somatostatin (SOM) Immunopositive Interneurons

In DG, SOM-immunopositive somata can be found in the hilus adjacent to the subgranular zone, in the deep hilus and in areas bordering CA3c stratum radiatum. The dendrites of SOM-immunopositive neurons which are covered by numerous long spines remain in the hilus with a few exceptions [65]. The axons project to the outer two-thirds of the molecular layer and form a terminal plexus with the outer one-third being denser than the middle one-third. In the inner molecular layer and the granule cell layer, there are a small number of radially running axons with nonvaricose. The main axon collaterals are often seen to cross the hippocampal fissure. Varicose collaterals in the hilus are sparse but occur consistently. The majority of axon collaterals in the molecular layer originate from ipsilateral hilar neurons [66], and a smaller proportion of axons originates from the contralateral hilus [66, 67]. According to the characteristic soma location and axonal and dendritic distribution, hilar SOM-immunopositive cells are likely to be identical to HIPP cells. It has been demonstrated that parvalbumin-, calretinin-, vasoactive intestinal polypeptide-, cholecystokinin-, substance P receptor-immunopositive interneurons receive innervation from somatostatin (SOM)-immunopositive boutons. Anatomical and electrophysiological data show that the main excitatory inputs of somatostatin-immunopositive HIPP interneurons originate from local principal cells [68]. Yuan et al. (2017) found another type of SOM-immunopositive cells in DG, i.e., the hilus-associated SOM-immunopositive interneurons. These hilar SOM-immunopositive cells provide perisomatic inhibition onto GABAergic cells in DG and project to the medial septum. Repetitive activation of glutamatergic inputs onto SOM-immunopositive cells induces long-lasting-depression (LTD) of synaptic transmission but long-term-potentiation (LTP) of synaptic signals in hilar interneurons. Thus, LTD in SOM-immunopositive cells may assist flow of spatial information from the entorhinal cortex to DG, while LTP in hilar interneurons may facilitate the temporal coordination of GCs with activity patterns governed by the medial septum [69].

Electron microscopic study of SOM-immunoreactive axon terminals shows that the majority of postsynaptic elements in the outer molecular layer are spines and spiny dendritic shafts, most likely belonging to granule cells [68]. The synapses are always symmetrical and are accompanied by an unstained asymmetrical synapse when terminating on a spine. Occasional synapses are formed on deep hilar neurons and on granule cell bodies. SOM-immunopositive dendrites are found to be spiny and received numerous asymmetrical synapses from mossy fiber terminals both along the shaft and on the spines [70]. The cell body and somatic spines are also contacted by mossy fiber terminals, although at a lower frequency. The cell bodies have typical features of interneurons, i.e., invaginated nuclei, asymmetric synaptic input, intranuclear rods, and numerous cytoplasmic organelles [65, 71].

Neuropeptide Y (NPY) -Immunopositive Neurons

There are four types of NPY immunopositive interneurons in DG; Type 1-3 NPY immunopositive interneurons are in the hilus, and Type 4 in the molecular layer of DG. Type 1 NPY immunopositive interneurons are large multipolar cells in the deep hilus (9%), Type 2 are medium-sized multipolar and fusiform hilar neurons (64%), and Type 3 are pyramidal shaped cells in the deep granule cell layer with long apical dendrites reaching the outer molecular layer (20%)[25, 72]. The Types 1 and 2 NPY-immunopositive interneurons are in the hilus or adjacent to the subgranular zone, contain somatostatin and give rise to the dense

NPY innervation of the dentate outer molecular layer. The NPY-immunopositive terminal density is moderate in the granule cell layer, but higher in the hilus [25, 72]. These interneurons do not send dendrites into the molecular layer, whereas the Type 3 NPY-immunopositive neurons have a prominent apical dendrite that ascends through the stratum moleculare often up to the hippocampal fissure or the pial surface. Their basal dendrites ramify within the hilus. The majority of fibers contributing to the axon plexus in the molecular layer likely originates from ipsilateral hilar neurons containing both NPY and SOM [73]. Some fibers may derive from the contralateral dentate hilus, as shown by retrograde labeling of hilar NPY-positive neurons [72]. Based on classical Golgi staining, the Type 3 pyramidal-shaped NPY immunopositive cells at the deep granule cell layer should be basket cells with a predominant innervation of hilar mossy cells because NPY-immunopositive terminal density in the hilus is higher than in the granule cell layer.

Electron microscopic study indicates that all types of NPY immuno-positive neurons are typical of interneurons, i.e., they have an infolded nuclear membrane, thick perinuclear cytoplasm rich in organelles, and a mixture of symmetrical and asymmetrical synaptic contact with the soma. Dendrites in the hilus are covered by numerous asymmetrical synapses, most of which appear to originate from mossy fibers. The pyramidal-shaped NPY cells have a dendritic tuft in the stratum moleculare, which are also covered by asymmetrical synapses. Further study suggests that some of the asymmetrical synapses originate from the entorhinal cortex and the commissural-associational pathway [70]. NPY immunopositive axon terminals in all layers form symmetrical synaptic contacts. Their postsynaptic targets are somata and dendrites of presumed mossy cells in the hilus [72, 74].

In humans, minute amounts of NPY are also expressed in dentate granule cells. NPYs target Y1 and Y2 receptors which are the most abundant NPY receptors expressed in DG. The former is localized postsynaptically, primarily on granule cell dendrites in the molecular layer and some interneurons, while the latter is presynaptic mediating inhibition of glutamate release. In humans, monkeys and mice, Y2 receptors are also present on mossy fibers [25]. Functionally, NPY suppresses depolarization-induced increases in intracellular Ca2+ concentrations in granule cells by inhibiting an N-type calcium current [75]. It exerts anticonvulsive actions mediated by Y2 receptors at mossy fiber terminals. Hilar interneurons containing NPY degenerate in temporal lobe epilepsy and in Alzheimer's disease and reduced levels of NPY in the dentate hilus are associated with depression. By activating Y1 receptors, NPY also exerts powerful neuroproliferative effects on subgranular zone progenitor cells, increasing the number of newly born granule cells in the adult DG [25, 76].

Vasoactive Intestinal Polypeptide (VIP)-Immunopositive Neurons

VIP-immunopositive cells are generally located near or in the granule cell layer, are highly heterogeneous and have a pyramidal-shaped soma with a rich basal dendritic arbor and a sparse apical dendritic tuft. In the deep hilus, a small number of VIP-immunopositive cells have multipolar dendrites which are long and cross the granule cell layer to enter the molecular layer, but their axon terminals project in the hilus with higher density in the ventral than in the dorsal hippocampus. The synaptic boutons are relatively small, and diffusely distributed in the neuropil with no obvious association with cell bodies. VIP-immunopositive axons in the granule cell layer are studded with large varicosities and appear at the apex of DG in clusters of varying diameters (100-200 μm). In the molecular layer, a smaller number of VIP-immunopositive axon collaterals contact the somata or proximal dendrites of VIP-immunopositive or other types of interneurons [23]. These cells have a main descending axon. Some VIP cells with soma and dendrites in the hilus also appear to contribute to the hilar axon collaterals. Several neurons that give rise to the clusters of large varicosities in the granule cell layer may have a soma-dendritic morphology and location similar to the cells with hilar projection [22]. In approximately two-thirds of morphologically reconstructed VIP-immunopositive cells, their axons ramify in the hilus. The remaining cells project their axons exclusively to the molecular layer (15%), to both the molecular layer and hilus (10%), or throughout the entire DG layers (8%)[77].

Electron microscopic study indicates that VIP-immunopositive interneuron axon terminals make symmetrical synapses and are immunopositive for GABA. The postsynaptic targets of the large varicose axon type are granule cell bodies and dendrites in the granule cell layer (GABA-immunonegative profiles). The neurons that project to the hilus innervate mostly GABAergic interneurons. The majority of targets of VIP-immunopositive cells that project to stratum moleculare also appear to be other interneurons [22].

For VIP-immunopositive neurons, there is a clear correlation between input-output features and neurochemical characteristics in DG. The basket type of VIP cells contains CCK but not calretinin (CR), whereas those projecting to the hilus are immunoreactive for CR but not for CCK [23]. The VIP-immunopositive cells that project to the hilus have a target selectivity complementary to that of some CCK-containing basket cells. Hilar collaterals of these CCK-immunopositive basket cells predominantly innervate the mossy cells [78], whereas the VIP-CR-immunopositive cells with hilar projection innervate mostly GABAergic interneurons. VIP- immunopositive basket cells account for only a small proportion of CCK-immunopositive basket cells in this region, and both the CCK- and the VIP-CCK immunopositive neurons represent basket cell populations that show no overlap with the PV- immunopositive neurons [79, 80].

Neurophysiological study indicates that VIP-immunopositive interneurons are recruited with a long latency in response to theta-band cortical inputs and preferentially innervate GABAergic interneurons over glutamatergic principal cells, so to control the DG output via disinhibition [75].

Cholecystokinin (CCK)-Immunopositive Neurons

CCK immunopositive neurons in the hilus of DG come from the molecular layer by the 12th postnatal day where they are horizontally oriented. These cells transform into tripolar and then to a vertical bipolar shape in the granular cell layer before settling at the interface between the granular cell layer and the hilus where they differentiate into typical pyramidal-shaped CCK immunopositive interneurons [24, 81]. Similar to Type 3 NPY-immunopositive interneurons, the majority of CCK-immunopositive neurons in DG are located in the deep granule cell layer. They have a pyramidal-shaped soma, a prominent apical dendrites branch in the stratum moleculare when running toward the pial surface, and basal dendrites penetrating the hilus. CCK-immunopositive cell bodies are extremely rare in stratum moleculare and the deep hilar region. Almost all CCK-immunopositive neurons in DG have a bitufted dendritic tree, i.e., one tuft of dendrites (apical) in stratum moleculare, and another (basal) in the hilus, thus allowing them to receive inputs both from the perforant path and from the local mossy fiber collaterals [22]. Their axon terminals project to the outer one-third of the granule cell layer, the adjacent narrow (20-50 μm thick) zone of the molecular layer and the deep hilus where axon terminals surround large unstained somata.

Electron microscopic study of CCK-immunopositive cell bodies and dendrites reveals that their dendrites in the hilus receive numerous synapses from mossy fiber terminals, whereas those in stratum moleculare are contacted by both asymmetric and symmetric synapses [76]. CCK- immunopositive boutons in the granule cell layer and in the adjacent region of stratum moleculare establish multiple symmetrical synaptic contacts with somata and proximal dendrites of granule cells, suggesting these cells are a specific subset of basket cells. The postsynaptic elements of CCK-immunopositive terminals or boutons in the deep hilar area are MC somata including those mossy cells with commissural-associational projections [78].

Neuronal Nitric Oxide Synthase (nNOS) Immunopositive Neurons (Or Neurons Stained for NADPH-Diaphorase)

Neuronal nitric oxide synthase (nNOS) immunopositive or NADPH-diaphorase-stained interneurons reside in all three layers of DG, the percentages of distribution in the molecular layer, granule cell layer and the hilus are 25.4%, 9.4% and 65.2%, respectively [82]. Almost every nNOS immunopositive cell expressed glutamic acid decarboxylase 67 (GAD67) or glutamic acid decarboxylase 65 (GAD65). At the deep granule cell layer, nNOS-immunopositive cell are similar to NPY or CCK immunopositive basket cells which have prominent apical dendrites crossing the stratum moleculare and several basal dendrites in the hilus. nNOS immunopositive cells in the deep hilus have generally large cell bodies and bitufted or multipolar dendritic trees with moderate spines. Cells in the granule cell layer have smaller, fusiform, or pyramidal-shaped somata and a radially running apical dendrite, which forms a tuft that often reaches the fissure or the pial surface. Basal dendrites have a few branches and run in the subgranular zone. Axonal staining is remarkably dense in the stratum moleculare, especially in the outer two-thirds, whereas the inner one-third displays a strong homogeneous staining. The hilus contains a smaller number of nNOS immunopositive axons [21].

Recent study suggests the existence of proliferative cells in the hilus or polymorphic layer of DG, i.e., the hilus is also a reservoir of progenitor cells in adult animals in addition to SGZ. These cells are mainly constituted by neural precursor cells, oligodendrocyte progenitor (OPCs), and neural progenitor cells (NPCs) being the most abundant. Proliferative mature astrocytes and Type 1-like cells are also part of the hilar proliferative pool. It seems that some of these cell populations are not similar to those in SGZ (García-Martinez et al., 2020).

THE STRATUM MOLECULARE (SM) OR THE MOLECULAR LAYER OF DG

Stratum moleculare is a relatively cell-free layer with a thickness of about 250 μm in the rat. It is occupied mainly by the dendrites of the dentate granule cells and fibers of the perforant path that originate in the entorhinal cortex and a variety of other extrinsic sources. In addition to glial cells, there are also different types of neurons such as the semilunar granule cells (SGCs) and interneurons in SM,

The Semilunar Granule Cells (SGCs)

This cell type is a morpho-functionally distinct class of hippocampal dentate projection neurons contributing to feedback inhibition and memory processing and is located in the inner molecular layer of DG of the rodent [81]. The SGCs activate hilar neurons, i.e., MCs and interneurons, which in turn lead to long-lasting inhibition of GCs [84-86]. Morphologically, the number of primary dendrites, dendritic angle, and soma width and soma ratio are significantly higher in SGCs than GCs and can be used to categorize SGCs and GCs. In particular, the multiple primary dendrites observed in SGCs stands in stark contrast to the typical one to two apical dendrites observed in granule cell reconstructions [87]. Neurophysiological study indicates that SGCs maintain higher spontaneous inhibitory postsynaptic current (sIPSC) frequency than GCs from infancy through adulthood. sIPSC amplitude and cumulative charge transfer decline from infancy to adulthood and are not different between GCs and SGCs. GC input resistance is higher than in SGCs during infancy and adolescence, input resistance decreases with developmental age in GCs, while it progressively increases in SGCs [86]. The neuroanatomical and neurophysiological features and their distinct window of embryonic day 12–15 for the SGC development [88], enhanced excitatory drive [84], and distinct synaptic and extrasynaptic inhibitory currents [89] indicate that SGCs are distinct from GCs. Functionally, SGCs may be feedback inhibition of GCs, gate dentate activity, and contribute to memory processing [84, 90]. Other neurons in the SM include Type 4 NPY-immunopositive interneurons with small multipolar cell bodies [25, 72], CCK [81, 91], nNOS [21] and cannabinoid receptor type 1 (CB1 R) immunopositive cells.

Glial Cells in DG

Microglia

Microglial development in DG takes place with the microenvironmental changes associated with neurogenesis, gliogenesis, angiogenesis, and synaptogenesis. The primary rat dentate neuroepithelium is distinguishable at pregnancy day 17. At pregnancy day 19, ameboid microglial (AM) type 3 (cells with the pleomorphic cell body and filopodia and/or pseudopodia), and cell types in transition from AM to primitive ramified microglia (PRM) appear in the developing hilus in the temporal levels of DG. The cells are generally located next to the vessels. Similar cells are rarely observed at the midposterior levels. At pregnancy day19, microglial cell precursors are located on both sides of the dentate migration path linking the secondary dentate matrix with the forming DG. At pregnancy day 21, a few PRM are seen just deep to the suprapyramidal blade of the granule cell layer and in the hilus next to blood vessels. At both ages, AM type 3 and cell types in transition from AM to PRM are also observed in close relation to blood vessels at the border of the primary dentate neuroepithelium. Neither AM nor PRM are observed in the developing granule cell layer at pregnancy day 19 and 21 [92].

At birth, rat DG contains much fewer microglial cells than Ammon's horn. At P0, microglia are confined to the hilu of DG. The majority of cells are AM cells. At P3, the outer part of the stratum moleculare is invaded by cell processes from microglia distributed in the stratum lacunosum-moleculare of CA1 area. On P6, PRM cell bodies appear for the first time in the dentate molecular layer. From the second postnatal week, PRM cells appear in all layers of DG and are progressively transformed into resting microglia (ReM) cells. At P9, microglia show a remarkable association with blood vessels in the hilus. Microglia are also seen lining up along the deep side of the dentate granule cell layer and preferentially in the suprapyramidal blade of the granule cell layer. In the stratum moleculare, PRM cells and reactive microglia appear in the outer two-thirds but rarely seen in the inner one-third. From P12, PRM cells gradually transformed into ReM cells, and the microglial population of the reactive cell type increased in the stratum moleculare. In the hilus, microglial cells spread out in all part. Between P15 and P18, microglial cells appear along the basal part of both the supra- and infra- pyramidal blades of granule cell layer. Microglial cell processes are observed among the granular cell bodies of the suprapyramidal blade from P12 and the infrapyramidal blades from P15. At P18, microglial cell bodies are rarely observed in granule cell layer, but appear gradually in the inner one-third of the stratum moleculare, in particular in the supragranular blade [93]. Kimoto et al. (2009) observed a significant increase in the number of ionized calcium-binding adapter molecule 1 (Iba1 a microglial marker)-immunopositive microglia in DG of 1-, 2-, and 4-week-old mice as compared with 8-week-old animals [94].

Hierarchical cluster and discriminant analysis of the multimodal morphometric features of microglia reveal two main morphological phenotypes of microglia in the outer and middle thirds of molecular layer of DG (MolDG) of 20-month-old Swiss albino mice. Type I presents a less complex and branching pattern and smaller convex hull volume than type II. The number of cells with type I morphotype is much greater than the number of cells with morphotype II. The type II microglia do not seem to be affected by environment or age, whereas the type I microglia of the same region have their complexity values significantly reduced in the old animals, regardless of the environment where they are kept. Furthermore, there are differential microglial morphological changes in the molecular layer of dorsal and ventral regions of aged mice, suggesting that type I and type II microglia may have different physiological roles [95].

In the aged (10-12-year-old) dog, the processes of microglia are hypertrophied in DG, but not in CA1. Moreover, Iba-1immunopositive cells in DG in the aged dog is higher than in the adult (2-3-year-old) dog [96]. Microglia distribution also shows a strain-specific difference. For instance, among eight widely used inbred strains (C57BL/6J, A/J, BALB/c, C3H/HeJ, FVB, 129/SvJ, DBA/1, and DBA/2) and one outbred strain (ICR) mice, the number of microglia in the polymorphic layer of DG is highest in the C57BL/6 strain and lowest in the DBA/2 strain [97].

Functionally, microglia are essential prenatally in supporting neuronal survival and regulating apoptosis [98, 99]. Vacuolar sorting protein 35 (VPS35) deletion-induced increased microglial activity, impaired adult hippocampal neurogenesis, impaired dendritic morphology and reduced dendritic spine density and depressive-like behaviour. It suggests that microglia may play a pivotal role in the regulation of adult hippocampal neurogenesis and the survival/integration of newborn neurons in the adult hippocampus [100]. On the other hand, acutely ablate microglia from either postnatal day (P) 7 or 14 impacts briefly on the brain but that the long-lasting effects are minimal, suggesting that neonatal microglia may be dispensable in the establishment of hippocampal brain function [101].

Astrocytes

Development of astroglial precursors in the embryonic hamster and mouse brain originate in the ventricular germinative zone of the hippocampus as early as the 13th [102] and 15th [103] gestational day respectively, near the fimbria and migrate tangentially through the subpial area towards DG, and persist until early postnatal stage. The differentiation of precursor cells to astrocytes occurs after their final settlement in DG. NSCs residing within SGZ of the postnatal and adult DG generate a small proportion of astrocytes [11].

Morphological [104-106], electrophysiological [107, 108], and molecular biological [109] studies have suggested a heterogeneity of astrocytes in the central nervous system (CNS). Astrocytes are labelled by glial fibrillary acidic protein (GFAP) and S100β. In DG, astrocytes show regional, laminar and circuit-specific distribution [110-113]. Only 80% of S100 immunopositive cells are GFAP immunopositive, all GFAP immunopositive cells are S100 immunopositive in DG of C57BL/6J mice [112]. S100β-negative astrocytes are located mainly in the hilus of the dorsal and ventral DG [114]. Astrocytes in the rat DG are the protoplasmic type and classified into six subtypes based on the location of their somata; i.e., astrocytes in the polymorph layer, in the subgranular zone, in the granular cell layer, at the border of the granular cell layer and the molecular layer, in the molecular layer, and subjacent to the pia surface [115]. In different layers of DG, astrocytes have higher density at the ventral than dorsal level [112]. In the molecular layer of rat DG, the astrocytes come from the secondary radial glial cells in the subgranular zone [116], their distribution is influenced by the boundary separating the associational/commissural and perforant path afferents. There is a higher density of astrocyte somata at the inner/middle laminar boundary [113]. While earlier study suggests that astrocyte in the molecular layer of DG are stellate in appearance [117], polarized astrocytes in the molecular layer of DG, which may have import for the functioning of astrocytes are also observed [113]. In Long-Evans hooded rats, astrocytic process surface density and thickness in the dentate molecular layer is highest in the outer one-third of the molecular layer and progressively decreased as processes approached the granule cell layer. No glial density lamination pattern is detectable in the stratum radiatum of the CA1 region of the hippocampus, suggesting that different afferents in the three parts of molecular layer may affect astrocyte morphology and functions [118]. The thin processes of astrocytes from the subgranular zone to the inner molecular layer [115] and aggregations of astrocyte cell bodies near the pial surface, which corresponds to the outer one-third of the molecular layer where the frequency of the thickest processes is greatest [119] may further support the above laminar distribution of astrocytes. The number density of astrocytes in the granule cell layer of DG is significantly smaller than molecular layer or the hilus [112]. Both the number and volume fraction of astrocytic processes in the dentate molecular layer are substantially greater in senescent rats than young adult rats [118]. However, this result is inconsistent with a study showing a slight increase in the number of astrocytes, but a slight decrease in GFAP volume per astrocyte in the dentate molecular layer with aging [120]. Compared with adult (2-3 years of age) dogs, GFAP immunoreactivity decreases markedly in the molecular layer of DG in the aged (10-12 years of age) group. GFAP protein level in the aged DG is also reduced. However, GFAP immunoreactivity in the CA1-3 region is increased in all layers, and the cytoplasm of GFAP immunoreactive astrocytes is hypertrophied, GFAP level in the CA1-3 region is increased. It suggests the functional difference of astrocytes between DG and Ammon's horn of hippocampus [121]. Shetty et al. (2005) found that aging does not decrease the total number of astrocytes but fractions of astrocytes that express fibroblast growth factor (FGF-2 decline considerably by middle age [122]. Astrocyte distribution also shows a strain-specific difference. For instance, among eight widely used inbred strains (C57BL/6J, A/J, BALB/c, C3H/HeJ, FVB, 129/SvJ, DBA/1, and DBA/2) and one outbred strain (ICR) mice, the number of astrocyte in the polymorphic layer of DG is highest in the DBA/1 strain and lowest in the 129/SvJ strain [97]. Environment condition may also affect astrocyte morphology. Astrocytes from animals housed in an enriched environment demonstrate a reduced distance between filament branch points and an increase in astrocyte process complexity in the rat DG [123].

Functionally, astrocytes play diverse roles in DG including support and providing nutrition to neurons, uptake of neurotransmitter and modulation of synaptic plasticity, maintenance of ion homeostasis, participation in neuronal migration during development, involving in synthesis, clearance and even release of neuroactive amino acids as well as energy supply and the formation of blood-brain barrier. Further study may be needed to elucidate the roles of subtypes of astrocytes in different sublaminars of DG molecular layer. Aging on DG astrocytes or the role of astrocytes in aging may also need to be investigated in order to correlate these changes to reduced memory in aged population.

Oligodendrocytes

The oligodendrocyte precursor cells originate from the ventral ventricular zone and from the latero-basal plate of the diencephalon during embryogenesis and migrate throughout the developing CNS where they proliferate and differentiate [124-126]. Previous studies suggest that NSCs residing SGZ of the postnatal and adult DG do not normally produce oligodendrocytes, instead these cells predominantly generate Prox1-expressing dentate granule neurons, as well as a small proportion of astrocytes [11, 127]. However, recent work indicates that DCX+ neuronal progenitors contribute to new oligodendrocytes [128]. Age-dependent alteration in the expression of oligodendrocyte-specific protein (OSP) occurs in the gerbil hippocampus. In the 1-month-old gerbil, OSP immunoreactive cell bodies are primarily detected in the hilus of DG; the detection of OSP immunoreactive fibers in DG is uncommon. From 2- to 6 -month-old gerbil, the number of OSP immunoreactive cell bodies decrease in DG, whereas OSP immunoreactive fibers increase. No obvious changes of the number of OSP immunoreactive cell bodies occur from 6- to 24-month-old gerbil, however, OSP immunoreactive fibers are marginally increased in the polymorphic layer [129]. A significant decrease in the area of expression of 2',3'-cyclic nucleotide 3'-phosphodiesterase (CNPase)-immunopositive fibers is found in DG of 1-, 2-, and 4-week-old mice [94]. It suggests that there may exist a difference in the development of oligodendrocyte processes between gerbils and mice.

Oligodendrocytes form myelin, which is involved in the fast saltatory conduction of nerve impulses in CNS [130]. While a broader range of oligodendrocytes morphologies in different brain regions have been described in many of previous studies [131-134], Murtie et al. (2007) observe remarkably homogeneous morphometric parameters in the mouse frontal cortical oligodendrocytes by three-dimensional reconstructions and measurement of the total process length, surface area, internode length, number of primary processes, branch points and internodes [135]. Using transgenic mice expressing CNPase-enhanced green fluorescent protein, a three-dimensional reconstruction tool and analysis, three morphologically distinct types, i.e., ramified, stellar and smooth oligodendrocytes are demonstrated in the mouse DG [136]. The least complex 'smooth' cell represents the youngest oligodendrocyte that matures into the stellar type and eventually turns into the most complex ramified oligodendrocyte. Each subclass of oligodendrocytes is split into two subgroups, i.e., 'near blood vessels' and 'not near blood vessels' [136]. Those oligodendrocytes 'near blood vessels' are responsible for the transportation of iron from the blood to CNS given that oligodendrocytes are the main producers of transferrin, a protein involved in iron transport [137] and involved in integrin maturation and blood–brain barrier maintenance [138].

In different layers of DG, the hilus has a high oligodendrocyte density, especially in the vicinity of the granule cell layer, suggesting that these oligodendrocytes may derive from the DG neurogenetic region, i.e., SGZ [132, 136]. Of different subtypes, ramified cells are present mostly in the hilus, stellar and smooth cells are distributed equally among the various regions. As few myelinated fibers are located in the hilus, the densely populated ramified cells with the longest processes suggest that these cells may myelinate axons outside the hilus and regulate axonal information processes in the molecular layer of DG or in the stratum lucidum and stratum lacunosum-moleculare of the CA3 area where myelinated fibers are located [136].

Functionally, oligodendrocytes in the hippocampus are implicated in a number of diseases. In particular, a number of abnormally expressed genes related to oligodendrocytes and myelin function have been demonstrated in schizophrenia [139]. Furthermore, atrophy of the myelinated fibers and swelling of oligodendrocytes processes have been described in patients with schizophrenia [140].

Neuron Glial Antigen (NG) 2 (NG2) or Platelet-Derived Growth Factor Receptor a (PDGFRα) Immunopositive Cells

NG2 immunopositive cells are also called PDGFRα immunopositive cells, as all NG2 glial cells are co-expressed PDGFRα [141]. These cells are found in grey and white matter tracts of the developing and adult CNS and have previously been assumed to represent oligodendrocyte precursor cells. New work using transgenic mice has shown that NG2 cells generate oligodendrocytes, protoplasmic astrocytes and in some instance neurons in vivo [142, 143]. In the hilus of DG, NG2 glia appear to remain at a constant low level from postnatal day 10 (P10) to P90, co-expression of NG2 and S100β is very low (3%) and constant throughout development [141]. However, in adult mice, NG2- oligodendrocyte progenitor (OPCs) is about 54% of all hilar proliferating cells compared to 11% in SGZ, represent a robust population of proliferative cells and are key to provide new oligodendrocytes to the hilar region in the adult stage [144]. These hilar $NG2^+$ cells are closer to interneurons and that both cell types receive inputs from the same populations of excitatory neurons, suggesting that hilar NG2 cells are regulated by DG neuronal activity [145].

Conclusion

In the granule cell layer of DG, densely packed granule cells in the suprapyramidal and infrapyramidal blades form a "V"- or "U"- shaped structure. The suprapyramidl blade develops earlier than infrapyramidal blade with long dendritic branches and more dendritic spines. The pyramidal basket cells are parvalbumin-, cholesystokinin (CCK) - vasoactive intestinal polypeptide (VIP)-, type 3 neuropeptide Y- or nitric oxide synthase (nNOS)- immunopositive, and located at the inner part of the granular cell layer and negatively regulate activity of granule cells. Mossy cells, like granule cells, are glutamatergic neurons and are main cells in the hilus of DG. Different subtypes of dentate interneurons are distributed in all three layers of DG. Semilunar granule cells (SGCs) which located in the inner molecular layer of DG, are morpho-functionally distinct class of dentate projection neurons, contribute to DG feedback inhibition and memory processing. In the stratum moleculare, the apical dendrites of granule cells receive three main sources of afferents, i.e., lateral and medical performant pathways and associational/commissural fibers which divide the stratum moleculare into outer, middle and inner molecular layers. The different afferent activities in the three sublayers of the stratum moleculare result in characteristic sublaminar distribution of microglia, astrocytes, and oligodendrocytes in the outer, middle and inner molecular layers, suggesting that these glial cells may also be involved in spatial and non-spatial memory. NG2 cells are main hilar proliferating cells to provide new oligodendrocytes to the hilar region in the adult stage, may receive excitatory inputs from neurons to form local circuits. The dorsal and ventral differences in their axonal projections from mossy cells, glial cell distribution throughout DG support different functional roles of dorsal and ventral DG. The residing of different type of cells at the various developmental stages in the subgranular zones suggests that DG is one of the most sensitive regions to different brain insults, in particular, radiation exposure, and is involved in pathogenesis of different neurological and neuropsychological disorders.

Further study of different laminar and sublaminar circuit-specific participation of glial cells in learning and memory processing may provide evidence for better understand the roles of different types and subtypes of glial cells in the regulation DG neuronal activity, memory formation and involvement in disease genesis.

REFERENCES

[1] Amaral, D.G., Scharfman, H.E., Lavenex, P. 2007. The dentate gyrus: fundamental neuroanatomical organization (dentate gyrus for dummies). *Prog. Brain Res.* 163, 3-22.

[2] Humphrey, T., 1967. The development of the human hippocampal fissure. *J. Anat.* 101, 655-676.

[3] Seress, L., 1992. Morphological variability and developmental aspects of monkey and human granule cells: Differences between the rodent and primate dentate gyrus. In: Ribak, C.E., Gall, C.M., Mody, I. (Eds.), The Dentate Gyrus and Its Role in Seizures. *Epilepsy Res. Suppl.* 7, 3-28.

[4] Arnold, S.E., Trojanowski, J.Q., 1996. Human fetal hippocampal development: I. Cytoarchitecture, myeloarchitecture and neuronal morphologic features. *J. Comp. Neurol.* 367, 274-292.

[5] Seress, L., 1988. Interspecies comparison of the hippocampal formation shows increased emphasis on the regio superior in the Ammon's horn of the human brain. *J. Hirnforsch.* 29, 335-340.

[6] Seress, L., Abrahám, H., Tornóczky, T., Kosztolányi, G. 2001. Cell formation in the human hippocampal formation from mid-gestation to the late postnatal period. *Neuroscience* 105(4), 831-43.

[7] Bayer, S.A., 1980. The development of the hippocampal region in the rat. I. Neurogenesis examined with 3H-thymidine autoradiography. *J. Comp. Neurol.* 190, 87-114.

[8] Bayer, S.A., 1982. Changes in the total number of dentate granule cells in juvenile and adult rats: A correlated volumetric and H3-thymidine autoradiographic study. *Exp. Brain Res.* 46, 315-323.

[9] Rakic, P., Nowakowski, R.S., 1981. The time of origin of neurons in the hippocampal region of the rhesus monkey. *J. Comp. Neurol.* 196, 99-128

[10] Kornack, D.R., Rakic, P., 1999. Continuation of neurogenesis in the hippocampus of the adult macaque monkey. *Proc. Natl. Acad. Sci.* USA 96, 5768-5773.

[11] Eriksson, P.S., Perfilieva, E., Björk-Eriksson, T., Alborn, A.M., Nordborg, C., Peterson, D.A., Gage, F.H. 1998. "Neurogenesis in the adult human hippocampus". *Nat. Med.* 4 (11), 1313–7.

[12] Bayer, S.A., Altman, J. 2008. *The Human Brain During The Early First Trimester. Atlas of Human Central Nervous System Development.* Book 5. Appendix, p. 497.

[13] Claiborne, B.J., Amaral, D.G., Cowan, WM. 1990. A quantitative three-dimensional analysis of granule cell dendrites in the rat dentate gyrus. *J. Comp. Neurol.* 302, 206–219.

[14] West, M.J., Slomianka, L., Gundersen, H.J.G. 1991. Unbiased stereological estimation of the total number of neurons in the subdivisions of the rat hippocampus using the optical fractionator. *Anat. Rec.* 231, 482–497.

[15] Rapp, P.R., & Gallagher, M. 1996. Preserved neuron number in the hippocampus of aged rats with spatial learning deficits. *Proc. Natl. Acad. Sci.* USA 93, 9926–9930.

[16] Frimmel, G., Ost, H.M., Wenzel, J. 1975. Quantitative studies on the neuron structure of the rat fascia dentate. *Z Mikrosk Anat Forsch.* 89(3), 495-511.

[17] Desmond, N.L., & Levy, W.B. 1985. Granule cell dendritic spine density in the rat hippocampus varies with spine shape and location. *Neurosci. Lett.* 54, 219–224.

[18] Wenzel, J., Stender, G., Duwe, G. 1981. Development of neuron structure of the fascia dentata in the rat. Neurohistologico-morphometric, ultrastructural and experimental study. *J. Hirnforsch.* 22(6), 629-83.

[19] Ribak, C.E., Seress, L.J. 1983. Five types of basket cell in the hippocampal dentate gyrus: a combined Golgi and electron microscopic study. *Neurocytol.* 12(4), 577-97.

[20] Seress, L., Pokorny, J. 1981. Structure of the granular layer of the rat dentate gyrus. A light microscopic and Golgi study. *J. Anat.* 133, 181–195.

[21] Valtschanoff, J.G., Weinberg, R.J., Kharazia, V.N., Schmidt, H.H., Nakane, M., Rustioni, A. 1993. Neurons in rat cerebral cortex that synthesize nitric oxide: NADPH diaphorase histochemistry, NOS immunocytochemistry, and colocalization with GABA. *Neurosci. Lett.* 157(2), 157-61.

[22] Freund, T.F., & Buzsaki, G. 1996. Interneurons of the hippocampus. *Hippocampus* 6, 347–470.

[23] Hajos, N., Acsidy, L., Freund, T.F. 1996 Target selectivity and neurochemical characteristics of VIP-immunoreactive interneurons in the rat dentate gyrus. *Eur. J. Neurosci.* 8,1415-1431.

[24] Morozov, Y.M., Ayoub, A.E., Rakic, P.J. 2006. Translocation of synaptically connected interneurons across the dentate gyrus of the early postnatal rat hippocampus. *Neurosci.* 26(19), 5017-27.

[25] Sperk, G., Hamilton, T., Colmers, W.F. 2007. Neuropeptide Y in the dentate gyrus. *Prog. Brain Res.* 163, 285-97.

[26] von Bohlen Und Halbach O. 2007. Immunohistological markers for staging neurogenesis in adult hippocampus. *Cell Tissue Res.* 329(3), 409-20.

[27] Zhang, J., & Jiao, J. 2015. Molecular biomarkers for embryonic and adult neural stem cell and neurogenesis. *Biomed. Res. Int.* 2015:727542.

[28] Gonçalves, J.T., Schafer, S.T., Gage, F.H. 2016. Adult neurogenesis in the hippocampus: From stem cells to behavior. *Cell* 167(4), 897-914.

[29] van Praag, H., Schinder, A.F., Christie, B.R., Toni, N., Palmer, T.D., Gage, F.H. 2002. Functional neurogenesis in the adult hippocampus. *Nature* 415,1030–4.

[30] Laplagne, D.A., Espósito, M.S., Piatti, V.C., Morgenstern, N.A., Zhao, C., van Praag, H., Gage, F.H., Schinder, A.F. 2006. Functional convergence of neurons generated in the developing and adult hippocampus. *PLoS Biol.* 4, e409.

[31] Soriano, E., & Frotscher, M. 1993. GABAergic innervation of the rat fascia dentata: a novel type of interneuron in the granule cell layer with extensive axonal arborization in the molecular layer. *J. Comp. Neurol.* 334(3), 385-96.

[32] Hosp, J.A., Struber, M., Yanagawa, Y., Obata, K., Vida, I., Jonas, P., Bartos, M. 2014. Morphophysiological criteria divide dentate gyrus interneurons into classes. *Hippocampus* 24,189–203.

[33] Yu, J., Swietek, B., Proddutur, A., Santhakumar, V. 2015. Dentate total molecular layer interneurons mediate cannabinoid-sensitive inhibition. *Hippocampus* 25(8), 884-9.

[34] Amaral, D. 1978. A Golgi study of cell types in the hilar region of the hippocampus in the rat. *J. Comp. Neurol.* 182(5), 851–914.
[35] Henze, D.A., & Buzsaki, G. 2007. Hilar mossy cells: functional identification and activity in vivo. *Prog. Brain Res.* 163,199–216.
[36] Sloviter, R.S., Bumanglag, A.V., Schwarcz, R., Frotscher, M. 2012. Abnormal dentate gyrus network circuitry in temporal lobe epilepsy. In: Noebels JL, Avoli M, Rogawski MA, Olsen RW, Delgado-Escueta AV, editors *Jasper's basic mechanisms of the epilepsies* [Internet]. 4. National Center for Biotechnology Information (US); Bethesda: 2012. 454–469.
[37] Jinde, S., Zsiros, V., Nakazawa, K. 2013. Hilar mossy cell circuitry controlling dentate granule cell excitability. *Front. Neural Circ.* 7, 14.
[38] Scharfman, H.E., Myers, C.E. 2013. Hilar mossy cells of the dentate gyrus: a historical perspective. *Front. Neural Circ.* 6, 106.
[39] Scharfman, H.E. 2016. The enigmatic mossy cell of the dentate gyrus. *Nat. Rev. Neurosci.*17, 562–575.
[40] Scharfman, H.E. 1992. Differentiation of rat dentate neurons by morphology and electrophysiology in hippocampal slices: granule cells, spiny hilar cells and aspiny 'fast-spiking' cells. *Epilepsy Res. Suppl.* 7, 93-109.
[41] Scharfman, H.E. 1999.The role of nonprincipal cells in dentate gyrus excitability and its relevance to animal models of epilepsy and temporal lobe epilepsy. *Adv. Neurol.* 79, 805–820.
[42] Scharfman, H., & Schwartzkroin, P. 1988. Electrophysiology of morphologically identified mossy cells of the dentate hilus recorded in guinea pig hippocampal slices. *J. Neurosci.* 8, 3812–3821
[43] Halasy, K., Somogyi, P. 1993. Subdivisions in the multiple GABAergicinnervation of granule cells in the dentate gyrus of the rat hippocampus. *Eur. J. Neurosci.* 5, 411-429.
[44] Han, Z.S., Buhl, E.H., Lorinczi, Z., Somogyi, P. 1993. A high degree of spatial selectivity in the axonal and dendritic domains of

physiologically identified local-circuit neurons in the dentate gyrus of the rat hippocampus. *Eur. J. Neurosci.* 5, 395-410.

[45] Houser, C.R. 2007. Interneurons of the dentate gyrus: an overview of cell types, terminal fields and neurochemical identity. *Prog. Brain Res.* 163, 217–232.

[46] Morgan, R.J., Santhakumar, V., Soltesz, I. 2007. Modeling the dentate gyrus. *Prog. Brain Res.* 163, 639–658.

[47] Liu, Y., Fujise, N., Kosaka, T. 1996. Distribution of calretinin immunoreactivity in the mouse dentate gyrus. I. General description. *Exp. Brain Res.* 108(3), 389-403.

[48] Tang, F.R., Chia, S.C., Jiang, F.L, Ma, D.L., Chen, P.M., Tang, Y.C. 2006. Calcium binding protein immunopositive neurons in the gliotic hippocampus of the mouse model of epilepsy with special reference to their afferents from the medial septum and nucleus of the diagonal band of Broca. *Neuroscience* 140(4), 1467-1479.

[49] Blasco-Ibáñez, J.M., & Freund, T.F. 1997. Distribution, ultrastructure, and connectivity of calretinin-immunoreactive mossy cells of the mouse dentate gyrus. *Hippocampus* 7(3), 307-20.

[50] Scharfman, H.E. 2018. Advances in understanding hilar mossy cells of the dentate gyrus. *Cell Tissue Res.* 373(3), 643-652.

[51] Botterill, J.J., Gerencer, K.J., Vinod, K.Y., Alcantara-Gonzalez, D., Scharfman, H.E. 2021. Dorsal and ventral mossy cells differ in their axonal projections throughout the dentate gyrus of the mouse hippocampus. *Hippocampus* 31(5), 522-539.

[52] Scharfman, H.E. 2007. The CA3 "backprojection" to the dentate gyrus. *Prog. Brain Res.* 163, 627–637.

[53] Deller, T., Katona, I., Cozzari, C., Frotscher, M., Freund, T.F. 1999. Cholinergic innervation of mossy cells in the rat fascia dentata. *Hippocampus* 9, 314–320.

[54] Sloviter, R.S. 1994. The functional organization of the hippocampal dentate gyrus and its relevance to the pathogenesis of temporal lobe epilepsy. *Ann. Neurol.* 35, 640–654.

[55] Ratzliff, A.H., Howard, A.L., Santhakumar, V., Osapay, I., Soltesz, I. 2004. Rapid deletion of mossy cells does not result in a hyperexcitable dentate gyrus: implications for epileptogenesis. *J. Neurosci.* 24, 2259–2269.

[56] GoodSmith, D., Chen, X., Wang, C., Kim, S.H., Song, H., Burgalossi, A., Christian, K.M., Knierim, J.J. 2017. Spatial representations of granule cells and mossy cells of the dentate gyrus. *Neuron* 93, 677–690.

[57] Senzai, Y., & Buzsaki, G. 2017. Physiological properties and behavioral correlates of hippocampal granule cells and mossy cells. *Neuron* 93, 691–704.

[58] Botterill, J.J., Lu, Y.L., LaFrancois, J.J., Bernstein, H.L., Alcantara-Gonzalez, D., Jain, S., Leary, P., Scharfman, H.E. 2019. An excitatory and epileptogenic effect of dentate gyrus mossy cells in a mouse model of epilepsy. *Cell Rep.* 29(9), 2875-2889.

[59] Bernstein, H.L., Lu, Y.L., Botterill, J.J., Scharfman, H.E. 2019. Novelty and novel objects increase c-Fos immunoreactivity in mossy cells in the mouse dentate gyrus. *Neural Plast.* 2019, 1815371.

[60] Botterill, J.J., Vinod, K.Y., Gerencer, K.J., Teixeira, C.M., LaFrancois, J.J., Scharfman, H.E. 2021. Bidirectional regulation of cognitive and anxiety-like behaviors by dentate gyrus mossy cells in male and female mice. *J. Neurosci.* 41(11), 2475-2495

[61] Buckmaster, P.S., & Schwartzkroin, P.A. 1995. Interneurons and inhibition in the dentate gyrus of the rat in vivo. *J. Neurosci.* 15, 774-789.

[62] Buckmaster, P.S., & Schwarzkroin, P.A. 1995. Physiological and morphological heterogeneity of dentate gyrus-hilus interneurons in the gerbil hippocampus in vivo. *Eur. J. Neurosci.* 7, 1393-1402.

[63] Savanthrapadian, S., Meyer, T., Elgueta, C., Booker, S.A., Vida, I., Bartos, M.J. 2014. Synaptic properties of SOM- and CCK-expressing cells in dentate gyrus interneuron networks. *Neurosci.* 34(24), 8197-209.

[64] Raza, S.A., Albrecht, A., Çalışkan, G., Müller, B., Demiray, Y.E., Ludewig, S., Meis, S., Faber, N., Hartig, R., Schraven, B., Lessmann, V., Schwegler, H., Stork, O. 2017. HIPP neurons in the dentate gyrus mediate the cholinergic modulation of background context memory salience. *Nat. Commun.* 8(1), 189.

[65] Leranth, C., Malcolm, A.J., Frotscher, M. 1990. Afferent and efferent synaptic connections of somatostatin-immunoreactive neurons in the rat fascia dentata. *J. Comp. Neurol.* 295, lll-122.

[66] Bakst, I., Avendano, C., Morrison, J.H., Amaral, D.G. 1986. An experimental analysis of the origins of somatoscatin-like immunoreactivity in the dentate gyrus of the rat. *J. Neurosci.* 6, 1452-1462.

[67] Deller, T., Nitsch, R., Frotscher, M. 1995. Phaseulus vulgaris-leucoagglutinin tracing of commissural fibers to the rat dentate gyrus: evidence for a previously unknown commissural projection to the outer molecular layer. *J. Comp. Neurol.* 352, 55-68.

[68] Katona, I., Acsády, L., Freund, T.F. 1999. Postsynaptic targets of somatostatin-immunoreactive interneurons in the rat hippocampus. *Neuroscience* 88(1), 37-55.

[69] Yuan., M., Meyer, T., Benkowitz, C., Savanthrapadian, S., Ansel-Bollepalli, L., Foggetti, A., Wulff, P., Alcami, P., Elgueta, C., Bartos, M. 2017. Somatostatin-positive interneurons in the dentate gyrus of mice provide local- and long-range septal synaptic inhibition. *Elife* 6, e21105.

[70] Leranth, C., & Frotscher, M. 1987. Cholinegic innervation of hippocampal GAD- and somatostatin-immunoreactive commissural neurons. *J. Comp. Neurol.* 261, 33-47.

[71] Gulyis, A.I., Gorcs, T.J., Freund, T.F. 1990. Innervation of different peptide-containing neurons in the hippocampus by GABAergic septa1 afferents. *Neuroscience* 37, 31-44.

[72] Deller, T., & Leranth, C. 1990. Synaptic connections of neuropeptide-Y (NPY) immunoreactive neurons in the hilar area of the rat hippocampus. *J. Comp. Neurol.* 300, 433-447.

[73] Kohler, C., Eriksson, L.G., Davies, S., Chan-Palay, V. 1987. Co-localization of neuropeptide tyrosine and somatostatin immunoreactivity in neurons of individual subfields of the rat hippocampal region. *Neurosci. Lett.* 78, 1-6.

[74] Milner, T.A., & Veznedaroglu, E. 1992. Ultrastructural localization of neuropeptide-Y-like immunoreactivity in the rat hippocampal formation. *Hippocampus* 2, 107-1 26.

[75] McQuiston, A.R., Petrozzino, J.J., Connor, J.A., Colmers, W.F. 1996. Neuropeptide Y1 receptors inhibit N-type calcium currents and reduce transient calcium increases in rat dentate granule cells. *J. Neurosci.* 15, 1422-1429.

[76] Vezzani, A., & Sperk, G. 2004. Overexpression of NPY and Y2 receptors in epileptic brain tissue: an endogenous neuroprotective mechanism in temporal lobe epilepsy? *Neuropeptides* 38(4), 245-52.

[77] Wei, Y.T., Wu, J.W., Yeh, C.W., Shen, H.C., Wu, K.P., Vida, I., Lien, C.C. 2021. Morpho-physiological properties and connectivity of vasoactive intestinal polypeptide-expressing interneurons in the mouse hippocampal dentate gyrus. *J. Comp. Neurol.* Jan 23. doi: 10.1002/cne.25116. Online ahead of print.

[78] Leranth, C., & Frotscher, M. 1986. Synaptic connections of cholecystokinin immunoreactive neurons and terminals in the rat fascia dentata: a combined light and electron microscopic study. *J. Comp. Neurol.* 254, 51-64.

[79] Gulyais, A.I., Toth, K., Danos, P., Freund, T.F. 1991. Subpopulations of GABAergic neurons containing parvalbumin, calbindin D28k, and cholecystokinin in the rat hippocampus. *J. Comp. Neurol.* 312, 371-378.

[80] Acsddy, L, Arabadzisz, D., Freund, T.F. 1996. Correlated morphological and neurochemical features indentify different subsets of VIP-immunoreactive interneurons in rat hippocampus. *Neuro-science* 73: 299-3 15.

[81] Morozov, Y.M., & Freund, T.F. 2003. Postnatal development and migration of cholecystokinin-immunoreactive interneurons in rat hippocampus. *Neuroscience* 120(4), 923-39.

[82] Liang, Z., Zhang, L., Wang, X., Gao, F., Wang, X., Zhou, S., Yu, S., Zhan, R.Z. 2013. Distribution and neurochemical features of neuronal nitric oxide synthase-expressing interneurons in the rat dentate gyrus. *Brain Res.* 1505,11-21.

[83] García-Martinez, Y., Sánchez-Huerta, K.B., Pacheco-Rosado, J. 2020. Quantitative characterization of proliferative cells subpopulations in the hilus of the hippocampus of adult Wistar rats: an integrative study. *J. Mol. Histol.* 51(4), 437-453.

[84] Larimer, P., & Strowbridge, B.W. 2010. Representing information in cell assemblies: persistent activity mediated by semilunar granule cells. *Nat. Neurosci.* 13, 213–222.

[85] Williams, P.A., Larimer, P., Gao, Y., Strowbridge, B.W. 2007. Semilunar granule cells: glutamatergic neurons in the rat dentate gyrus with axon collaterals in the inner molecular layer. *J. Neurosci.* 27,13756– 13761.

[86] Gupta, A., Proddutur, A., Chang, Y.J., Raturi, V., Guevarra, J., Shah, Y., Elgammal, F.S., Santhakumar, V. 2020. Dendritic morphology and inhibitory regulation distinguish dentate semilunar granule cells from granule cells through distinct stages of postnatal development. *Brain Struct. Funct.* 225(9), 2841-2855.

[87] Thind, K.K., Ribak, C.E., Buckmaster, P.S. 2008. Synaptic input to dentate granule cell basal dendrites in a rat model of temporal lobe epilepsy. *J. Comp. Neurol.* 509,190–202.

[88] Save, L., Baude, A., Cossart, R. 2019. Temporal embryonic origin critically determines cellular physiology in the dentate gyrus. *Cereb. Cortex.* 29(6), 2639-2652.

[89] Gupta, A., Elgammal, F.S., Proddutur, A., Shah, S., Santhakumar, V. 2012. Decrease in tonic inhibition contributes to increase in dentate semilunar granule cell excitability after brain injury. *J. Neurosci.* 32(7), 2523-37.

[90] Walker, M.C., Pavlov, I., Kullmann, D.M. 2010. A 'sustain pedal' in the hippocampus? *Nat. Neurosci.* 13,146–148.

[91] Gall, C., Berry, L.M., L A Hodgson, L.A. 1986. Cholecystokinin in the mouse hippocampus: localization in the mossy fiber and dentate commissural systems. *Exp. Brain Res.* 62(2), 431-7.

[92] Dalmau, I., Finsen, B., Tønder, N., Zimmer, J., González, B., Castellano, B. 1997. Development of microglia in the prenatal rat hippocampus. *J. Comp. Neurol.* 377(1), 70-84.

[93] Dalmau, I., Finsen, B., Zimmer, J., González, B., Castellano, B. 1998. Development of microglia in the postnatal rat hippocampus. *Hippocampus* 8(5), 458-74.

[94] Kimoto, H., Eto, R., Abe, M., Kato, H., Araki, T. 2009. Alterations of glial cells in the mouse hippocampus during postnatal development. *Cell Mol. Neurobiol.* 29(8), 1181-9

[95] de Oliveira, T.C.G., Carvalho-Paulo, D., de Lima, C.M., de Oliveira, R.B., Santos Filho, C., Diniz, D.G., Bento Torres Neto, J., Picanço-Diniz, C.W. 2020. Long-term environmental enrichment reduces microglia morphological diversity of the molecular layer of dentate gyrus. *Eur. J. Neurosci.* 52(9), 4081-4099.

[96] Hwang, I.K., Lee, C.H., Li, H., Yoo, K.Y., Choi, J.H., Kim, D.W., Kim, D.W., Suh, H.W., Won, M.H. 2008. Comparison of ionized calcium-binding adapter molecule 1 immunoreactivity of the hippocampal dentate gyrus and CA1 region in adult and aged dogs. *Neurochem. Res.* 33(7), 1309-15.

[97] Kim, J.W., Nam, S.M., Yoo, D.Y., Jung, H.Y., Hwang, I.K., Seong, J.K., Yoon, Y.S. 2018. Strain-specific differential expression of astrocytes and microglia in the mouse hippocampus. *Brain Behav.* 8(5), e00961.

[98] Tremblay, M.È., Lowery, R.L., Majewska, A.K. 2010. Tremblay MÈ, Microglial interactions with synapses are modulated by visual experience. *PLoS Biol.* 8(11), e1000527.

[99] Squarzoni, P., Oller, G., Hoeffel, G., Pont-Lezica, L., Rostaing, P., Low, D., Bessis, A., Ginhoux, F., Garel, S. 2014. Microglia

modulate wiring of the embryonic forebrain. *Cell Rep.* 8(5), 1271-9.

[100] Appel, J.R., Ye, S., Tang, F., Sun, D., Zhang, H., Mei, L., Xiong, W.C. 2018. Increased microglial activity, impaired adult hippocampal neurogenesis, and depressive-like behavior in microglial VPS35-depleted mice. *J. Neurosci.* 38(26), 5949-5968.

[101] Soch, A., Sominsky, L., Younesi, S., De Luca, S.N., Gunasekara, M., Bozinovski, S., Spencer, S.J. 2020. The role of microglia in the second and third postnatal weeks of life in rat hippocampal development and memory. *Brain Behav. Immun.* 88, 675-687.

[102] Sievers, J., Hartmann, D., Pehlemann, F.W., Berry, M. 1992. Development of astroglial cells in the proliferative matrices, the granule cell layer, and the hippocampal fissure of the hamster dentate gyrus. *J. Comp. Neurol.* 320(1), 1-32

[103] Yuasa, S. 2001. Development of astrocytes in the mouse hippocampus as tracked by tenascin-C gene expression. *Arch. Histol. Cytol.* 64(2),149-58.

[104] Bailey, M.S., & Shipley, M.T. 1993. Astrocyte subtypes in the rat olfactory bulb: morphological heterogeneity and differential laminar distribution. *J. Comp. Neurol.* 328,501–526.

[105] Walz, W., & Lang, M.K. 1998. Immunocytochemical evidence for a distinct GFAP-negative subpopulation of astrocytes in the adult rat hippocampus. *Neurosci, Lett,* 257,127–130.

[106] Emsley, J.G., & Macklis, J.D. 2006. Astroglial heterogeneity closely reflects the neuronal-defined anatomy of the adult murine CNS. *Neuron Glia Biol.* 2,175–186.

[107] McKhann, G.M. 2nd, D'Ambrosio. R., Janigro. D. 1997. Heterogeneity of astrocyte resting membrane potentials and intercellular coupling revealed by whole-cell and gramicidin-perforated patch recordings from cultured neocortical and hippocampal slice astrocytes. *J. Neurosci.* 17, 6850–6863.

[108] Walz, W. 2000. Controversy surrounding the existence of discrete functional classes of astrocytes in adult gray matter. *Glia* 31, 95–103.

[109] Doyle, J.P., Dougherty, J.D., Heiman, M., Schmidt, E.F., Stevens, T.R., Ma, G., Bupp, S., Shrestha, P., Shah, R.D., Doughty, M.L., Gong, S., Greengard, P., Heintz, N. 2008. Application of a translational profiling approach for the comparative analysis of CNS cell types. *Cell* 135, 749–762.

[110] Isaacs, K.R., Sirevaag, A.M., Marks, A.E., Chang, F.L., Greenough, W.T. 1993. A method for quantification of astrocytic processes reveals laminar differences in the dentate gyrus but not in CA1 of the hippocampal formation. *J. Neurosci. Methods* 48(1-2),141-8.

[111] Rapp, P.R., Stack, E.C., Gallagher, M. 1999. Morphometric studies of the aged hippocampus: I. Volumetric analysis in behaviorally characterized rats. *J. Comp. Neurol.* 403, 459–470.

[112] Ogata, K., & Kosaka, T. 2002. Structural and quantitative analysis of astrocytes in the mouse hippocampus. *Neuroscience* 113, 221–233.

[113] Bushong, E.A., Martone, M.E., Ellisman, M.H. 2003. Examination of the relationship between astrocyte morphology and laminar boundaries in the molecular layer of adult dentate gyrus *J. Comp. Neurol.* 462(2), 241-51.

[114] Jinno, S. 2011. Regional and laminar differences in antigen profiles and spatial distributions of astrocytes in the mouse hippocampus, with reference to aging. *Neuroscience* 180,41-52.

[115] Kosaka, T., & Hama, K. 1986. Three-dimensional structure of astrocytes in the rat dentate gyrus. *J. Comp. Neurol.* 249(2), 242-60.

[116] Brunne, B., Zhao, S., Derouiche, A., Herz, J., May, P., Frotscher, M., Bock, H.H. 2010. Origin, maturation, and astroglial transformation of secondary radial glial cells in the developing dentate gyrus. *Glia* 58(13),1553-69.

[117] Patrylo, P.R., & Nowakowski, R.S. 1994. Morphology and distribution of astrocytes in the molecular layer of the dentate gyrus in NZB/BlNJ, Dreher, and C57BL/6J mice. *Glia* 10, 1–9.

[118] Geinisman, Y., Bondareff, W., Dodge. J. 1978. Hypertrophy of astroglial processes in the dentate gyrus of the senescent rat. *Am. J. Anat.,* 153, 537-544

[119] Kishi, K., Stanfield, B., Cowan, W. 1978. A note on the distribution of glial cells in the molecular layer of the dentate gyrus. *Brain Res. Bull.*, 4, 35-41.

[120] Pilegaard, K., & Ladefoged, O. 1996. Total number of astrocytes in the molecular layer of the dentate gyrus of rats at different ages. *Anal. Quant. Cytol. Histol.* 18(4), 279-85.

[121] Hwang, I.K., Choi, J.H., Li, H., Yoo, K.Y., Kim, D.W., Lee, C.H., Yi, S.S., Seong, J.K., Lee, I.S., Yoon, Y.S., Won, M.H. 2008. Changes in glial fibrillary acidic protein immunoreactivity in the dentate gyrus and hippocampus proper of adult and aged dogs. *J. Vet Med. Sci.* 70(9), 965-9.

[122] Shetty, A.K., Hattiangady, B., Shetty, G.A. 2005. Stem/progenitor cell proliferation factors FGF-2, IGF-1, and VEGF exhibit early decline during the course of aging in the hippocampus: role of astrocytes. *Glia* 51(3),173-86.

[123] Salois, G., Smith, J.S. 2016. Housing complexity alters GFAP-immunoreactive astrocyte morphology in the rat dentate gyrus. *Neural Plast.* 2016, n3928726.

[124] Timsit, S., Martinez, S., Allinquant, B., Peyron, F., Puelles, L. & Zalc, B. (1995) Oligodendrocytes originate in a restricted zone of the embryonic ventral neural tube defined by DM-20 mRNA expression. *J. Neurosci.,* 15, 1012–1024.

[125] Miller, R.H. (1996) Oligodendrocyte origins. *Trends Neurosci.,* 19, 92–96

[126] He, W., Ingraham, C., Rising, L., Goderie, S. & Temple, S. (2001) Multipotent stem cells from the mouse basal forebrain contribute GABAergic neurons and oligodendrocytes to the cerebral cortex during embryogenesis. *J. Neurosci.,* 21, 8854–8862.

[127] Gil V, Bichler Z, Lee JK, Seira O, Llorens F, Bribian A, Morales R, Claverol-Tinture E, Soriano E, Sumoy L, et al. Developmental

expression of the oligodendrocyte myelin glycoprotein in the mouse telencephalon. *Cereb Cortex* 2010; 20:1769-79.

[128] Klein, B., Mrowetz, H., Kreutzer, C., Rotheneichner, P., Zaunmair, P., Lange, S., Coras, R., Couillard-Despres, S., Rivera, F.J., Aigner, L. 2020. DCX^+ neuronal progenitors contribute to new oligodendrocytes during remyelination in the hippocampus. *Sci. Rep.* 10(1), 20095.

[129] Lee HA, Park JH, Kim DW, Lee CH, Hwang IK, Kim H, Shin MC, Cho JH, Lee JC, Noh Y, Kim SS, Won MH, Ahn JH. Age-dependent alteration in the expression of oligodendrocyte-specific protein in the gerbil hippocampus. *Mol Med Rep.* 2018 Mar;17(3):3615-3620.

[130] Baumann, N., & Pham-Dinh, D. 2001. Biology of oligodendrocyte and myelin in the mammalian central nervous system. *Physiol. Rev.* 81, 871-927.

[131] Ogawa, Y., Eins, S., Wolff, J.R. 1985. Oligodendrocytes in the pons and middle cerebellar peduncle of the cat. Topographical relations to neurons and transverse axon bundles. *Cell Tissue Res.* 240, 541–552.

[132] Berger, T., & Frotscher, M. 1994. Distribution and morphological characteristics of oligodendrocytes in the rat hippocampus in situ and in vitro: an immunocytochemical study with the monoclonal Rip antibody. *J. Neurocytol.* 23, 61–74.

[133] Butt AM, Colquhoun K, Tutton M, Berry M. 1994. Three-dimensional morphology of astrocytes and oligodendrocytes in the intact mouse optic nerve. *J Neurocytol.* 23:469–485.

[134] McIver, S.R., Lee, C.S., Lee, J.M., Green, S.H., Sands, M.S., Snider, B.J., Goldberg, M.P. 2005. Lentiviral transduction of murine oligodendrocytes in vivo. *J. Neurosci. Res.* 82, 397–403

[135] Murtie, J.C., Macklin, W.B., Corfas, G. 2007. Morphometric analysis of oligodendrocytes in the adult mouse frontal cortex. *J. Neurosci. Res.* 85, 2080–2086.

[136] Vinet J, Lemieux P, Tamburri A, Tiesinga P, Scafidi J, Gallo V, Sík A. Subclasses of oligodendrocytes populate the mouse hippocampus. *Eur J Neurosci.* 2010 Feb;31(3):425-38.

[137] Todorich, B., Zhang, X., Slagle-Webb, B., Seaman, W.E. & Connor, J.R. (2008) Tim-2 is the receptor for H-ferritin on oligodendrocytes. *J. Neurochem.,* 107, 1495–1505.

[138] Del Zoppo, G.J., Milner, R., Mabuchi, T., Hung, S., Wang, X., Koziol, J.A. 2006. Vascular matrix adhesion and the blood-brain barrier. *Biochem. Soc. Trans.,* 34, 1261–1266.

[139] Haroutunian, V., Katsel, P., Dracheva, S., Stewart, D.G., Davis, K.L. 2007. Variations in oligodendrocyte-related gene expression across multiple cortical regions: implications for the pathophysiology of schizophrenia. *Int. J. Neuropsychopharmacol.* 10, 565–573.

[140] Uranova, N.A., Vostrikov, V.M., Vikhreva, O.V., Zimina, I.S., Kolomeets, N.S., Orlovskaya, D.D. 2007. The role of oligodendrocyte pathology in schizophrenia. *Int. J. Neuropsycho-Pharmacol.* 10, 537–545.

[141] Moshrefi-Ravasdjani, B., Dublin, P., Seifert, G., Jennissen, K., Steinhäuser, C., Kafitz, K.W., Rose, C.R. 2017. Changes in the proliferative capacity of NG2 cell subpopulations during postnatal development of the mouse hippocampus. *Brain Struct. Funct.* 222(2), 831-847.

[142] Belachew, S., Chittajallu, R., Aguirre, A.A., Yuan, X., Kirby, M., Anderson, S., Gallo, V. 2003. Postnatal NG2 proteoglycan-expressing progenitor cells are intrinsically multipotent and generate functional neurons. *J. Cell Biol.* 161(1), 169-86

[143] Trotter, J., Karram, K., Nishiyama, A. 2010. NG2 cells: Properties, progeny and origin. *Brain Res. Rev.* 63(1-2), 72-82.

[144] Huang, W., Zhao, N., Bai, X., Karram, K., Trotter, J., Goebbels, S., Scheller, A., Kirchhof, F. 2014. Novel NG2-CreERT2 knock-in mice demonstrate heterogeneous diferentiation potential of NG2glia during development. *Glia* 62, 896–913.

[145] Mangin, J.M., Kunze, A., Chittajallu, R., Gallo, V. 2008. Satellite NG2 progenitor cells share common glutamatergic inputs with associated interneurons in the mouse dentate gyrus. *J. Neurosci.* 28(30), 7610-23.

In: The Dentate Gyrus
Editor: Feng-Ru Tang
ISBN: 978-1-68507-212-4

Chapter 3

AFFERENT AND EFFERENT OF THE DENTATE GYRUS AND THEIR NEUROPHYSIOLOGICAL ROLES

Jie Hua Xu**, PhD

Department of Human Anatomy and Histoembryology,
Xi'an Jiaotong University School of Basic Medical Sciences,
Key Laboratory of Environment and Genes Related to Diseases
(Xi'an Jiaotong University), Ministry of Education, Xi'an,
Shaanxi Province, The People's Republic of China

ABSTRACT

The dentate gyrus is the first input region of trisynaptic pathways of the hippocampus where all sensory modalities, including olfactory, vestibular, visual, auditory, and somatosensory inputs merge to form unique representation. The interaction or integration of different inputs may play a critical role in learning and memory. To understand the function of the dentate gyrus, we may have to firstly appreciate its anatomical neuronal connections. In this chapter, I summarized the

* Corresponding Author's Email: xujiehua@xjtu.edu.cn.

detailed afferent and efferent pathway of the dentate gyrus, including the connections related to both principal neurons and interneurons. The cell architecture of each sub-regions of the dentate gyrus and their chemical property (neurotransmitters) are then reviewed. The neurophysiological roles of the dentate gyrus are discussed in the last part of the chapter.

Keywords: hippocampus, dentate gyrus, entorhinal cortex, granule cell, mossy cell, afferent, efferent, neurophysiological roles, learning and memory

1. Introduction

The dentate gyrus (DG) is one of the important structures of the larger functional brain system called the hippocampal formation [1-3]. The brain processes, stores and retrieves relevant information from the environment. In the mammalian brain, the interaction between the hippocampal formation and the neocortex is important for this function [4-6]. The dentate gyrus is strongly involved in cognitive function. Animal experimental research and human study indicate that neurons in the dentate gyrus play an important role in learning and memory [7-9]. Abnormalities in hippocampal formation have been heavily implicated in the pathophysiology of schizophrenia. The dentate gyrus was shown to manifest an immature molecular profile in patients with schizophrenia as well as in various animal models of schizophrenia. More specifically, it is presumed that the dentate gyrus is involved in decorrelating the incoming information from layer II of the entorhinal cortex (pattern separation) and CA3 recurrent network is involved in the pattern completion [10-15]. In adult rodents, monkeys and humans, the dentate gyrus is also an area with neurogenesis [3, 16, 17].

Along with other parts of the hippocampal formation, the dentate gyrus forms a “banana-shaped structure” [1]. Morphologically, the dentate gyrus is subdivided into three distinct layers: molecular, granular, and polymorphic. The classic trisynaptic pathway plays a central role in information processing, and in this pathway, the dentate gyrus is the gateway to the hippocampus. Strong evidence suggests that the dentate gyrus receives diverse information from the environment and acts as a preprocessor of incoming information, preparing it for the subsequent processing in CA3 area of the hippocampus.

To unspecialized neurosurgeons or neurologists, anatomy of the hippocampal formation is very intricate and difficult to comprehend [2]. Recent studies of the structure, function, and plasticity of hippocampal dentate gyrus microcircuits have revealed many new connections, and suggested that the classic trisynaptic pathway comprises the excitatory cells (mostly stellate cells) in layer II of the entorhinal cortex, the granule cells in the dentate gyrus, and the pyramidal cells in CA3 and CA1 regions of the hippocampal formation [1, 18-21]. Granule cells, the main efferent cells of the dentate gyrus, send mossy fibers to CA3 area and innervate a small number of principal neurons and a disproportionally large number of interneurons [22, 23]. CA3 principal neurons then form recurrent excitatory network and send axons to CA1 area. The idea that the dentate gyrus-CA3 system performs the pattern separation and the pattern completion of the inputs to the hippocampus, operations needed for memory encoding and retrieval is supported by theoretical work, as well as anatomical, physiological, and behavioral experiments.

In this chapter, I focus on reviewing the detailed microcircuit (including both intrinsic and extrinsic connections) of the dentate gyrus, as well as its relevant physiological roles.

2. Afferent of the Dentate Gyrus

2.1. Cortical Afferent of the Dentate Gyrus

2.1.1. Entorhinal Input to the Dentate Gyrus

The major input of the dentate gyrus and also the main input of the hippocampus and the subiculum is from the entorhinal cortex. Fibers originating mainly from neurons located in layers II and III of the entorhinal cortex, with a smaller component from the deeper layers of the entorhinal cortex are the main input to the dentate gyrus, which is referred to as the so-called perforant pathway. Neuronal origin of the perforant pathway has been considered coming exclusively from the stellate cells in layer II and the pyramidal neurons in layer III of the entorhinal cortex. However, there are studies indicating that many other cell types, such as GABAergic neurons, also project to the dentate gyrus and other hippocampal sub-regions [24, 25].

All sub-regions of the hippocampal formation receive the input of the perforant pathway [26-32]. The axons of the neurons in the entorhinal cortex pass through the underlying white matter and the angular bundle, cross the pyramidal cell layer of the subiculum, traverse the hippocampal fissure, and finally, part of them enters the dentate gyrus and part of them is distributed to the molecular layer of the subiculum and the hippocampus. In addition to the typical perforant pathway, the entorhinal cortex axons also take alternative pathways to the other hippocampal sub-regions, such as passing through the stratum alveus before entering the hippocampus or traversing the molecular layers of the entorhinal cortex and the pre- and parasubiculum. Therefore, the term perforant pathway nowadays encompasses all of the projection systems from the entorhinal cortex to the hippocampal formation [32]. In this chapter, I will focus on the afferent to the dentate gyrus.

While the dentate gyrus is considered being an exclusive target of the perforant pathway initially, the entorhinal cortex also projects to the other hippocampal sub-regions, such as CA1, CA2, and CA3, as well as the subiculum [30-32]. The axons to the dentate gyrus originate from layer II of the entorhinal cortex [31, 33-36]. There is evidence indicating that a minor component of the axons of the perforant pathway is from the layer IV to layer VI of the entorhinal cortex [27]. The perforant pathway axons terminate to the outer two thirds of the molecular layer of the dentate gyrus, where asymmetric synapses are formed [37]. The asymmetric synapses occur mainly on the dendritic spines of the granule cells of dentate gyrus, a minor proportion of the perforant pathway axons terminates on parvalbumin-immunopositive interneurons [38]. In the outer two thirds of the molecular layer of dentate gyrus, the perforant pathway asymmetric synapses account for at least 85% of the total population of synapses in this layer [37].

The characteristics of the entorhinal input to the dentate gyrus are summarized as the followings:

1. The outer one third of the molecular layer of the dentate gyrus receives the axons from the lateral entorhinal area (LEA) and the middle one third of the molecular layer receives axons from the medial entorhinal area (MEA) [30, 32, 39-41]. Using anterograde transport of tritiated amino acids, the perforant pathway is suggested to be subdivided into lateral, intermediate, and medial components [31, 41]. The intermediate component of the perforant pathway is from the intermediate entorhinal area and project to the molecular layer between the projections from the LEA and MEA. However, the study conducted with the anterograde tracer PHA-L indicates that there is probably not a discrete intermediate perforant pathway. Rather, the perforant pathway is organized in such a way that, as the position of the neurons of origin moves from lateral to medial in the LEA or MEA, the densest portion of the terminal field shifts from the outer to inner molecular layer [42].
2. The lateral and medial components of the perforant pathway may also distribute their fibers differentially along the transverse axis of the dentate gyrus, with the lateral component preferentially terminates to the suprapyramidal blade of the dentate gyrus, whereas the medial component either does not show a preference or predominantly targets the infrapyramidal blade [41]. Using PHA-L as a tracer, it has been shown that the entire transverse extent of the molecular layer of the dentate gyrus receive projections from both LEA and MEA, although the termination does have a topography relating to the lateral to medial axis of origin inside the entorhinal cortex. The suprapyramidal blade almost exclusively receives terminations from the lateral

component of LEA, whereas the infrapyramidal blade preferentially receives terminations from the more medial component of LEA. The suprapyramidal blade receives heavy terminations from lateral and caudal components of MEA, whereas the infrapyramidal blade receives denser termination from the medial components of MEA. In the dentate gyrus, there is no cells found projecting back to the entorhinal cortex. The neurotransmitter used in the perforant pathway is glutamate [43]. For those from the lateral perforant pathway, it may also be enkephalin immunopositive, whereas those from the medial pathway, it may be cholecystokinin (CCK) immunopositive [44].

2.1.2. Presubiculum and Parasubiculum Inputs to the Dentate Gyrus

The dentate gyrus also receives projections from the presubiculum and parasubiculum [26]. Axons from these regions enter the molecular layer of the dentate gyrus first, and then bifurcate in a region that is located between the lateral and medial components of the perforant pathway terminations. The axons from the presubiculum tend to be thicker than those from the entorhinal cortex. These axons give rise to collaterals with a radial course in the molecular layer of dentate gyrus. The precise targets and neurotransmitter used by these axons are still unknown. Based on the fact that the anterior thalamic nucleus provides the only direct innervation to presubiculum. These fibers may offer a potential link for communication of the anterior thalamus and the dentate gyrus.

2.1.3. CA3 Input to the Dentate Gyrus

The mossy fibers from the granule cells of the dentate gyrus innervate CA3 pyramidal neurons. This is the main output of the dentate gyrus. Meanwhile, CA3 also project back to the dentate gyrus [45, 46]. Animal experimental studies indicate that the hilus of dentate gyrus receives collateral projections from CA3 pyramidal neurons [47, 48] and the collateral projections terminate in the inner molecular layer (IML) of the ventral pole of the hippocampal formation [48]. Based on a variety of subtle differences in the dendritic organization of the pyramidal neurons in different part of CA3, CA3 is subdivided into CA3a, CA3b and CA3c. Most of the collateral projections to the dentate gyrus arise from CA3c, with fewer from CA3b and CA3a. However, the recurrent collaterals between CA3a–CA3b pyramidal neurons and CA3c pyramidal neurons can make it possible for CA3a–CA3b to influence the dentate gyrus via the CA3c [45]. In addition, in the hilus, mossy cells and interneurons are innervated by axons from CA3 pyramidal neurons [49-51]. CA3c axons modulates the mossy cells which in turn project to granule cells and interneurons to excite and/or inhibit granule cells. This circuit may be involved in the pattern separation process. Axons from CA3 pyramidal neurons, in particular from ventral CA3c, cross the granule cell layer and collateralized in the inner molecular layer of the dentate gyrus. These axons exhibit numerous varicosities, suggesting that they innervate dentate gyrus granule cells and other cells. Therefore, the CA3c pyramidal neurons of ventral hippocampus may provide the most CA3 input to the dentate gyrus to regulate the activity of the granule cells [47].

2.2. Subcortical Afferent of the Dentate Gyrus

Subcortical inputs to the dentate gyrus originate mainly from the septal nuclei, the supramamillary region of the posterior hypothalamus, and several monoaminergic nuclei in the brain stem, especially the locus coeruleus and the raphe nuclei.

2.2.1. Projections from the Septal Region

The septal inputs to the hippocampal formation was demonstrated in the early 1950s [52, 53], and subsequent studies further confirm the projection [54-63]. Neurons from the medial septal nucleus and the nucleus of the diagonal band of Broca project to hippocampal formation. The axons from the septal region travel to the hippocampal formation via three routes: the fimbria, dorsal fornix, and supracallosal stria. The axons from the amygdaloid complex travel to the hippocampal formation via a ventral pathway. All sub-regions of the hippocampal formation receive the septal axons terminals and the fibers in the dentate gyrus are particularly prominent. In the dentate gyrus, septal fibers heavily innervate the polymorphic layer, particularly in a narrow infragranular band, and terminate more lightly in the molecular layer.

The septal projection to the dentate gyrus and other parts of the hippocampal formation is topographically organized. Cells located medially in the medial septal nucleus tend to project preferentially to septal or dorsal levels of the hippocampal formation, whereas cells located laterally in the septal area tend to project temporally in the hippocampal formation [64-67]. Retrograde tracer studies have demonstrated, that septal levels of the dentate gyrus and other hippocampal fields obtain most of their cholinergic input from the nucleus of the diagonal band whereas temporal levels of the areas receive their cholinergic innervation primarily from the medial septal nucleus [54]. The ventral septal pathway to the hippocampal formation appears to arise mainly from the nucleus of the diagonal band of Broca [57, 60].

As fimbrial transections led to a substantial loss of histochemical staining of the degradative enzyme acetyl-cholinesterase, Lewis and Shute [68] proposed that the septohippocampal projection was cholinergic. Combined immunohistochemical staining of the specific cholinergic marker choline acetyl-transferase with retrograde tracer techniques showed that 30-50% of the cells in the medial septal nucleus and 50-75% of the cells in the nucleus of the diagonal band that project to the hippocampal formation are cholinergic [54, 69, 70]. Retrograde tracing studies verified that only the part of the septal neurons that terminate to the hippocampal formation are cholinergic. Many of the septal neurons that terminate to the dentate gyrus and other hippocampal sub-regions contain glutamic acid decarboxylase and are presumably GABAergic [71]. These GABAergic terminals target the dentate gyrus and also the sub-regions of the hippocampus, with an obvious preference for the GABAergic interneurons [72]. Many of the GABAergic interneurons that receive GABAergic septal terminals are also immunoreactive for cholecystokinin, somatostatin, or VIP [73] or contain one of the calcium binding proteins (calretinin, calbindin, or parvalbumin) [72, 74].

2.2.2. Projections from the Supramammillary Region

The dentate gyrus also receives input from the hypothalamus. The main hypothalamic projection to the dentate gyrus is from a subset of big neurons in the supramammillary area which cap and partially surround the mammillary nuclei of the mammillary body [36, 75-80]. Heavy projection from the supramammillary area terminates in the inner molecular layer of the dentate gyrus whereas only light projection is found in the hilus of the dentate gyrus. Further study indicated two distinct neurochemical pathways from the supramammillary nucleus to the dentate gyrus. The first pathway originates from neurons in the lateral region of the supramammillary nucleus and innervates the supragranular layer of the dorsal dentate gyrus and, to a much lesser extent, the ventral dentate gyrus. This pathway displays a unique dual phenotype for GABAergic and glutamatergic neurotransmission. Axon terminals contain markers of GABAergic neurotransmission, including the synthesizing enzyme of GABA, glutamate decarboxylase 65, and the vesicular GABA transporter and also a marker of glutamatergic neurotransmission, the vesicular glutamate transporter 2. The second pathway originates from neurons in the most posterior and medial part of the supramammillary nucleus and innervates exclusively the inner molecular layer of the ventral dentate gyrus and the CA2/CA3a pyramidal cell layer of the hippocampus. The axon terminals from the medial part of the supramammillary nucleus contain the vesicular glutamate transporter 2 only [81].

In addition to the neurons in the supramammillary region, there are other neurons scattered in several hypothalamic nuclei (many of which are in a perifornical or within the lateral hypothalamic area) that project to the hippocampal formation too. These neurons constitute a sizable input to the hippocampal formation. However, it is difficult to study their projection due to the diffuse distribution pattern and lack of any distinctive biochemical marker. A subset of these neurons demonstrates alpha-melanocyte stimulating hormone-like immunoreactivity and project diffusely to different parts of the hippocampal formation [82]. This supramammillary-dentate gyrus pathway is also immunoreactive for substance P [83-85].

2.2.3. Monoaminergic Projections from the Brain Stem

A particularly prominent noradrenergic projection to the dentate gyrus is from the pontine nucleus locus coeruleus [86-93]. The noradrenergic axons project mainly to the hilus of the dentate gyrus. In addition, the serotonergic projections that originates from several subdivisions of the raphe nuclei also terminate heavily in the hilus, but the projection tends to be limited to the subgranular zone [94]. Halasy et al. [95] have shown that the raphe serotonergic fibers preferentially terminate on a class of interneurons in the dentate gyrus that primarily influence the distal dendrites of the granule cells. However, as with the cholinergic projection, many of the cells in the raphe nuclei that project to the hippocampal formation appear to be non-serotonergic [96, 97]. Therefore, both serotonin- and non-serotonin-containing neurons in the raphe nucleus innervate the dentate gyrus. Study indicated that these projections may be crossed but not bilateral. The dentate gyrus also receives a minor and diffusely distributed dopaminergic projection mainly from cells located in the ventral tegmental area [98]. The dopaminergic fibers terminate mainly in the hilus of the dentate gyrus.

3. Efferent of the Dentate Gyrus

3.1. Efferent from the Granule Cells of the Dentate Gyrus

The dentate gyrus gives rise to the main extrinsic projections, the unmyelinated mossy fibers, to the CA3 area of the hippocampus. In CA3, the mossy fiber has few collaterals. The mossy fibers have characteristic large (3-6 μm in diameter) presynaptic varicosities /CA3 pyramidal cell contacts (mossy fiber expansions) which are distributed at approximately

140um intervals [99]. The axons extend throughout the full transverse extent of the CA3 field regardless of the location of their origin from the granule cells. Proximal to CA3, the infrapyramidal bundle is formed by mossy fibers traveling deep to the pyramidal cell layer; the intrapyramidal bundle is formed by fibers projecting within the pyramidal cell layer; whereas the suprapyramidal bundle are formed by other fibers taking a course superficial to the pyramidal cell layer, which is the major constituent of stratum lucidum. All the bundles project to the stratum lucidum and stop at the CA3/ CA2 border.

The mossy fiber presynaptic expansion forms a unique synaptic complex with an equally intricate postsynaptic process, the thorny excrescence of dendrites of CA3 pyramidal neurons. These spine-like processes are large, multi-lobulated entities (with as many as 16 branches) that are surrounded by a single mossy fiber expansion. As many as 37 synaptic contacts can be formed between a single mossy fiber expansion and a single CA3 pyramidal cell dendrite [100]. Based on the large size and proximal dendritic formation of the mossy fiber synapse, granule cells play a vital role in regulating the activity of hippocampal pyramidal cells although their mossy fibers innervate relatively few pyramidal neurons [101]. It have been estimated that in the stratum lucidum, each mossy fiber has approximately 14 synaptic expansions along its course. Based on the fact that each of expansion contacts only one single pyramidal cell (or at most two dendrites from adjacent pyramidal cells), only 14-28 pyramidal neurons are likely to be influenced by one granule cell [99]. In contrast, one CA3 pyramidal cell may receive contacts from about 50 granule cells.

Based on the lamellar trajectory, the mossy fibers remain as approximately the same septotemporal level in the stratum lucidum as the cells of origin [67, 99, 102, 103]. Mossy fibers from the septal pole of dentate gyrus make an abrupt temporal turn near the CA3/CA2 border and in turn extend for 1 mm or more toward the temporal pole. It suggests that the most distal portion of CA3 area may be influenced by granule cells from a much wider septotemporal extent of the dentate gyrus than the proximal portions of CA3 area. They might, therefore, form a special class of integrator CA3 cells. By using in vivo intracellular techniques, Acsady et al. verified that mossy fibers traveled temporally for 2–3 mm and typical mossy fiber expansions along this portion of their trajectory were found [1, 22].

Like other principal intrinsic networks of the rat hippocampal formation, the mossy fibers use glutamate as a primary neurotransmitter [83]. However it is now clear that some mossy fibers also use opiate peptides such as dynorphin as a neurotransmitter [105-110].

3.2. Efferent from the Polymorphic Neurons of Dentate Gyrus

The inner third of the molecular layer of the dentate gyrus receives projections that originate exclusively from cells in the polymorphic layer [46, 67, 111-115]. The origin of this projection is from both the ipsilateral and the contralateral sides, it is called the associational/commissural projection. The majority of terminals of this pathway form asymmetric excitatory synaptic terminals on spines of the granule cell dendrites [116, 117]. Many of these axons originate from the large mossy cells of the polymorphic layer, and individual mossy cell contributes a projection to both ipsilateral associational and contralateral commissural projections [46, 113, 114, 118, 119]. Because the mossy cells are immunoreactive for glutamate [120], it is likely that they release this excitatory transmitter substance at their terminals within the associational/commissural zone of the molecular layer. The projections from one septotemporal lamella of the polymorphic layer of dentate gyrus to the molecular layer are widely distributed. The projection at the level of original lamella appears to be obviously lighter than that to more distant lamella of the dentate gyrus [21]. The granule cells give dense innervation to the mossy cells at the same lamella, and mossy cells in turn send their associational/ commissural fibers to granule cells located at distant lamella of the dentate gyrus. The associational and commissural fibers also contact the dendritic shafts and spines of GABAergic basket cells [121, 122]. Thus, the associational and commissural projections from the polymorphic layer may function both as a feed-forward excitatory and inhibitory pathways. As the somatostatin/GABA pathway has a limited distribution pattern, mossy fiber collaterals projecting on somatostatin/GABA neurons in the polymorphic layer may lead predominantly to a direct inhibition of granule cells at the same septotemporal lamella and to either inhibition or excitation (via the ipsilateral associational connection component) at distant lamella of the dentate gyrus [21]. It is a significant contradiction to the lamellar notion of hippocampal information processing that the hippocampal cortex seems to be organized in parallel lamellae, both with regard to the neuronal and the vascular system. By means of this lamellar organization, small strips of the hippocampal cortex may operate as independent functional units, although excitatory and inhibitory transverse connections may modify the behaviour of the neighbouring lamellae [123].

While previous studies suggest that mossy cells in the dorsal and ventral dentate gyrus have similar patterns of termination in the inner one-third of the dentate molecular layer, recent reports indicate that axonal projections of mossy cells in these two regions are considerably different. In the ventral dentate gyrus, a dense band of mossy cell fibers is present in the inner one-fourth of the molecular layer and extended bilaterally throughout the rostral-caudal extent of dentate gyrus. Whereas in the dorsal dentate gyrus, the mossy cell fibers may also expand into the middle molecular layer and form a distinct band. These findings suggest that mossy cells in the dorsal and ventral dentate gyrus differ in the distribution of their axonal projections and possibly their function [124]. The surprising difference in dorsal and ventral mossy cell projections should therefore be considered when evaluating dorsal–ventral differences in dentate gyrus function [125].

In the commissural component, a few presumably GABAergic neurons also contribute to its formation [126-128], but the exact targeting area for these cells are not known.

4. Intrinsic Connection of the Dentate Gyrus

4.1. Projections from the Granule Cells

The mossy fibers from the granule cells of the dentate gyrus not only innervate CA3 pyramidal neurons they also innervate neurons in the polymorphic layer of the dentate gyrus by collateral branches. Within the polymorphic layer, each principal mossy fiber (which is on the order of 0.2-0.5 μm in diameter) gives rise to about seven thinner collaterals [99]. The mossy fiber collaterals present two types of synaptic varicosities. Throughout the axonal collateral plexus of a single granule cell, there are about 160 small (approximately 2 μm) varicosities, and they form contacts on spines and dendritic shafts of neurons located in the polymorphic layer [99]. There are usually single, larger (3-5 μm), irregularly shaped varicosities at the end of each of the collateral branches similar to the mossy fiber terminals found in the CA3. It is verified that the mossy fiber collateral terminals in the polymorphic layer establish contacts with the proximal dendrites of the mossy cells, the basal dendrites of the pyramidal basket cells, and other unidentified cells [118, 129, 130].

4.2. Projections from Basket Cells and Other "GABAergic" Interneurons

In the dentate gyrus, different basket cells are located close to the granule cell layer. Their axons form dense terminal plexus around granule cells. The chemical feature of this basket plexus are GABAergic and these GABAergic axons form symmetric, presumably inhibitory contacts on the cell bodies and shaft of apical dendrites of the granule cells [131]. There is ample evidence that these GABAergic basket neurons in the polymorphic layer are themselves innervated by GABAergic terminals [132, 133]. Golgi-stained axonal plexuses analysis of single basket cells indicates that axons extend on average 400 μm in the transverse axis of the dentate gyrus and about 1.1 mm in the septotemporal axis [134]. It is conceivable that a single basket cell can influence over a very large number of granule cells although their numbers are much less than the granule cells.

A second inhibitory input to granule cells is originating from the axo-axonic or chandelier cells located in the molecular layer of the dentate gyrus [135-137]. These projections form symmetric synapses exclusively with the axon initial segment of dentate granule cells.

Using the antibody against the peptide somatostatin, another intrinsic projection from somatostatin immunopositive neurons which scattered throughout the polymorphic layer are demonstrated to project to the granule cells [126, 138]. In the outer two thirds of the molecular layer, there is a dense plexus of somatostatin immunopositive fibers and terminals. It is verified that somatostatin immunopositive cells (SOM) located in the polymorphic layer, which are co-localized with GABA, are the main source of this plexus of fibers and terminals in the molecular layer. These somatostatin immunopositive fibers contact on the distal dendrites of the granule cells, provide the third inhibitory control of granule cell activity [126, 139].

In addition, there are vasoactive intestinal polypeptide-expressing (VIP) interneurons preferentially targeting other interneurons in several brain regions. In the mouse dentate gyrus, VIP interneurons are highly heterogeneous based on their morpho-physiological characteristics. In approximately two-thirds of morphologically VIP cells, their axons ramify in the hilus. The remaining cells project their axons exclusively to the molecular layer (15%), to both the molecular layer and hilus (10%), or throughout the entire dentate gyrus layers (8%). These VIP-immunopositive fibers preferentially innervate GABAergic interneurons over glutamatergic principal neurons [140].

5. Specific Neurophysiological Roles of the Cells in the Dentate Gyrus and Its Associated Disorders

5.1. Neurophysiological Roles of the Granule Cells

The low firing rate of the physiological activity of granule cells of the dentate gyrus play a vital role in the memory and emotion process. As discussed above, the granule cells do not directly innervate each other and are extensively inhibited by several classes of resident inhibitory interneurons. Hence, the majority of granule cells are basally silent, only a small subset of granule cells fires upon activation by the excitatory inputs from the entorhinal cortex [1, 101, 141-144]. These attributes underlie the sparse coding pattern in the dentate gyrus. The inputs from the cortical areas are encoded in non-overlapping populations of granule cells that functionally represent specific contextual engrams. The sparse coding pattern enables the dentate gyrus to complete pattern separation, a key function during memory coding and processing [145]. Pattern separation by the granule cells of dentate gyrus involves memory formation and memory retrieval of both emotional and cognitive contexts and emotional dysfunction could be induced by impairment in pattern separation of emotional memory [146]. Anxiety [147-149], post-traumatic stress disorder [150-152] and depression, both in humans and in rodent models [147, 149, 153] are related to emotional memory dysfunction and deficit in pattern separation.

There are evidences that granule cells are involved in the pathological process of depression and stress and reduced dentate gyrus activity was demonstrated in chronic mild stress rat model of depression [154]. The marked atrophy in the dendrites of the granule cells was found in rats subjected to stress [155].

The whole function of the dentate gyrus, including information encoding, spatial pattern separation, temporal information integration, and remote memory function are mainly dependent on the role of granule cells (please refer to the section 6 for details).

5.2. Neurophysiological Roles of Cholecystokinin (CCK) Immunopositive Basket Cells

The CCK immunopositive basket cells are a subtype of interneurons which synthesize and release high levels of CCK and therefore are highly immunopositive to the neuropeptide. The physiological activity of these cells is firing accommodating spikes at moderate frequencies with relatively high membrane input resistance [156]. Postsynaptic expression of calcium-impermeable GluR2-containing AMPA receptors may account for the lack of synaptic plasticity at these basket cells [157]. The extensive distribution of CCK in the brain, in particular, the limbic system, including the hippocampus in addition to the gastrointestinal system strongly suggests its neuromodulator effect on behavior [158]. Based on its high expression in limbic regions, numerous experimental data suggest that CCK plays a crucial role in inducing anxiety and fear behaviors. Pharmacological experiments suggest that CCK-2 receptors mediate anxiety [159]. Intriguingly, CCK-2 receptor is expressed on parvalbumin (PV) immunopositive cells in the dentate gyrus, suggesting that the neuroendocrine communication between the hippocampal basket cells is critical in fear and anxiety. Moreover, CCK immunopositive interneurons unidirectionally inhibit PV immunopositive basket cells through GABA-A receptors to suppress their fast spiking activity [160].

5.3. Neurophysiological Roles of PV Immunopositive Basket Cells

The basket cells that express the calcium-binding protein PV share some profound similarities with the CCK immunopositive basket cells. Their morphology and localization within the subgranular zone are similar between these interneurons. Both neuronal types provide perisomatic inhibition to the granule cells. Nevertheless, the physiological properties as well as the neuromodulators affecting PV basket neurons are substantially different from the neighboring CCK basket cells [156]. PV basket cells are rapidly recruited by excitatory synaptic inputs, generate high-frequency trains of action potentials, discharge single action potentials phase-locked to fast network oscillations and provide fast, stable and timed inhibitory output onto their target cells. PV immunopositive basket cells express postsynaptic AMPA receptor composed mainly of GluR1 and GluR4 subunits. Expression of low levels of the calcium-impermeable GluR2 facilitates the fast deactivation kinetics of PV basket cells [161] and confers these cells the ability to accommodate long-term potentiation (LTP) and postsynaptic plasticity events [162]. PV immunopositive basket cells are regulated by different neuromodulators, and their inhibitory activity is tightly regulated by the CCK basket cells.

The PV basket cells in the dentate gyrus have been implicated in depression, yet very few studies directly investigated their function in stress, depression and action of antidepressants. Recent study indicated that the activity of PV basket cells plays a major role in the behavioral response to novelty and stress. Activation of the Kv3.1 channel in PV basket cells may represent a target for the development of cell-type specific, fast-acting antidepressants [163].

5.4. Neurophysiological Roles of Mossy Cells

As the unique excitatory interneurons, mossy cells are residing in the hilar region of the dentate gyrus. They are innervated mostly by the granule cells but also by local interneurons [164]. Both PV and CCK basket cells give dense innervation to the hilar mossy cells [165]. The mossy cells are innervated heavily by the granule cells through massive dendritic spines, which is uncommon among interneuron populations [20]. Recent study indicates that mossy cells–granule cells synapses undergo a presynaptic, NMDA-receptor-independent form of LTP that requires postsynaptic brain-derived neurotrophic factor (BDNF)/TrkB and presynaptic cyclic AMP (cAMP)/PKA signaling. This LTP is input specific and selectively expressed at mossy cells–granule cells synapses, but not at the disynaptic inhibitory loop. By increasing the excitation/inhibition balance, mossy cells–granule cells LTP enhances granule cells output at the associative mossy cells–granule cells recurrent circuit and may contribute to dentate-dependent forms of learning and epilepsy [166]. Notably, BDNF signaling in the dentate gyrus is essential for the behavioral effects after chronic selective serotonin reuptake inhibitors (SSRIs) [167]. Indeed, mossy cells express both p11 and SMARCA3, which are crucial for the response to chronic SSRIs [168]. Reciprocally, the mossy cells also excite inhibitory interneurons, as seen in targeted deletion and optogenetic studies [169, 170]. Overall, it is likely that mossy cells dynamically regulate granule cells activity in the dentate gyrus. This is further confirmed using chemogenetics to study the mossy cell interaction with the radial neural stem cells in the dentate gyrus [171]. Mossy cells project to the progenitor cells and mossy cell activation bidirectionally modulates stem cell activation. High mossy cell excitation increases stem cell activity, whereas moderate mossy cell activation increases stem cell quiescence through dominant indirect inhibition mediated by local interneurons. Moreover, chronic ablation of mossy cells results in stem cell depletion [171].

The mossy cells typically make synapses upon the proximal dendritic spines of the granule cells. These axons terminate on local or distal granule cells [20]. Such a network of local and distal synapses may underlie a connectivity along the longitudinal axis of the dentate gyrus. This type of wiring enables the integration of the functions mediated by the diverse parts of the dentate gyrus. The integration of information by local and distal synapses of the mossy cells may allow the integration of cognitive and emotional behaviors. The role of mossy cells in mood modulation has also been established by several studies. Targeted mossy cells degeneration resulted in induced anxiety [169], and acute stress resulted in a transient mossy cells inhibition [172]. A recent study indicates that the mossy cells are inhibited by unpredicted stress and regain activity after chronic SSRIs treatment. Moreover, chemogenetic inhibition of mossy cell activity impaired SSRIs-induced antidepressant effect, and induction of mossy cell activity induced SSRIs-mediated neurogenesis [173].

6. Neurophysiological Roles of the Dentate Gyrus

One of the unique features of the hippocampal formation is that many of its connections are unidirectional. Thus, the entorhinal cortex provides the major input to the dentate gyrus via fibers called the perforant path (refer to section 2.1). However, the dentate gyrus does not have reciprocal projections to the entorhinal cortex. Given that the entorhinal cortex provides the main source of the cortical sensory information, and it also projects heavily to the dentate gyrus, it is reasonable to consider that as the first station for information processing, the dentate gyrus is involved in the formation of episodic memories. Moreover, the unique neuroanatomy of the dentate gyrus suggests that it performs a specific information-processing from the entorhinal cortex and ultimately conveys the synthetic information to CA3 area of the hippocampus.

The input of the dorsal dentate gyrus from the perforant path can be divided into medial and lateral components. The medial component processes spatial information and the lateral component processes nonspatial (e.g., objects, odors) information [32, 174]. The rats with dorsal dentate gyrus lesions did not affect the recognition for a change within object feature configuration and object recognition tasks. However, they have a deficit in recognition for a change within object-spatial feature configuration, complex object-place feature configuration and spatial recognition tasks. It suggests that the dorsal dentate gyrus supports object-place and complex object-place feature information via a conjunctive encoding process. Further studies indicated that the perforant pathway input into the dorsal dentate gyrus through the medial component mediates spatial information via activation of NMDA receptors, whereas those through lateral component mediates both visual object information and spatial information via activation of opioid receptors. These results are suggesting an important role for the dorsal dentate gyrus in supporting object-place conjunctive processes.

A single granule cell in the dentate gyrus may be activated by different sensory inputs, including vestibular, olfactory, visual, auditory, and somatosensory, as well as higher order integration of sensory stimuli [175]. However, it remains unknown whether these sensory inputs via conjunctive encoding have a memory representation within the dentate gyrus. One possible role of the dentate gyrus in processing all sensory information may be to provide sensory markers to demarcate a spatial location, so that the dentate gyrus can mediate spatial information more efficiently.

It has been suggested that the pattern separation is facilitated by sparse connections in the mossy fiber system, which connects dentate granular cells to dorsal CA3 pyramidal neurons [12, 176, 177]. The dorsal dentate gyrus-lesioned rats demonstrate deficits similar to complete hippocampal lesions when tested on a working memory version of the radial eight-arm maze [178-181] and on the Morris water maze task [182-185]. Based on their experimental study, Gilbert et al. (2001) conclude that lesions of the dorsal dentate gyrus decrease the efficiency of spatial pattern separation, which results in impairments on trials with increased spatial proximity and similarity among working memory representations. Thus, the dorsal dentate gyrus may function to encode and to separate events in space producing spatial pattern separation. Such spatial pattern separation ensures that new highly processed sensory information is organized within the hippocampus, which in turn enhances the possibility of encoding and temporarily remembering one spatial location as separate from another. Deficits for spatial tasks of dentate gyrus-lesioned rat may also indicate an increased interference and impairment in the utilization of a spatial pattern separation process [186, 187]. In addition to the spatial pattern separation on the same horizontal plane, it has been revealed that the dentate gyrus is also associated with height or slope (vertical space) related spatial pattern separation [188-192]. Spatial pattern separation of the dentate gurus is also observed in clinic investigation on human beings. Deficits of spatial separation were found in hypoxic subjects [19] and older impaired adults [193, 194] when compared to normal controls and young unimpaired adults respectively.

The mechanism of the spatial pattern separation of dentate gyrus is still unclear so far. Ablation of the new born granule cells using low-dose X-irradiation in the sub-granular area of dentate gyrus could interfere the spatial pattern separation, suggesting that the new born neurons in the dentate gyrus may play a role in spatial pattern separation [195]. It is supported by studies showing reduced spatial pattern separation after ablation of young granule cells in transgenic mouse models [196].

Computational model of neurogenesis indicates that the dentate gyrus contributes to a temporal associative integration process for events presented within the same time frame [197]. The behavioral test in rats suggests that selective colchicine-induced dentate gyrus lesions are capable of disrupting the formation of temporal associations between spatial events [198, 199]. These results suggest that neurogenesis may play an important role in time-based remote memory.

Recognition of an object is associated with place (including both horizontal and vertical), shape (geometry) and surface characteristics (such as color). The separation of shape and spatial pattern separation of the dentate gyrus are verified by experimental study showing that the dentate gyrus-lesioned rats display a pattern separation for the shades of grey context across the shades of grey spectrum, but at a lower level compared with controls [200, 201]. These data indicated that dentate gyrus play a role in pattern separation for the shades of grey context across the shades of grey spectrum.

The dorsal dentate gyrus may play an important role in combining object and place information via conjunctive encoding [202]. The experimental study in the dentate gyrus-lesioned rats indicates that the dorsal dentate gyrus plays an important role in object-context recognition at short retention intervals; and it also plays an important role in object recognition at long retention intervals, but not at short retention intervals [203].

Rats with the dentate gyrus lesions demonstrate impairments in the ability to acquire the cue–context associations compared with the controls, suggesting that the dentate gyrus may play an important role in conjunctive encoding of space paired with olfactory information [204]. In addition, the ventral dentate gyrus is verified to be involved in the odor separation function. Rats with the ventral dentate gyrus lesion show a decreased efficiency of odor-based pattern separation, which results in impairments on trials with increased odor proximity and similarity among working memory representations [205]. Because odors represent an important feature to be processed during social recognition test, there would be a possibility that the ventral but not the dorsal dentate gyrus would play an important role in supporting a social recognition process. Indeed, lesions of the ventral but not dorsal dentate gyrus, resulted in a deficit in social recognition. The result suggests that lesion of the ventral dentate gyrus may disrupt social recognition memory [206].

The dentate gyrus also plays an important role in reward value separation. In reward value shifts experiment, the sham-lesioned and control rats displayed a graded decrease in runway velocities following decrease in reward value, suggesting a pattern separation process. In contrast, the ventral dentate gyrus-lesioned rats continued to maintain runway velocities regardless of the reward value-shifts. The maintained runway velocity seems not due to hyperactivity of animals, but could be due to the fact that the ventral dentate gyrus is part of a decision-making circuitry to predict goal relevant reward outcomes [207]. It indicates the important role of ventral dentate gyrus in reward value pattern separation.

The dentate gyrus receives many cortical and subcortical inputs, processes them and then transmits the primarily processed information to CA3 which in turn send to CA1 area of hippocampus for further processing and interpretation. The intricate functional processes, including memory formation, its retrieval, and the modulation of emotional mood are with great correlation with the dentate gyrus.

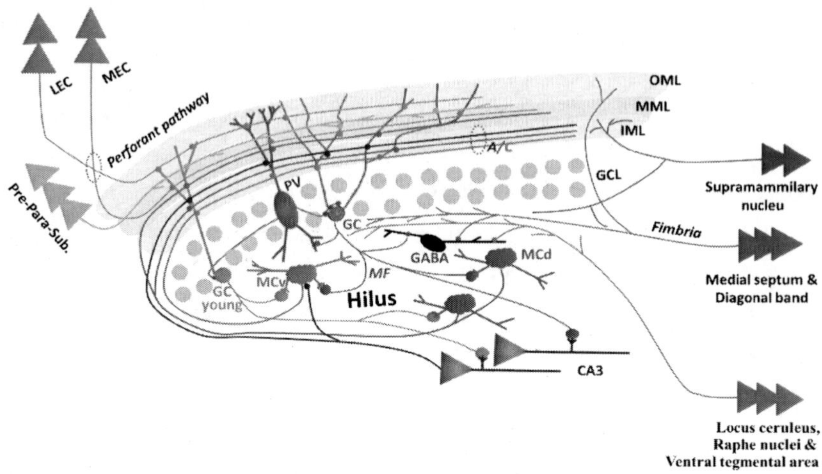

A/C: associational/commissural projection; GABA: GABAergic interneurons; GC: granule cell; GCL: granular cell layer; IML: inner molecular layer; LEC: lateral entorhinal cortex; MCd: mossy cell in dorsal dentate gyrus; MCv: mossy cell in ventral dentate gyrus; MEC: medial entorhinal cortex; MF: mossy fiber; MML: middle molecular layer; OML: outer molecular layer; Pre-Para-Sub: presubiculum and parasubiculum; PV: parvalbumin immunopositive interneuron.

Figure 1. The extrinsic connections of the dentate gyrus.

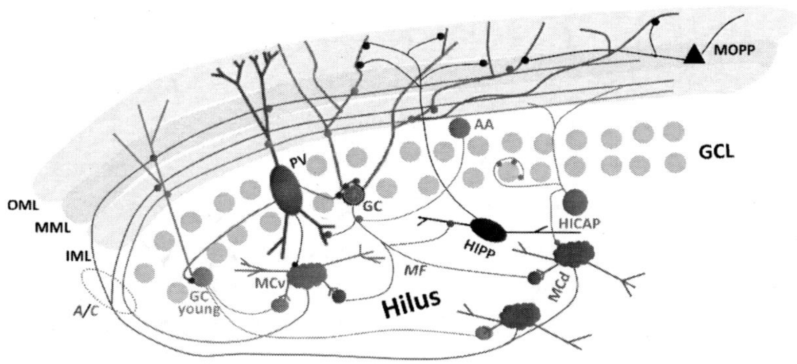

AA, axo-axonic cell; A/C, associational/commissural projection; GC, granule cell; GCL, granular cell layer; HICAP, interneurons with a hilar cell body with axon targeting the commissural/associational pathway; HIPP, hilar cells that project to the terminal zone of the perforant path; IML, inner molecular layer; MCd, mossy cell in dorsal dentate gyrus; MCv, mossy cell in ventral dentate gyrus; MF, mossy fiber; MML, middle molecular layer; MOPP, molecular layer perforant path-associated cell; OML, outer molecular layer; PV, parvalbumin immunopositive interneuron.

Figure 2. The intrinsic connections of the dentate gyrus.

The afferent, efferent fibers and intrinsic connection of the dentate gyrus are the basis of its function. Any factors that alter the network connection may influence the processing system of dentate gyrus and result in cognitive or emotional problems, such as dementia, depression, anxiety. The extrinsic and intrinsic connections of the dentate gyrus are summarized in Figure 1 and Figure 2 respectively.

CONCLUSION

Extensive animal experimental studies have demonstrated the afferent and efferent, extrinsic and intrinsic neural pathways of the dentate gyrus. The characteristic laminar, septal and temporal, superapyramidal and infrapyramidal distribution patterns of the dentate gyrus connections suggest that different parts of the dentate gyrus may play different roles in the learning and memory processing, pattern separation, and pathological disease genesis. Further study in the following areas may still be needed: 1) complex intrinsic connections among the granule cells, mossy cells and different subtypes of interneurons in the dentate gyrus; 2) plasticity, physiological and pathophysiological roles of different types or subtypes of ion channels such as K(v)7 and K(ir)6 channels, G protein-gated inwardly rectifying K^+ (GIRK) channels, K(v)3.1/K(v)3.2 Kv4, M-type (KCNQ2/3) K^+ channels, N-, P/Q- and R-type Ca(2+) channels and voltage-gated Na^+ channels as any changes of these ion channels may affect neural pathway activity; 3) interaction of each neural pathway with laminal and sublaminar distributed astrocytes, oligodendrocytes and microglial cells in the dentate gyrus as glial reaction in each sublaminar pathway may significantly affect neural pathway activity; 4) functional study of each neural pathway may reveal novel therapeutic approaches to treat dentate gyrus-related neurological and neuropsychological disorders.

REFERENCES

[1] Amaral, D. G., Scharfman, H. E., Lavenex, P. 2007. The dentate gyrus: fundamental neuroanatomical organization (dentate gyrus for dummies). *Prog. Brain Res.* 163, 3-22.

[2] Destrieux, C., Bourry, D., Velut, S. 2013. Surgical anatomy of the hippocampus. *Neurochirurgie* 59, 149-58.

[3] Parmar, S. K., Pruthi, N., Ravindranath, R., Ravindranath, Y., Somanna, S., Philip, M. 2018. Anatomical variations of the temporomesial structures in normal adult brain - A Cadaveric Study. *J. Neurosci. Rural. Pract.* 9, 317-25.

[4] Buzsáki, G. 1989. Two-stage model of memory trace formation: a role for "noisy" brain states. *Neuroscience* 31, 551-70.

[5] Squire, L. R. 1992. Memory and the hippocampus: a synthesis from findings with rats, monkeys, and humans. *Psychol. Rev.* 99, 195-231.

[6] McClelland, J. L., McNaughton, B. L., O'Reilly, R. C. 1995. Why there are complementary learning systems in the hippocampus and neocortex: insights from the successes and failures of connectionist models of learning and memory. *Psychol. Rev.* 102, 419-57.

[7] Dey, J., Alam, M. T., Chandra, S., Gandhi, S., Tripathi, P. P. 2019. Recalibrating the existence of new neurons in adult brain. *ACS Chem. Neurosci.* 10, 2091-3.

[8] Eichenbaum, H. 1999. Conscious awareness, memory and the hippocampus. *Nat. Neurosci.* 2, 775-6.

[9] Su, S., Qi, T., Su, B., Gu, H., Wang, J., Yang, L. 2014. Tooth loss inhibits neurogenesis in the dentate gyrus of adult mice. *Neural. Regen. Res.* 9, 1606-9.

[10] Marr, D. 1971. Simple memory: a theory for archicortex. *Philos. Trans. R. Soc. Lond. B. Biol. Sci.* 262, 23-81.

[11] Treves, A., & Rolls, E. T. 1994. Computational analysis of the role of the hippocampus in memory. *Hippocampus* 4, 374-91.

[12] Rolls, E. T., & Kesner, R. P. 2006. A computational theory of hippocampal function, and empirical tests of the theory. *Prog. Neurobiol.* 79, 1-48.

[13] Yassa, M. A., & Stark, C. E. 2011. Pattern separation in the hippocampus. *Trends Neurosci*, 34, 515-25.

[14] Myers, C. E., & Scharfman, H. E. 2009. A role for hilar cells in pattern separation in the dentate gyrus: a computational approach. *Hippocampus* 19, 321-37.

[15] Knierim, J. J., & Neunuebel, J. P. 2016. Tracking the flow of hippocampal computation: Pattern separation, pattern completion, and attractor dynamics. *Neurobiol. Learn. Mem.* 129, 38-49.

[16] Eriksson, P. S., Perfilieva, E., Björk-Eriksson, T., Alborn, A. M., Nordborg, C., Peterson, D. A., Gage, F. H. 1998. Neurogenesis in the adult human hippocampus. *Nat. Med.* 4, 1313-7.

[17] Treves, A., Tashiro, A., Witter, M. P., Moser, E. I. 2008. What is the mammalian dentate gyrus good for? *Neuroscience* 154, 1155-72.

[18] Jonas, P., & Lisman, J. 2014. Structure, function, and plasticity of hippocampal dentate gyrus microcircuits. *Front Neural. Circuits* 8, 107.

[19] Kesner, R. P. 2018. An analysis of dentate gyrus function (an update). *Behav. Brain Res.* 354, 84-91.

[20] Scharfman, H. E. 2016. The enigmatic mossy cell of the dentate gyrus. *Nat. Rev. Neurosci.* 17, 562-75.

[21] Amaral, D. G., & Witter, M. P. 1989. The three-dimensional organization of the hippocampal formation: a review of anatomical data. *Neuroscience* 31, 571-91.

[22] Acsády, L., Kamondi, A., Sík, A., Freund, T., Buzsáki, G. 1998. GABAergic cells are the major postsynaptic targets of mossy fibers in the rat hippocampus. *J. Neurosci.* 18, 3386-403.

[23] Henze, D. A., Wittner, L., Buzsáki, G. 2002. Single granule cells reliably discharge targets in the hippocampal CA3 network in vivo. *Nat. Neurosci.* 5, 790-5.

[24] Caballero-Bleda, M., & Witter, M. P. 1993. Regional and laminar organization of projections from the presubiculum and parasubiculum to the entorhinal cortex: an anterograde tracing study in the rat. *J. Comp. Neurol.* 328, 115-29.

[25] Germroth, P., Schwerdtfeger, W. K., Buhl, E. H. 1989. GABAergic neurons in the entorhinal cortex project to the hippocampus. *Brain Res.* 494, 187-92.

[26] Köhler, C. 1985. Intrinsic projections of the retrohippocampal region in the rat brain. I. The subicular complex. *J. Comp. Neurol.* 236, 504-22.

[27] Köhler, C. 1985. A projection from the deep layers of the entorhinal area to the hippocampal formation in the rat brain. *Neurosci. Lett.* 56, 13-9.

[28] Köhler, C. 1986. Intrinsic connections of the retrohippocampal region in the rat brain. II. The medial entorhinal area. *J. Comp. Neurol.* 246, 149-69.

[29] Köhler, C. 1988. Intrinsic connections of the retrohippocampal region in the rat brain: III. The lateral entorhinal area. *J. Comp. Neurol.* 271, 208-28.

[30] Steward, O. 1976. Topographic organization of the projections from the entorhinal area to the hippocampal formation of the rat. *J. Comp. Neurol.* 167, 285-314.

[31] Steward, O., & Scoville, S. A. 1976. Cells of origin of entorhinal cortical afferents to the hippocampus and fascia dentata of the rat. *J. Comp. Neurol.* 169, 347-70.

[32] Witter, M. P., Groenewegen, H. J., Lopes da Silva, F. H., Lohman, A. H. 1989. Functional organization of the extrinsic and intrinsic circuitry of the parahippocampal region. *Prog. Neurobiol.* 33, 161-253.

[33] Ruth, R. E., Collier, T. J., Routtenberg, A. 1982. Topography between the entorhinal cortex and the dentate septotemporal axis in rats: I. Medial and intermediate entorhinal projecting cells. *J. Comp. Neurol.* 209, 69-78.

[34] Ruth, R. E., Collier, T. J., Routtenberg, A. 1988. Topographical relationship between the entorhinal cortex and the septotemporal axis of the dentate gyrus in rats: II. Cells projecting from lateral entorhinal subdivisions. *J. Comp. Neurol.* 270, 506-16.

[35] Schwartz, S. P., & Coleman, P. D. 1981. Neurons of origin of the perforant path. *Exp. Neurol.* 74, 305-12.

[36] Segal, M., & Landis, S. 1974. Afferents to the hippocampus of the rat studied with the method of retrograde transport of horseradish peroxidase. *Brain Res.* 78, 1-15.

[37] Nafstad, P. H. 1967. An electron microscope study on the termination of the perforant path fibres in the hippocampus and the fascia dentata. *Z. Zellforsch Mikrosk Anat.* 76, 532-42.

[38] Zipp, F., Nitsch, R., Soriano, E., Frotscher, M. 1989. Entorhinal fibers form synaptic contacts on parvalbumin-immunoreactive neurons in the rat fascia dentata. *Brain Res.* 495, 161-6.

[39] Hjorth-Simonsen, A. 1972. Projection of the lateral part of the entorhinal area to the hippocampus and fascia dentata. *J. Comp. Neurol.* 146, 219-32.

[40] Witter, M. P. 1993. Organization of the entorhinal-hippocampal system: a review of current anatomical data. *Hippocampus.* 3 Spec No, 33-44.

[41] Wyss, J. M. 1981. An autoradiographic study of the efferent connections of the entorhinal cortex in the rat. *J. Comp. Neurol.* 199, 495-512.

[42] Witter, M. P. 2007. The perforant path: projections from the entorhinal cortex to the dentate gyrus. *Prog. Brain Res.* 163, 43-61.

[43] Fonnum, F. 1970. Topographical and subcellular localization of choline acetyltransferase in rat hippocampal region. *J. Neurochem.* 17, 1029-37.

[44] Fredens, K., Stengaard-Pedersen, K., Larsson, L. I. 1984. Localization of enkephalin and cholecystokinin immuno-reactivities in the perforant path terminal fields of the rat hippocampal formation. *Brain Res.* 304, 255-63.

[45] Scharfman, H. E. 2007. The CA3 “backprojection” to the dentate gyrus. *Prog. Brain Res.* 163, 627-37.

[46] Shi, Y., Grieco, S. F., Holmes, T. C., Xu, X. 2019. Development of Local Circuit Connections to Hilar Mossy Cells in the Mouse Dentate Gyrus. *eNeuro.* 6(2).

[47] Li, X. G., Somogyi, P., Ylinen, A., Buzsáki, G. 1994. The hippocampal CA3 network: an in vivo intracellular labeling study. *J. Comp. Neurol.* 339, 181-208.

[48] Ishizuka, N., Weber, J., Amaral, D. G. 1990. Organization of intrahippocampal projections originating from CA3 pyramidal cells in the rat. *J. Comp. Neurol.* 295, 580-623.

[49] Scharfman, H. E. 1994. EPSPs of dentate gyrus granule cells during epileptiform bursts of dentate hilar “mossy” cells and area CA3 pyramidal cells in disinhibited rat hippocampal slices. *J. Neurosci.* 14, 6041-57.

[50] Scharfman, H. E. 1994. Evidence from simultaneous intracellular recordings in rat hippocampal slices that area CA3 pyramidal cells innervate dentate hilar mossy cells. *J. Neurophysiol.* 72, 2167-80.

[51] Kneisler, T. B., & Dingledinem R. 1995. Synaptic input from CA3 pyramidal cells to dentate basket cells in rat hippocampus. *J. Physiol.* 487, 125-46.

[52] Daitz, H. M., & Powell, T. P. 1954. Studies of the connexions of the fornix system. *J. Neurol. Neurosurg. Psychiatry.* 17, 75-82.

[53] Morin, F. 1950. An experimental study of hypothalamic connections in the guinea pig. *J. Comp, Neurol*, 92, 193-213.

[54] Amaral, D. G., & Kurz, J. 1985. An analysis of the origins of the cholinergic and noncholinergic septal projections to the hippocampal formation of the rat. *J. Comp, Neurol*, 240, 37-59.

[55] Baisden, R. H., Hoover, D. B., Cowie, R. J. 1979. Retrograde demonstration of hippocampal afferents from the interpeduncular and reuniens nuclei. *Neurosci. Lett.* 13, 105-9.

[56] Fibiger, H. C. 1982. The organization and some projections of cholinergic neurons of the mammalian forebrain. *Brain Res.* 257, 327-88.

[57] Gage, F. H., Björklund, A., Stenevi, U. 1984. Cells of origin of the ventral cholinergic septohippocampal pathway undergoing compensatory collateral sprouting following fimbria-fornix transection. *Neurosci. Lett.* 44, 211-6.

[58] Meibach, R. C., & Siegel, A. 1975. The origin of fornix fibers which project to the mammillary bodies in the rat: a horseradish peroxidase study. *Brain Res.* 88, 508-12.

[59] Meibach, R. C., & Siegel, A. 1977. Efferent connections of the septal area in the rat: an analysis utilizing retrograde and anterograde transport methods. *Brain Res.* 119, 1-20.

[60] Milner, T. A., & Amaral, D. G. 1984. Evidence for a ventral septal projection to the hippocampal formation of the rat. *Exp Brain Res.* 55, 579-85.

[61] Mosko, S., Lynch, G., Cotman, C. W. 1973. The distribution of septal projections to the hippocampus of the rat. *J. Comp. Neurol.* 152, 163-74.

[62] Swanson, L. W. 1977. The anatomical organization of septo-hippocampal projections. *Ciba Found. Symp.* 58, 25-48.

[63] Swanson, L. W., & Cowan, W. M. 1977. An autoradiographic study of the organization of the efferent connections of the hippocampal formation in the rat. *J. Comp. Neurol.* 172, 49-84.

[64] Gaykema, R. P., Luiten, P. G., Nyakas, C., Traber, J. 1990. Cortical projection patterns of the medial septum-diagonal band complex. *J. Comp. Neurol.* 293, 103-24.

[65] Nyakas, C., Luiten, P. G., Spencer, D. G., Traber, J. 1987. Detailed projection patterns of septal and diagonal band efferents to the hippocampus in the rat with emphasis on innervation of CA1 and dentate gyrus. *Brain Res. Bull* 18, 533-45.

[66] Siegel, A., & Tassoni, J. 1971. Differential efferent projections from the ventral and dorsal hippocampus of the cat. *Brain Behav. Evol.* 4, 185-200.

[67] Swanson, L. W., Wyss, J. M., Cowan, W. M. 1978. An autoradiographic study of the organization of intrahippocampal association pathways in the rat. *J. Comp. Neurol.* 181, 681-715.

[68] Lewis, P. R., & Shute, C. C. 1967. The cholinergic limbic system: projections to hippocampal formation, medial cortex, nuclei of the ascending cholinergic reticular system, and the subfornical organ and supra-optic crest. *Brain* 90, 521-40.

[69] Wainer, B. H., Levey, A. I., Mufson, E. J., Mesulam, M. M. 1984. Cholinergic systems in mammalian brain identified with antibodies against choline acetyltransferase. *Neurochem. Int.* 6, 163-82.

[70] Wainer, B. H., Levey, A. I., Rye, D. B., Mesulam, M. M., Mufson, E. J. 1985. Cholinergic and non-cholinergic septohippocampal pathways. *Neurosci. Lett.* 54, 45-52.

[71] Köhler, C., Chan-Palay, V., Wu, J. Y. 1984. Septal neurons containing glutamic acid decarboxylase immunoreactivity project to the hippocampal region in the rat brain. *Anat. Embryol* (Berl). 169, 41-4.

[72] Freund, T. F., & Antal, M. 1988. GABA-containing neurons in the septum control inhibitory interneurons in the hippocampus. *Nature* 336, 170-3.

[73] Gulyás, A. I., Görcs, T. J., Freund, T. F. 1990. Innervation of different peptide-containing neurons in the hippocampus by GABAergic septal afferents. *Neuroscience* 37, 31-44.

[74] Acsády, L., Halasy, K., Freund, T. F. 1993. Calretinin is present in non-pyramidal cells of the rat hippocampus--III. Their inputs from the median raphe and medial septal nuclei. *Neuroscience* 52, 829-41.

[75] Dent, J. A., Galvin, N. J., Stanfield, B. B., Cowan, W. M. 1983. The mode of termination of the hypothalamic projection to the dentate gyrus: an EM autoradiographic study. *Brain Res.* 258, 1-10.

[76] Haglund, L., Swanson, L. W., Köhlerm C. 1984. The projection of the supramammillary nucleus to the hippocampal formation: an immunohistochemical and anterograde transport study with the lectin PHA-L in the rat. *J. Comp. Neurol.* 229, 171-85.

[77] Riley, J. N., & Moore, R. Y. 1981. Diencephalic and brainstem afferents to the hippocampal formation of the rat. *Brain Res. Bull* 6, 437-44.

[78] Vertes, R. P. 1992. PHA-L analysis of projections from the supramammillary nucleus in the rat. *J. Comp. Neurol*. 326, 595-622.

[79] Wyss, J. M., Swanson, L. W., Cowan, W. M. 1979. Evidence for an input to the molecular layer and the stratum granulosum of the dentate gyrus from the supramammillary region of the hypothalamus. *Anat. Embryol* (Berl). 156, 165-76.

[80] Wyss, J. M., Swanson, L. W., Cowan, W. M. 1979. A study of subcortical afferents to the hippocampal formation in the rat. *Neuroscience* 4, 463-76.

[81] Soussi, R., Zhang, N., Tahtakran, S., Houser, C. R., Esclapez, M. 2010. Heterogeneity of the supramammillary-hippocampal pathways: evidence for a unique GABAergic neurotransmitter phenotype and regional differences. *Eur. J. Neurosci*. 32, 771-85.

[82] Köhler, C., Haglund, L., Swanson, L. W. 1984. A diffuse alpha MSH-immunoreactive projection to the hippocampus and spinal cord from individual neurons in the lateral hypothalamic area and zona incerta. *J. Comp. Neurol*. 223, 501-14.

[83] Davies, S., & Köhler, C. 1985. The substance P innervation of the rat hippocampal region. *Anat. Embryol* (Berl). 173, 45-52.

[84] Gall, C., & Selawski, L. 1984. Supramammillary afferents to guinea pig hippocampus contain substance P-like immunoreactivity. *Neurosci. Lett*. 51, 171-6.

[85] Borhegyi, Z., & Leranth, C. 1997. Substance P innervation of the rat hippocampal formation. *J. Comp. Neurol*. 384, 41-58.

[86] Haring, J. H., & Davis, J. N. 1983. Topography of locus ceruleus neurons projecting to the area dentata. *Exp. Neurol*. 79, 785-800.

[87] Haring, J. H., & Davis, J. N. 1985. Differential distribution of locus coeruleus projections to the hippocampal formation: anatomical and biochemical evidence. *Brain Res*. 325, 366-9.

[88] Haring, J. H., & Davis, J. N. 1985. Retrograde labeling of locus coeruleus neurons after lesion-induced sprouting of the coeruleohippocampal projection. *Brain Res.* 360, 384-8.

[89] Koda, L. Y., Schulman, J. A., Bloom, F. E. 1978. Ultrastructural identification of noradrenergic terminals in rat hippocampus: unilateral destruction of the locus coeruleus with 6-hydroxydopamine. *Brain Res.* 145, 190-5.

[90] Koda, L. Y., Wise, R. A., Bloom, F. E. 1978. Light and electron microscopic changes in the rat dentate gyrus after lesions or stimulation of the ascending locus coeruleus pathway. *Brain Res.* 144, 363-8.

[91] Moore, R. Y., Ziegler, B., Bayer, S. A. 1978. Monoamine neuron innervation of the hippocampal formation: alteration by neonatal irradiation. *Exp. Neurol.* 60, 318-26.

[92] Pickel, V. M., Segal, M., Bloom, F. E. 1974. A radioautographic study of the efferent pathways of the nucleus locus coeruleus. *J. Comp. Neurol.* 155, 15-42.

[93] Swanson, L. W., & Hartman, B. K. 1975. The central adrenergic system. An immunofluorescence study of the location of cell bodies and their efferent connections in the rat utilizing dopamine-beta-hydroxylase as a marker. *J. Comp. Neurol.* 163, 467-505.

[94] Conrad LC, Leonard CM, Pfaff DW. 1974. Connections of the median and dorsal raphe nuclei in the rat: an autoradiographic and degeneration study. *J. Comp. Neurol.* 156, 179-205.

[95] Halasy, K., Miettinen, R., Szabat, E., Freund, T. F. 1992. GABAergic Interneurons are the Major Postsynaptic Targets of Median Raphe Afferents in the Rat Dentate Gyrus. *Eur. J. Neurosci.* 4, 144-53.

[96] Köhler, C., & Steinbusch, H. 1982. Identification of serotonin and non-serotonin-containing neurons of the mid-brain raphe projecting to the entorhinal area and the hippocampal formation. A combined immunohistochemical and fluorescent retrograde tracing study in the rat brain. *Neuroscience* 7, 951-75.

[97] Montone, K. T., Fass, B., Hamill, G. S. 1988. Serotonergic and nonserotonergic projections from the rat interpeduncular nucleus to the septum, hippocampal formation and raphe: a combined immunocytochemical and fluorescent retrograde labelling study of neurons in the apical subnucleus. *Brain Res. Bull* 20, 233-40.

[98] Swanson, L. W. 1982. The projections of the ventral tegmental area and adjacent regions: a combined fluorescent retrograde tracer and immunofluorescence study in the rat. *Brain Res. Bull* 9, 321-53.

[99] Claiborne, B. J., Amaral, D. G., Cowan, W. M. 1986. A light and electron microscopic analysis of the mossy fibers of the rat dentate gyrus. *J. Comp. Neurol.* 246, 435-58.

[100] Chicurel, M. E., & Harris, K. M. 1992. Three-dimensional analysis of the structure and composition of CA3 branched dendritic spines and their synaptic relationships with mossy fiber boutons in the rat hippocampus. *J. Comp. Neurol.* 325, 169-82.

[101] Amaral, D. G., Ishizuka, N., Claiborne, B. 1990. Neurons, numbers and the hippocampal network. *Prog. Brain Res.* 83, 1-11.

[102] Gaarskjaer, F. B. 1978. Organization of the mossy fiber system of the rat studied in extended hippocampi. II. Experimental analysis of fiber distribution with silver impregnation methods. *J. Comp. Neurol.* 178, 73-88.

[103] Gaarskjaer, F. B. 1978. Organization of the mossy fiber system of the rat studied in extended hippocampi. I. Terminal area related to number of granule and pyramidal cells. *J. Comp. Neurol.* 178, 49-72.

[104] Storm-Mathisen, J., & Fonnum, F. 1972. Localization of transmitter candidates in the hippocampal region. *Prog. Brain. Res.* 36, 41-58.

[105] Gall, C. 1984. The distribution of cholecystokinin-like immunoreactivity in the hippocampal formation of the guinea pig: localization in the mossy fibers. *Brain Res.* 306, 73-83.

[106] Gall, C., & Moore, R. Y. 1984. Distribution of enkephalin, substance P, tyrosine hydroxylase, and 5-hydroxytryptamine

immunoreactivity in the septal region of the rat. *J. Comp. Neurol.* 225, 212-27.

[107] McGinty, J. F., Henriksen, S J., Goldstein, A., Terenius, L., Bloom, F. E. 1983. Dynorphin is contained within hippocampal mossy fibers: immunochemical alterations after kainic acid administration and colchicine-induced neurotoxicity. *Proc. Natl. Acad. Sci. USA* 80, 589-93.

[108] McGinty, J. F., van der Kooy, D., Bloom, F. E. 1984. The distribution and morphology of opioid peptide immunoreactive neurons in the cerebral cortex of rats. *J. Neurosci.* 4, 1104-17.

[109] Roberts, G. W., Allen, Y., Crow, T. J., Polak, J. M. 1983. Immunocytochemical localization on neuropeptides in the fornix of rat, monkey and man. *Brain Res.* 263, 151-5.

[110] van Daal, J. H., Zanderink, H. E., Jenks, B. G., van Abeelen, J. H. 1989. Distribution of dynorphin B and methionine-enkephalin in the mouse hippocampus: influence of genotype. *Neurosci. Lett.* 97, 241-4.

[111] Blackstad, T. W. 1956. Commissural connections of the hippocampal region in the rat, with special reference to their mode of termination. *J. Comp. Neurol.* 105, 417-537.

[112] Laurberg, S. 1979. Commissural and intrinsic connections of the rat hippocampus. *J. Comp. Neurol.* 184, 685-708.

[113] Laurberg, S., & Sørensen, K. E. 1981. Associational and commissural collaterals of neurons in the hippocampal formation (hilus fasciae dentatae and subfield CA3). *Brain Res.* 212, 287-300.

[114] Swanson, L. W., Sawchenko, P. E., Cowan, W. M. 1981. Evidence for collateral projections by neurons in Ammon's horn, the dentate gyrus, and the subiculum: a multiple retrograde labeling study in the rat. *J. Neurosci.* 1, 548-59.

[115] Zimmer, J. 1971. Ipsilateral afferents to the commissural zone of the fascia dentata, demonstrated in decommissurated rats by silver impregnation. *J. Comp. Neurol.* 142, 393-416.

[116] Kishi, K., Stanfield, B. B., Cowan, W. M. 1980. A quantitative EM autoradiographic study of the commissural and associational connections of the dentate gyrus in the rat. *Anat. Embryol* (Berl). 160, 173-86.

[117] Laatsch, R. H., Cowan, W. M. 1966. Electron microscopic studies of the dentate gyrus of the rat. I. Normal structure with special reference to synaptic organization. *J. Comp. Neurol.* 128, 359-95.

[118] Ribak, C. E., Seress, L., Amaral, D. G. 1985. The development, ultrastructure and synaptic connections of the mossy cells of the dentate gyrus. *J. Neurocytol.* 14, 835-57.

[119] Frotscher, M., Seress, L., Schwerdtfeger, W. K., Buhl, E. 1991. The mossy cells of the fascia dentata: a comparative study of their fine structure and synaptic connections in rodents and primates. *J. Comp. Neurol.* 312, 145-63.

[120] Soriano, E., & Frotscher, M. 1994. Mossy cells of the rat fascia dentata are glutamate-immunoreactive. *Hippocampus* 4, 65-9.

[121] Frotscher, M., & Zimmer, J. 1983. Commissural fibers terminate on non-pyramidal neurons in the guinea pig hippocampus -- a combined Golgi/EM degeneration study. *Brain Res.* 265, 289-93.

[122] Seress, L., & Ribak, C. E. 1984. Direct commissural connections to the basket cells of the hippocampal dentate gyrus: anatomical evidence for feed-forward inhibition. *J. Neurocytol.* 13, 215-25.

[123] Andersen, P., Bliss, T. V. P., Skrede, K. K. 1971. Lamellar organization of hippocampal excitatory pathways. *Experimental Brain Research* 13, 222-38.

[124] Houser, C. R., Peng, Z., Wei, X. 2021. Mossy cells in the dorsal and ventral dentate gyrus differ in their patterns of axonal projections. *J. Neurosci.* 41(5), 991-1004.

[125] Botterill, J. J., Gerencer, K. J., Vinod, K. Y., Alcantara-Gonzalez, D. 2021. Dorsal and ventral mossy cells differ in their axonal projections throughout the dentate gyrus of the mouse hippocampus. *Hippocampus* 31(5), 522-39.

[126] Bakst, I., Avendano, C., Morrison, J. H., Amaral, D. G. 1986. An experimental analysis of the origins of somatostatin-like

immunoreactivity in the dentate gyrus of the rat. *J. Neurosci.* 6, 1452-62.

[127] Ribak, C. E., Seress, L., Peterson, G. M., Seroogy, K. B., Fallon, J. H., Schmued, L. C. 1986. A GABAergic inhibitory component within the hippocampal commissural pathway. *J. Neurosci.* 6, 3492-8.

[128] Seress, L., & Ribak, C. E. 1983. GABAergic cells in the dentate gyrus appear to be local circuit and projection neurons. *Exp. Brain Res.* 50, 173-82.

[129] Ribak, C. E., & Seress, L. 1983. Five types of basket cell in the hippocampal dentate gyrus: a combined Golgi and electron microscopic study. *J. Neurocytol.* 12, 577-97.

[130] Scharfman, H. E., Kunkel, D. D., Schwartzkroin, P. A. 1990. Synaptic connections of dentate granule cells and hilar neurons: results of paired intracellular recordings and intracellular horseradish peroxidase injections. *Neuroscience* 37, 693-707.

[131] Kosaka, T., Hama, K., Wu, J. Y. 1984. GABAergic synaptic boutons in the granule cell layer of rat dentate gyrus. *Brain Res.* 293, 353-9.

[132] Misgeld, U., & Frotscher, M. 1986. Postsynaptic-GABAergic inhibition of non-pyramidal neurons in the guinea-pig hippocampus. *Neuroscience* 19, 193-206.

[133] Savanthrapadian, S., Meyer, T., Elgueta, C., Booker, S. A., Vida, I., Bartos, M. 2014. Synaptic properties of SOM- and CCK-expressing cells in dentate gyrus interneuron networks. *J. Neurosci.* 34, 8197-209.

[134] Struble, R. G., Desmond, N. L., Levy, W. B. 1978. Anatomical evidence for interlamellar inhibition in the fascia dentata. *Brain Res.* 152, 580-5.

[135] Kosaka, T. 1983. Axon initial segments of the granule cell in the rat dentate gyrus: synaptic contacts on bundles of axon initial segments. *Brain Res.* 274, 129-34.

[136] Soriano, E., & Frotscher, M. 1989. A GABAergic axo-axonic cell in the fascia dentata controls the main excitatory hippocampal pathway. *Brain Res*. 503, 170-4.

[137] Han, Z. S., Buhl, E. H., Lörinczi, Z., Somogyi, P. 1993. A high degree of spatial selectivity in the axonal and dendritic domains of physiologically identified local-circuit neurons in the dentate gyrus of the rat hippocampus. *Eur. J. Neurosci*. 5, 395-410.

[138] Morrison, J. H., Benoit, R., Magistretti, P. J., Ling, N., Bloom, F. E. 1982. Immunohistochemical distribution of pro-somatostatin-related peptides in hippocampus. *Neurosci. Lett*. 34, 137-42.

[139] Halasy, K., & Somogyi, P. 1993. Subdivisions in the multiple GABAergic innervation of granule cells in the dentate gyrus of the rat hippocampus. *Eur. J. Neurosci*. 5, 411-29.

[140] Wei, Y. T., Wu, J. W., Yeh, C. W., Shen, H. C., Wu, K. P., Vida, I. 2021. Morpho-physiological properties and connectivity of vasoactive intestinal polypeptide-expressing interneurons in the mouse hippocampal dentate gyrus. *J. Comp. Neurol*. 529, 2658-75.

[141] West, M. J., Slomianka, L., Gundersen, H. J. 1991. Unbiased stereological estimation of the total number of neurons in thesubdivisions of the rat hippocampus using the optical fractionator. *Anat. Rec*. 231, 482-97.

[142] Pernía-Andrade, A. J., & Jonas, P. 2014. Theta-gamma-modulated synaptic currents in hippocampal granule cells in vivo define a mechanism for network oscillations. *Neuron* 81, 140-52.

[143] Diamantaki, M., Frey, M., Berens, P. 2016. Sparse activity of identified dentate granule cells during spatial exploration. *Elife* 5, e20252.

[144] Senzai, Y., & Buzsáki, G. 2017. Physiological Properties and Behavioral Correlates of Hippocampal Granule Cells and Mossy Cells. *Neuron* 93, 691-704.e5.

[145] Bakker, A., Kirwan, C. B., Miller, M., Stark, C. E. 2008. Pattern separation in the human hippocampal CA3 and dentate gyrus. *Science* 319, 1640-2.

[146] Jacobs, B. L., van Praag, H., Gage, F. H. 2000. Adult brain neurogenesis and psychiatry: a novel theory of depression. *Mol. Psychiatry* 5, 262-9.

[147] Anacker, C., & Hen, R. 2017. Adult hippocampal neurogenesis and cognitive flexibility - linking memory and mood. *Nat. Rev. Neurosci.* 18, 335-46.

[148] Balderston, N. L., Mathur, A., Adu-Brimpong, J., Hale, E. A., Ernst, M., Grillon, C. 2017. Effect of anxiety on behavioural pattern separation in humans. *Cogn. Emot.* 31, 238-48.

[149] Gandy, K., Kim, S., Sharp, C., Dindo, L., Maletic-Savatic, M., Calarge, C. 2017. Pattern Separation: A Potential Marker of Impaired Hippocampal Adult Neurogenesis in Major Depressive Disorder. *Front. Neurosci.* 11, 571.

[150] Kheirbek, M. A., Klemenhagen, K. C., Sahay, A., Hen, R. 2012. Neurogenesis and generalization: a new approach to stratify and treat anxiety disorders. *Nat. Neurosci.* 15, 1613-20.

[151] Liberzon, I., & Abelson, J. L. 2016. Context Processing and the Neurobiology of Post-Traumatic Stress Disorder. *Neuron* 92, 14-30.

[152] Lange, I., Goossens, L., Michielse, S., Bakker, J., Lissek, S., Papalini, S., Verhagen, S., Leibold, N., Marcelis, M., Wichers, M., Lieverse, R., van Os, J., van Amelsvoort, T., Schruers, K. 2017. Behavioral pattern separation and its link to the neural mechanisms of fear generalization. *Soc. Cogn. Affect Neurosci.* 12, 1720-9.

[153] Dillon, D. G., & Pizzagalli, D. A. 2018. Mechanisms of Memory Disruption in Depression. *Trends Neurosci.* 41, 137-49.

[154] Airan, R. D., Meltzer, L. A., Roy, M., Gong, Y., Chen, H., Deisseroth, K. 2007. High-speed imaging reveals neurophysiological links to behavior in an animal model of depression. *Science* 317, 819-23.

[155] Bessa, J. M., Ferreira, D., Melo, I., Marques, F., Cerqueira, J. J., Palha, J. A., Almeida, O. F., Sousa, N. 2009. The mood-improving actions of antidepressants do not depend on neurogenesis but are

associated with neuronal remodeling. *Mol. Psychiatry* 14, 764-73, 39.

[156] Bartos, M., & Elgueta, C. 2012. Functional characteristics of parvalbumin- and cholecystokinin-expressing basket cells. *J. Physiol.* 590, 669-81.

[157] Nissen, W., Szabo, A., Somogyi, J., Somogyi, P., Lamsa, K. P. 2010. Cell type-specific long-term plasticity at glutamatergic synapses onto hippocampal interneurons expressing either parvalbumin or CB1 cannabinoid receptor. *J. Neurosci.* 30, 1337-47.

[158] Vanderhaeghen, J. J., Signeau, J. C., Gepts, W. 1975. New peptide in the vertebrate CNS reacting with antigastrin antibodies. *Nature* 257, 604-5.

[159] Wang, H., Wong, P. T., Spiess, J., Zhu, Y. Z. 2005. Cholecystokinin-2 (CCK2) receptor-mediated anxiety-like behaviors in rats. *Neurosci. Biobehav. Rev.* 29, 1361-73.

[160] Armstrong, C., & Soltesz, I. 2012. Basket cell dichotomy in microcircuit function. *J. Physiol.* 590, 683-94.

[161] Geiger, J. R., Melcher, T., Koh, D. S., Sakmann, B., Seeburg, P. H., Jonas, P., Monyer, H. 1995. Relative abundance of subunit mRNAs determines gating and Ca2+ permeability of AMPA receptors in principal neurons and interneurons in rat CNS. *Neuron* 15, 193-204.

[162] Lamsa, K. P., Heeroma, J. H., Somogyi, P., Rusakov, D. A., Kullmann, D. M. 2007. Anti-Hebbian long-term potentiation in the hippocampal feedback inhibitory circuit. *Science* 315, 1262-6.

[163] Medrihan, L., Umschweif, G., Sinha, A., Reed, S., Lee, J., Gindinova, K., Sinha, S. C., Greengard, P., Sagi, Y. 2020. Reduced Kv3.1 Activity in Dentate Gyrus Parvalbumin Cells Induces. Vulnerability to Depression. *Biol. Psychiatry* 88, 405-14.

[164] Frazier, C. J. 2007. Endocannabinoids in the dentate gyrus. *Prog. Brain Res.* 163, 319-37.

[165] Acsády, L., Katona, I., Martínez-Guijarro, F. J., Buzsáki, G., Freund, T. F. 2000. Unusual target selectivity of perisomatic

inhibitory cells in the hilar region of the rat hippocampus. *J. Neurosci.* 20, 6907-19.

[166] Hashimotodani, Y., Nasrallah, K., Jensen, K. R., Chávez, A. E., Carrera, D., Castillo, P. E. 2017. LTP at Hilar Mossy Cell-Dentate Granule Cell Synapses Modulates Dentate Gyrus Output by Increasing Excitation/Inhibition Balance. *Neuron* 95, 928-43.e3.

[167] Russo-Neustadt, A. A., & Chen, M. J. 2005. Brain-derived neurotrophic factor and antidepressant activity. *Curr. Pharm. Des.* 11, 1495-510.

[168] Oh, Y. S., Gao, P., Lee, K. W., Ceglia, I., Seo, J. S., Zhang, X., Ahn, J. H., Chait, B. T., Patel, D. J., Kim, Y., Greengard, P. 2013. SMARCA3, a chromatin-remodeling factor, is required for p11-dependent antidepressant action. *Cell* 152, 831-43.

[169] Jinde, S., Zsiros, V., Jiang, Z., Nakao, K., Pickel, J., Kohno, K., Belforte, J. E., Nakazawa, K. 2012. Hilar mossy cell degeneration causes transient dentate granule cell hyperexcitability and impaired pattern separation. *Neuron* 76, 1189-200.

[170] Hsu, T. T., Lee, C. T., Tai, M. H., Lien, C. C. 2016. Differential Recruitment of Dentate Gyrus Interneuron Types by Commissural Versus Perforant Pathways. *Cereb. Cortex* 26, 2715-27.

[171] Yeh, C. Y., Asrican, B., Moss, J., Quintanilla, L. J., He, T., Mao, X., Cassé, F., Gebara, E., Bao, H., Lu, W., Toni, N., Song, J. 2018. Mossy Cells Control Adult Neural Stem Cell Quiescence and Maintenance through a Dynamic Balance between Direct and Indirect Pathways. *Neuron* 99, 493-510.e4.

[172] Moretto, J. N., Duffy, Á. M., Scharfman, H. E. 2017. Acute restraint stress decreases c-fos immunoreactivity in hilar mossy cells of the adult dentate gyrus. *Brain Struct. Funct.* 222, 2405-19.

[173] Oh, S. J., Cheng, J., Jang, J. H., Arace, J., Jeong, M., Shin, C. H., Park, J., Jin, J., Greengard, P., Oh, Y. S. 2020. Hippocampal mossy cell involvement in behavioral and neurogenic responses to chronic antidepressant treatment. *Mol. Psychiatry* 25, 1215-28.

[174] Hargreaves, E. L., Rao, G., Lee, I., Knierim, J. J. 2005. Major dissociation between medial and lateral entorhinal input to dorsal hippocampus. *Science* 308, 1792-4.

[175] Hunsaker, M. R., Mooy, G. G., Swift, J. S., Kesner, R. P. 2007. Dissociations of the medial and lateral perforant path projections into dorsal DG, CA3, and CA1 for spatial and nonspatial (visual object) information processing. *Behav. Neurosci.* 121, 742-50.

[176] Rolls, E. T. 1996. A theory of hippocampal function in memory. *Hippocampus* 6, 601-20.

[177] O'Reilly, R. C., & McClelland, J. L. 1994. Hippocampal conjunctive encoding, storage, and recall: avoiding a trade-off. *Hippocampus* 4, 661-82.

[178] Emerich, D. F., & Walsh, T. J. 1989. Selective working memory impairments following intradentate injection of colchicine: attenuation of the behavioral but not the neuropathological effects by gangliosides GM1 and AGF2. *Physiol. Behav.* 45, 93-101.

[179] McLamb, R. L., Mundy, W. R., Tilson, H. A. 1988. Intradentate colchicine disrupts the acquisition and performance of a working memory task in the radial arm maze. *Neurotoxicology* 9, 521-8.

[180] Tilson, H. A., Rogers, B. C., Grimes, L., Harry, G. J., Peterson, N. J., Hong, J. S., Dyer, R. S. 1987. Time-dependent neurobiological effects of colchicine administered directly into the hippocampus of rats. *Brain Res.* 408, 163-72.

[181] Walsh, T. J., Schulz, D. W., Tilson, H. A., Schmechel, D. E. 1986. Colchicine-induced granule cell loss in rat hippocampus: selective behavioral and histological alterations. *Brain Res.* 398, 23-36.

[182] Jeltsch, H., Bertrand, F., Lazarus, C., Cassel, J. C. 2001. Cognitive performances and locomotor activity following dentate granule cell damage in rats: role of lesion extent and type of memory tested. *Neurobiol. Learn. Mem.* 76, 81-105.

[183] Nanry, K. P., Mundy, W. R., Tilson, H. A. 1989. Colchicine-induced alterations of reference memory in rats: role of spatial versus non-spatial task components. *Behav. Brain Res.* 35, 45-53.

[184] Sutherland, R. J., Whishaw, I. Q., Kolb, B. 1983. A behavioural analysis of spatial localization following electrolytic, kainate- or colchicine-induced damage to the hippocampal formation in the rat. *Behav. Brain. Res.* 7, 133-53.

[185] Xavier, G. F., Oliveira-Filho, F. J., Santos, A. M. 1999. Dentate gyrus-selective colchicine lesion and disruption of performance in spatial tasks: difficulties in "place strategy" because of a lack of flexibility in the use of environmental cues? *Hippocampus* 9, 668-81.

[186] McDonald, R. J., & White, N. M. 1995. Hippocampal and nonhippocampal contributions to place learning in rats. *Behav. Neurosci.* 109, 579-93.

[187] Morris, A. M., Churchwell, J. C., Kesner, R. P., Gilbert, P. E. 2012. Selective lesions of the dentate gyrus produce disruptions in place learning for adjacent spatial locations. *Neurobiol. Learn. Mem.* 97, 326-31.

[188] Miniaci, M. C., Scotto, P., Bures, J. 1999. Place navigation in rats guided by a vestibular and kinesthetic orienting gradient. *Behav. Neurosci.* 113, 1115-26.

[189] Kesner, R. P., Kirk, R. A., Yu, Z., Polansky, C., Musso, N. D. 2016. Dentate gyrus supports slope recognition memory, shades of grey-context pattern separation and recognition memory, and CA3 supports pattern completion for object memory. *Neurobiol. Learn. Mem.* 129, 29-37.

[190] Hayman, R., Verriotis, M. A., Jovalekic, A., Fenton, A. A., Jeffery, K. J. 2011. Anisotropic encoding of three-dimensional space by place cells and grid cells. *Nat. Neurosci.* 14, 1182-8.

[191] Savelli, F., & Knierim, J. J. 2011. Coming up: in search of the vertical dimension in the brain. *Nat. Neurosci.* 14, 1102-3.

[192] Kesner, R. P., & Rolls, E. T. 2015. A computational theory of hippocampal function, and tests of the theory: new developments. Neurosci. *Biobehav. Rev.* 48, 92-147.

[193] Holden, H. M., Hoebel, C., Loftis, K., Gilbert, P. E. 2012. Spatial pattern separation in cognitively normal young and older adults. *Hippocampus* 22, 1826-32.

[194] Reagh, Z. M., & Yassa, M. A. 2014. Object and spatial mnemonic interference differentially engage lateral and medial entorhinal cortex in humans. *Proc. Natl. Acad. Sci. USA* 111, E4264-73.

[195] Clelland, C. D., Choi, M., Romberg, C., Clemenson, G. D., Jr., Fragniere. A., Tyers, P., Jessberger, S., Saksida, L. M., Barker, R. A., Gage, F. H., Bussey, T. J. 2009. A functional role for adult hippocampal neurogenesis in spatial pattern separation. *Science* 325, 210-3.

[196] Nakashiba, T., Cushman, J. D., Pelkey, K. A., Renaudineau, S., Buhl, D. L., McHugh, T. J., Rodriguez, Barrera. V., Chittajallu, R., Iwamoto, K. S., McBain, C.J., Fanselow, M. S., Tonegawa, S. 2012. Young dentate granule cells mediate pattern separation, whereas old granule cells facilitate pattern completion. *Cell* 149, 188-201.

[197] Aimone, J. B., Wiles, J., Gage, F. H. 2006. Potential role for adult neurogenesis in the encoding of time in new memories. *Nat. Neurosci.* 9, 723-7.

[198] Morris, A. M., Curtis, B. J., Churchwell, J. C., Maasberg, D. W., Kesner, R. P. 2013. Temporal associations for spatial events: the role of the dentate gyrus. *Behav Brain Res*. 256, 250-6.

[199] Rangel, L. M., Alexander, A. S., Aimone, J. B., Wiles, J., Gage, F. H., Chiba, A. A., Quinn, L. K. 2014. Temporally selective contextual encoding in the dentate gyrus of the hippocampus. *Nat. Commun*. 5, 3181.

[200] Spanswick, S. C., & Sutherland, R. J. 2010. Object/context-specific memory deficits associated with loss of hippocampal granule cells after adrenalectomy in rats. *Learn. Mem*. 17, 241-5.

[201] Eacott, M. J., & Norman, G. 2004. Integrated memory for object, place, and context in rats: a possible model of episodic-like memory? *J. Neurosci*. 24, 1948-53.

[202] Dellu, F., Fauchey, V., Le Moal, M., Simon, H. 1997. Extension of a new two-trial memory task in the rat: influence of environmental context on recognition processes. *Neurobiol. Learn. Mem.* 67, 112-20.

[203] Dees, R. L., & Kesner, R. P. 2013. The role of the dorsal dentate gyrus in object and object-context recognition. *Neurobiol. Learn. Mem.* 106, 112-7.

[204] Morris, A. M., Weeden, C. S., Churchwell, J. C., Kesner, R. P. 2013. The role of the dentate gyrus in the formation of contextual representations. *Hippocampus* 23, 162-8.

[205] Weeden, C. S., Hu, N. J., Ho, L. U., Kesner, R. P. 2014. The role of the ventral dentate gyrus in olfactory pattern separation. *Hippocampus* 24, 553-9.

[206] Maaswinkel, H., Baars, A. M., Gispen, W. H., Spruijt, B. M. 1996. Roles of the basolateral amygdala and hippocampus in social recognition in rats. *Physiol. Behav.* 60, 55-63.

[207] Kirk, R. A., Redmon, S. N., Kesner, R. P. 2017. The ventral dentate gyrus mediates pattern separation for reward value. *Behav. Neurosci.* 131, 42-5.

In: The Dentate Gyrus
Editor: Feng-Ru Tang

ISBN: 978-1-68507-212-4

Chapter 4

DENTATE GYRUS AS A BRAIN SENSOR FOR RADIATION EXPOSURE

Genevieve Saw*
Radiation Physiology Lab,
Singapore Nuclear Research and Safety Initiative,
National University of Singapore, Singapore

ABSTRACT

The hippocampal dentate gyrus plays a vital role in adult hippocampal neurogenesis as well as in learning and memory. It has been the site of an abundance of radiation studies in the brain suggesting its importance as a key structure that is extremely sensitive to radiation resulting in radiation-induced changes and is therefore a prime sensor for radiation exposure in the brain. Various cells types within the dentate gyrus are differentially sensitive to radiation exposure and exhibit varying reactions to different doses of radiation ranging from low to high. Profound changes have been seen in the dentate gyrus after radition exposure in areas involving neurogenesis, angiogenesis, inflammation and cognitive impairment. Cellular and molecular respones in cells post-irradiation are crucial as biomarkers in

* Corresponding Author's Email: genevievesaw@nus.edu.sg.

determining the dose of radiation absorbed and the correlating damage incurred. Biomarkers of radiation absorption and injury can be used as targets for the development of new radiation countermeasures.

Keywords: hippocampus, dentate gyrus, radiation, angiogenesis, biodosimetry

INTRODUCTION

The human brain is one of the largest and most complex organs in the human body comprising of more than 100 billion neurons [1]. The hippocampus is a structure in the brain within the medial temporal lobe [2] which plays an important role in the limbic system and is involved in learning, memory processing and emotions [3]. The three principle structures of the hippocampal formation are the hippocampus, dentate gyrus (DG) and subiculum and they are predominantly made up of glutamatergic principal neurons and inhibitory GABAergic neurons [4]. The DG is the site of most radiation studies in the brain. This suggests its prominence as a key structure that is sensitive to radiation and subject to radiation-related changes and thus has been suggested to be a brain sensor for radiation exposure. Studies have seen profound effects of radiation on adult hippocampal neurogenesis in the DG [5], angiogenesis [6], inflammation [7] and also cognitive impairment [8].

NEUROGENESIS IN THE DENTATE GYRUS

The DG of the hippocampus in mammals continuously generates new neurons even throughout adulthood [9] in a process known as adult hippocampal neurogenesis. Neurogenesis is the process by which new functional neurons are generated from neural stem cells (NSCs) [10]. The production of new neurons in the adult central nervous system (CNS) in the subventricular zone (SVZ) of the lateral ventricle and the subgranular zone (SGZ) of the DG in the hippocampus is one of the major breakthroughs in neuroscience research [11]. Adult hippocampal neurogenesis was first discovered in rodents [12] and subsequently confirmed in the human brain [13-15]. Since the discovery of adult hippocampal neurogenesis, research has been done to investigate the integration of these newborn neurons and how they contribute to learning and memory [16], behavioural functions and the potential role they may play in various diseases that affect the brain [17].

The DG receives input from the entorhinal cortex (EC) via the perforant path [18]. Excitatory projections from the EC to the DG play a crucial role in encoding new memories and thus are seen to be severely affected in patients with Alzheimer's disease (AD) contributing to the dysfunction of this pathology [19]. Animal model studies demonstrate the importance of hippocampal neurogenesis in the DG for normal cognitive function [7]. Recent studies have confirmed that learning and memory throughout adulthood is enabled by the activity of neural stem cells generated via adult hippocampal neurogenesis. Studies have shown that inhibition of neurogenesis interferes with memory function [20]. New granule neurons generated in adults plays a significant role in synaptic plasticity in the DG and the production and plasticity of these young neurons has an important role in hippocampal functions such as information processing and memory formation [21].

It has been established that radiation induces a myriad of cognitive impairments and dysfunction [8, 22, 23]. Children and adults who receive radiotherapy often experience progressive cognitive decline and severe learning and memory deficits [7]. The hippocampal formation plays a vital role in learning and memory, which are the functions that also happen to be the most prominently affected by radiation [24]. Neurogenic regions, such as the SVZ and DG are particularly sensitive to radiation exposure [25] and thus have the potential of acting as radiation sensors. An increase in γ-H2AX was seen in cell nuclei after targeted irradiation to the dorsal and ventral DG [26]. Targeted X-ray irradiation (0.25-2 Gy) to the hippocampal dorsal DG was also found to induce more profound effects as compared to whole-brain X-ray irradiation of the same dose

[5]. Serrano et al. (2021) found that spatial memory was not affected after whole-brain exposure but a deficit was seen after targeted irradiation (1 Gy) to the dorsal DG. At this dose, neurogenesis was also found to be more impacted as compared to whole-brain exposure [5].

Neural progenitor cells in the hippocampal DG are known to undergo apoptosis when exposed to radiation [27]. Radiation-induced changes in inflammatory cells and neuronal progenitors have been linked to cognitive deficits [28]. A study by Mizumatsu et al. (2003) showed that in adult male C57BL mice, whole-brain X-ray irradiation (2-10 Gy) brought about a reduction in proliferating cells (93-96%) and immature neurons (40-60%) in a dose-dependent manner [29] alluding to the extreme sensitivity of adult neurogenesis even to low doses of X-irradiation. Work in other animal models has also shown that exposure to therapeutic doses of irradiation induced apoptosis [30] and a reduction in stem/precursor cell differentiation into neurons within the hippocampus [31]. In addition, a study by Sienkiewicz et al. (1994) showed a decline in both neurogenesis and the performance in behavioural tests involving hippocampal function post-irradiation in a dose-dependent fashion [32] while a single dose of 10 Gy irradiation to the cranium of a mature rat was able to ablate hippocampal neurogenesis [31]. These studies support the notion that irradiation ablates hippocampal neurogenesis and this in turn contributes to cognitive impairments seen in patients post-radiotherapy indicating the sensitivity of the hippocampus, particularly the DG, to radiation.

Radiosensitivity of Different Subpopulation of Cells in the Dentate Gyrus

The DG is made up of three layers. The granule cell layer is the principal layer and it is made up of densely packed granule cells and a thickness of 4 to 8 neurons [33]. Granule cells are the most abundant neurons of the DG [34]. Studies have shown that dentate granule cell neurogenesis in the adult hippocampus is exceptionally vulnerable to low-dose ionising radiation as a single dose of 5 Gy X-ray irradiation was able to block cell proliferation and eliminate putative NPCs in the SGZ [35]. These results indicate that dentate granule cell neurogenesis in the mature hippocampal formation is vulnerable to the effects of low-dose ionising irradiation. In studies involving rabbits that were subjected to 4.5 Gy of whole-body or brain alone γ-irradiation, it was found that there were lesions in the nuclei of the mature granule cells [36] appearing as light spots and disappearing after 48 hours. In addition, when young adult-born granule cells were ablated by X-irradiation, there was an increase in spontaneous bursts of granule cell activity in the DG [37] suggesting a disinhibitory effect.

The granule cell layer encloses the polymorphic cell layer and the most abundant cell type here are mossy cells [33]. Mossy cells are a major population of excitatory interneurons in the dentate hilus and play an important role in the circuitry of the hippocampus, including neurogenesis, spatial navigation and memory [38]. Their dendrites are short and do not leave the hilus while their axons project into the layers of the DG synapsing with granule cells [39]. Exposing wild-type mice to clinically relevant doses of X-ray irradiation led to a significant decrease in the number of mossy cells as well as their activity, measured through the *c-Fos* marker [38].

The SGZ is a narrow layer of cells between the granule cell layer and the hilus of the DG characterised by an abundance of NSCs at various stages in their development [40]. It is estimated that 100-150 neurons are generated a day in the SGZ of adult rodents [41]. NPCs in the SGZ have prominent radial processes [41] and are known as type I progenitors. These type I progenitors give rise to type II progenitors which are highly proliferative and form aggregates between radial processes [42].

Neurogenic cells in the SGZ are particularly sensitive to ionising radiation and will undergo apoptosis after exposure to doses ranging from 0.4 Gy to 18 Gy [29, 30, 43-46]. Studies have shown that there is a significant decline in neurogenesis in the SGZ of the DG in young adult rats following exposure to 10 Gy radiation whereby radiation was found to significantly reduce the number of neuroblasts and differentiating neurons [28] marked by doublecortin (DCX), which serves as an index reflecting the ongoing generation of neurons, and is therefore an accurate indication of changes in adult neurogenesis [47]. A study by Li et al. (2016) found that adult hippocampal NPCs showed differential sensitivity to radiation in the absence of p53 [27] indicating that radiation-induced apoptosis of NPCs is p53-dependent. In addition, rampiril, an angiotensin-converting enzyme inhibitor (ACEI), was able to mitigate radiation-induced impairment of neurogenesis in the rat DG following 10 Gy whole-brain irradiation [48]. Human neural progenitor cells (hNPCs) exposed to low-dose irradiation showed changes in their development after 496 mGy radiation exposure while DNA repair and cell adhesion changes were observed at a much lower dose of 124 mGy of radiation [49]. This study elucidates the clinical phenotypes of impaired neuronal development induced by chronic low-dose irradiation. Similarly, mice exposed to low (0.1 Gy) or moderate (2 Gy) doses X-ray irradiation had changes in hippocampal neurogenesis due to DNA damage in neural progenitors [50]. These effects were found to be age-related possibly due to a redox imbalance in the hippocampus after radiation-induced stress.

Endothelial cells have also been found to undergo changes following radiation exposure. Radiation-induced inflammation is capable of permeabilising the endothelial barrier [51]. Human cardiac endothelial cells exposed to radiation doses of 0-10 Gy of ^{60}Co irradiation showed varying changes. Low-moderate doses (0.25 Gy and 0.5 Gy) showed very minor proteome changes while at higher doses (2 Gy and 10 Gy), DNA damage, inflammation and oxidative stress was observed [51]. Transcriptomic profiling suggests the involvement of IGFBP5 in the senescence of endothelial cells following chronic low dose irradiation [52]. After one week of exposure at a rate of 4.1 mGy/h, an early stress response was observed which then evolved into a more inflammation-related state which may be responsible for the radiation-induced premature senescence of endothelial cells [52]. There was also an observable increase in pyknotic cells, which are only found in the SGZ, post-irradiation of rabbit full-body and whole brain irradiation which peak at 5-7 hours then are no longer detectable after 24 hours [36]. However, it was observed that in older animals (27 months), these cells were relatively sparse [36]. At lower doses of 0.25 to 1 Gy, pyknotic cell numbers showed significant increases in a dose-dependent manner [53]. In another study by Saha et al. (2014) they noted that pyknotic cells became evident after low dose radiation exposure (0.24 Gy). This was regardless as to whether the dose was delivered as a single or split dose.

Glial cells refer to the non-neuronal cells in the brain which make up roughly 80% of the total cells in the human brain [54]. Glial cells in the DG consist of microglia, astrocytes and oligodendrocytes. Studies have shown that glial cells are differentially radiosensitive as compared to neurons in the hippocampus [36]. Radiation was found to induce microglial activation, characterised by an amoeboid morphology and proliferation in the cerebellum of rats 24 hours after irradiation of 6 Gy compared to non-irradiated controls [25]. Similarly, Conner et al. (2011) observed that microglia in irradiated rats exhibited an activated phenotype with processes that were shorter and wider than those in control animals [28]. The inflammatory response was quantified by measuring the release of cytokines, chemokines and growth factors post-irradiation. Compared to controls, vascular endothelial growth factor (VEGF), IL-6 and IL-8 all showed increases after radiation exposure [25]. This supports previous studies that show that 10 Gy irradiation induces a microglial inflammatory response [28]. Cobalt-60 (^{60}Co) irradiation of 0.5 Gy was also found to cause a long-term de-ramification of microglial processes in the DG [55] which indicates an amoieboid, phagocytic transition. Conversely, a lower dose of 0.063 Gy ^{60}Co irradiation brought about hyper-ramification. The effect of radiation on the morphology of microglia was more evident than on the number of microglia at low doses [55]. Tamoxifen has been shown to ameliorate radiation-induced brain injury by dampening the microglial inflammatory response in BV2 cells as well as *in vivo* in animals exposed to a single dose of 2-10 Gy of X-ray radiation [56]. Studies have also shown that a single radiation event has long-term effects on glial cells in a dose-dependent manner inducing a state of heightened immunity after high dose irradiation (0.125 Gy and 0.5 Gy) but conversely, a more neuroprotective state after low dose irradiation (0.063 Gy) [57]. In addition, selective inhibition of microglia-mediated neuroinflammation was found to alleviate radiation-induced cognitive impairment [58] possibly by restoring neurogenesis in the SGZ maintaining the DG integrity which suggesting a major role for microglia in radiation-induced cognitive impairment.

Astrocytes are the second major cell type that is involved in the inflammatory response to radiation exposure [59]. Neumann et al. (2020) found that cranial irradiation did not affect the activity and reactivity of astrocytes in an ischemic cortex. Astrocytes were still reactive and an upregulation of glial fibrillary acidic protein (GFAP) was seen [60] which suggests that irradiation did not affect the GFAP-immunoreactivity of astrocytes induced by ischemia. Morphological analysis shows significant dose-dependent differences in the number of astrocyte processes. ^{60}Co irradiation with 0.125 Gy and 0.5 Gy was able to decrease the number of processes and intersections between these processes in astrocytes in the DG as compared to 0.063 Gy and controls [55]. The length of their branches was also reduced. The data suggests that exposure to radiation brings about a decrease in the ramification and complexity of astrocytes. At these doses, the number of astrocytes did not show any change but indicate that there may be an increase in astrocyte numbers with higher doses of radiation [55]. In other study, GFAP levels after whole brain irradiation increased after a single high dose (20-45 Gy) of radiation but the same was not seen at lower doses (2 or 8 Gy) [61] indicative of the reactive gliosis and inflammation that increases with radiation dose. Immunohistochemical labelling of senescent cells in the irradiated human brain showed that upon exposure to cranial radiation therapy, astrocytes become senescent [62]. This radiation-induced senescence was found to be ameliorated by Δ133p53, an inhibitory isoform of p53, which is reduced in irradiated astrocytes [62]. Cell senescence is a primary inducing factor for age-related neurodegenerative diseases [63]. Astrocyte senescence is heavily implicated in AD, as it contributes to Aβ accumulation, tau hyperphosphorylation, and the deposition of neurofibrillary tangles (NFTs) [63], suggesting that radiation-induced changes may ultimate underlie AD progression.

Studies on the effects of radiation on oligodendrocytes seem to suggest that X-ray radiation exposure leads to a loss of oligodendrocyte progenitor cells (OPCs) as well as demyelination over time [64]. Oligodendrocytes associated with myelination are likely damaged by radiation-induced apoptosis leading to a depletion which may then cause delays in myelination of axons [65]. The oligodendrocytes in the hilus appear to be one of the most affected cell populations other than the NPCs in the SGZ [66] suggesting an increase in immunoreactivity after radiation which may be associated with the pathogenesis of radiation injury. This was similarly seen in the spinal cord of adult rats where oligodendrocytes underwent radiation-induced apoptosis [67]. Whole-brain irradiation (25 Gy) of mice showed a stark decrease in the number of oligodendrocytes from as soon as 24 hours post-irradiation in an age-dependent manner [68]. Irradiation of mature oligodendrocytes cultured from rat pups resulted in a significant increase in apoptotic cells as compared to control [69]. Overall, these studies elucidate the sensitivity of oligodendrocytes to radiation leading to apoptosis.

RADIATION AND DG ANGIOGENESIS

It has come to light that blood vessels are an integral part of stem cell niches, including those in the adult brain with the two major neurogenic niches being the SVZ and the hippocampus [70]. NSCs are surrounded in a specialised niche filled with cell-cell and cell-microenvironment interactions regulating their proliferation and fate [6]. Blood vessels have been found to control the function of NSCs in these areas by acting as conduits for blood-borne substances impacting the activity of NSCs [71] and regulating NSC properties during development as well as throughout adulthood [72]. In adult neurogenic niches, NSCs inhabit a specialised microenvironment in which they interact with a variety of other cell types influencing their behaviour. The vasculature in both the SGZ and SVZ is extremely organised, forming a unique architecture compared to other non-neurogenic regions [71] with a dense network of interconnected blood vessels providing substrates for NSCs [73]. Studies have shown that stem cells in the SVZ as well as their progeny are coupled to blood vessels in a specialised vascular niche [74] which is a crucial microenvironment for the support of these cells and their progeny.

All radiation is harmful to vascular systems bringing about a number of vascular pathologies [6]. Changes in the vasculature of the brain have been found to contribute to impairments in learning and memory after radiation exposure [75]. Cranial irradiated patients were also found to develop vascular abnormalities later in life increasing their risk of cerebral ischemia [60].

Evidence has shown that gamma rays promote angiogenesis and increase metastasis by increasing the expression of pro-angiogenic factors such as VEGF, IL-6 and basic fibroblast growth factor (bFGF) in both human and murine cells as well as in primary endothelial and fibroblast cells *in vitro* [76]. In the brains of young rats (P14), cranial irradiation of 8 Gy saw changes in the neurovascular niche whereby there was an increase in the distance between microvessels and DCX-positive cells 6 hours post-irradiation and also between microvessels and Ki-67-positive cells 1 week post-irradiation [77]. There was also a decrease in pericyte coverage by 17% 6 hours after radiation exposure [77]. Hippocampal microvessels exposed to ^{56}Fe ions at doses of 0 to 2 Gy also showed a loss of endothelial cells in the hippocampal CA1 region [78]. However mice that received 4 Gy ^{56}Fe ions showed a repopulation following an initial rapid loss of endothelial cells. None of these changes were seen in the DG [78], suggesting that the vascular topological differences between these areas may account for the variation in dose response.

RADIATION-INDUCED BIOMARKER CHANGES

Radiation induces a myriad of changes in cell density, morphology and secretion [79]. The first step in medical management of radiation exposure is determining the dosage of radiation received. The levels of radiation exposure can be assessed by looking at cell viability, chromosome aberrations [80] and also metabolites in biological fluids [81]. The levels of gene and protein expression are also valid biomarkers for radiation [80]. Peripheral blood cell counts post-irradiation are useful indicators of the dose of radiation absorbed [81] as a diagnostic tool determining radiation exposure. Neutrophils in peripheral blood exposed to radiation showed an increase in the severity of neutropenia and thrombocytopenia [81].

Chromosomal aberrations occur post-irradiation after single and double stranded DNA breaks resulting in a repair process that forms a dicentric chromosome (an unstable chromosome with two centromeres) [82]. Thus, the dicentric cytogenetic assay is a well-accepted biodosimetry assay after a radiation emergency.

Exposure to radiation also triggers cascades of molecular and cellular responses in cells and tissues. Citrulline, a nitrogen end product of glutamate metabolism in small-bowel enterocytes, has also been identified as a potential biomarker for radiation-induced gastrointestinal (GI) damage reflecting enterocyte mass [81]. The correlation between epithelial cell loss caused by radiation and levels of citrulline has been well studied in mice [83, 84].

Biomarkers of radiation-induced brain damage are crucial as this is the dose-limiting factor in radiotherapy [85]. Damage to the brain ranges from neurocognitive deficits to tissue necrosis [86]. There is currently no validated biomarker to measure the dose of radiation absorbed by the brain after ionising radiation exposure or a nuclear event [87]. However, studies have also observed an increase in cerebrospinal fluid (CSF) oxysterols in plasma as a potential marker of radiation exposure to the CNS [88]. Whole brain radiotherapy also appeared to reduce the levels of CSF Hypocretin (Orexin A) levels suggesting its use as a biomarker for brain damage following radiotherapy [89]. In a study by Fernström et al. (2018), they found that the levels of inflammatory markers such as IL-16, IL-15 and Monocyte Chemoattractant Protein-1 (MCP-1/CCL2) were higher in the CSF 3 months after prophylactic cranial irradiation (PCI) compared to controls [86]. Other markers such as Growth Associated Protein 43 (GAP-43) and Synaptosome Associated Protein 25 (SNAP-25) also showed the same trend. Contrastingly, brevican and neurocan leves decreased after PCI [86]. This study shows the effect of cranial radiotherapy on extracellular matrix (ECM)-related proteins allowing for a better understanding of the mechanisms underlying the negative side effects that occur after radiotherapy.

Conclusion

The hippocampal dentate gyrus plays a vital role in adult hippocampal neurogenesis as well as in learning and memory. It has been the site of an abundance of radiation studies in the brain suggesting its importance as a key structure that is extremely sensitive to radiation resulting in radiation-induced changes and is therefore a prime sensor for radiation exposure in the brain. Various cells types within the dentate gyrus are differentially sensitive to radiation exposure and exhibit varying reactions to different doses of radiation ranging from low to high. Profound changes have been seen in the dentate gyrus after radition exposure in areas involving neurogenesis, angiogenesis, inflammation and cognitive impairment.

The hippocampal DG is crucial for adult hippocampal neurogenesis and memory formation. A majority of radiation studies done on brains seem to focus most on the DG alluding to its sensitivity and importance as a sensor for radiation exposure in the brain. The different cell types within the DG show differential sensitivities to radiation exposure eliciting a myriad of responses. We see that exposure to radiation substantially reduces the number of NPCs within the SGZ from doses of as low as 0.1 Gy, while endothelial cells and pyknotic cells show changes after exposure to 0.25 Gy and 0.24 Gy of radiation respectively. The most targeted areas and cells of radiation-induced apoptosis are the NPCs in the SGZ and the oligodendrocytes in the hilus. Glial cells appear to show differential radiosensitivity with oligodendrocytes seeming to be the most sensitive to radiation in terms of apoptosis and cell death. Microglia on the other hand are found to proliferate more and are activated after exposure to low doses of radiation from as low as 0.063 Gy and are therefore the most sensitive cells to radiation. Astrocytes the most subtle changes with a mere morphological change as their endings and intersections are reduced after exposure to 0.125 Gy radiation but their numbers do not change as drastically. The studies infer DG sensitivity to radiation indicating a prime role for the DG as a radiation sensor. Further studies should be done with even lower doses of radiation to determine the ultimate dose to which cells in the DG are sensitive to. Cellular and molecular respones in cells post-irradiation are crucial as biomarkers in determining the dose of radiation absorbed and the correlating damage incurred. Biomarkers of radiation absorption and injury can be used as targets for the development of new radiation countermeasures. An interesting area to explore would be to compare the changes in protein expression in the CSF after radiation exposure to that in blood after radiation exposureto see if any correlations can be made. This may aid in the detection of changes in the brain post-irradiation merely by checking for blood biomarkers allowing early detection of any serious underlying dysfunction in the brain.

REFERENCES

[1] Herculano-Houzel, S. (2009). The Human Brain in Numbers: A Linearly Scaled-up Primate Brain. *Frontiers in human neuroscience*, *3*, 31.

[2] Knierim, J. J. (2015). The Hippocampus. *Current biology*, *25*, R1116-R1121.

[3] Tatu, L. & Vuillier, F. (2014). *Structure and Vascularization of the Human Hippocampus The Hippocampus in Clinical Neuroscience*: Karger publishers, pp. 18-25.

[4] Fink, G. (2019). *Stress: Physiology, Biochemistry, and Pathology: Handbook of Stress Series*: Academic Press.

[5] Serrano, C., Dos Santos, M., Kereselidze, D., Beugnies, L., Lestaevel, P., Poirier, R. & Durand, C. (2021). Targeted Dorsal Dentate Gyrus or Whole Brain Irradiation in Juvenile Mice Differently Affects Spatial Memory and Adult Hippocampal Neurogenesis. *Biology*, *10*, 192.

[6] Capilla-Gonzalez, V., Bonsu, J. M., Redmond, K. J., Garcia-Verdugo, J. M. & Quiñones-Hinojosa, A. (2016). Implications of Irradiating the Subventricular Zone Stem Cell Niche. *Stem cell research*, *16*, 387-396.

[7] Monje, M. L. & Palmer, T. (2003). Radiation Injury and Neurogenesis. *Current opinion in neurology*, *16*, 129-134.

[8] Pazzaglia, S., Briganti, G., Mancuso, M. & Saran, A. (2020). Neurocognitive Decline Following Radiotherapy: Mechanisms and Therapeutic Implications. *Cancers*, *12*, 146.

[9] Gonçalves, J. T., Schafer, S. T. & Gage, F. H. (2016). Adult Neurogenesis in the Hippocampus: From Stem Cells to Behavior. *Cell*, *167*, 897-914.

[10] Ming, G. l. & Song, H. (2011). Adult Neurogenesis in the Mammalian Brain: Significant Answers and Significant Questions. *Neuron*, *70*, 687-702.

[11] Saw, G. & Tang, F. R. (2020). Epigenetic Regulation of the Hippocampus, with Special Reference to Radiation Exposure. *International journal of molecular sciences*, *21*, 9514.

[12] Altman, J. (1962). Are New Neurons Formed in the Brains of Adult Mammals? *Science* (New York, N.Y.), *135*, 1127-1128.

[13] Eriksson, P. S., Perfilieva, E., Björk-Eriksson, T., Alborn, A. M., Nordborg, C., Peterson, D. A. & Gage, F. H. (1998). Neurogenesis in the Adult Human Hippocampus. *Nature medicine*, *4*, 1313-1317.

[14] Roy, N. S., Wang, S., Jiang, L., Kang, J., Benraiss, A., Harrison-Restelli, C., Fraser, R. A., Couldwell, W. T., Kawaguchi, A. & Okano, H. (2000). *In Vitro* Neurogenesis by Progenitor Cells Isolated from the Adult Human Hippocampus. *Nature medicine*, *6*, 271-277.

[15] Knoth, R., Singec, I., Ditter, M., Pantazis, G., Capetian, P., Meyer, R. P., Horvat, V., Volk, B. & Kempermann, G. (2010). Murine Features of Neurogenesis in the Human Hippocampus across the Lifespan from 0 to 100 Years. *PloS one*, *5*, e8809.

[16] Covic, M., Karaca, E. & Lie, D. (2010). Epigenetic Regulation of Neurogenesis in the Adult Hippocampus. *Heredity*, *105*, 122-134.

[17] Denoth-Lippuner, A. & Jessberger, S. (2021). Formation and Integration of New Neurons in the Adult Hippocampus. *Nature reviews neuroscience*, 1-14.

[18] Witter, M. P. (2007). The Perforant Path: Projections from the Entorhinal Cortex to the Dentate Gyrus. *Progress in brain research*, *163*, 43-61.

[19] Savtchouk, I., Di Castro, M. A., Ali, R., Stubbe, H., Luján, R. & Volterra, A. (2019). Circuit-Specific Control of the Medial Entorhinal Inputs to the Dentate Gyrus by Atypical Presynaptic Nmdars Activated by Astrocytes. *Proceedings of the national academy of sciences*, *116*, 13602-13610.

[20] Winocur, G., Wojtowicz, J. M., Sekeres, M., Snyder, J. S. & Wang, S. (2006). Inhibition of Neurogenesis Interferes with Hippocampus-Dependent Memory Function. *Hippocampus*, *16*, 296-304.

[21] Snyder, J., Kee, N. & Wojtowicz, J. (2001). Effects of Adult Neurogenesis on Synaptic Plasticity in the Rat Dentate Gyrus. *Journal of neurophysiology*, *85*, 2423-2431.

[22] Haldbo-Classen, L., Amidi, A., Wu, L. M., Lukacova, S., Oettingen, G.v., Gottrup, H., Zachariae, R. & Høyer, M. (2019). Long-Term Cognitive Dysfunction after Radiation Therapy for Primary Brain Tumors. *Acta oncologica*, *58*, 745-752.

[23] Greene-Schloesser, D. & Robbins, M. E. (2012). Radiation-Induced Cognitive Impairment-from Bench to Bedside. *Neuro-oncology*, *14*, iv37-iv44.

[24] Warrington, J. P., Csiszar, A., Mitschelen, M., Lee, Y. W. & Sonntag, W. E. (2012). Whole Brain Radiation-Induced Impairments in Learning and Memory Are Time-Sensitive and Reversible by Systemic Hypoxia. *PloS one*, *7*, e30444.

[25] Zhou, K., Boström, M., Ek, C. J., Li, T., Xie, C., Xu, Y., Sun, Y., Blomgren, K. & Zhu, C. (2017). Radiation Induces Progenitor Cell Death, Microglia Activation, and Blood-Brain Barrier Damage in the Juvenile Rat Cerebellum. *Scientific reports*, *7*, 1-14.

[26] Dos Santos, M., Kereselidze, D., Gloaguen, C., Benadjaoud, M., Tack, K., Lestaevel, P. & Durand, C. (2018). Development of Whole Brain Versus Targeted Dentate Gyrus Irradiation Model to Explain Low to Moderate Doses of Exposure Effects in Mice. *Scientific reports*, *8*, 1-12.

[27] Li, Y. Q., Cheng, Z. & Wong, S. (2016). Differential Apoptosis Radiosensitivity of Neural Progenitors in Adult Mouse Hippocampus. *International journal of molecular sciences*, *17*, 970.

[28] Conner, K. R., Forbes, M. E., Lee, W. H., Lee, Y. W. & Riddle, D. R. (2011). At1 Receptor Antagonism Does Not Influence Early Radiation-Induced Changes in Microglial Activation or Neurogenesis in the Normal Rat Brain. *Radiation research*, *176*, 71-83.

[29] Mizumatsu, S., Monje, M. L., Morhardt, D. R., Rola, R., Palmer, T. D. & Fike, J. R. (2003). Extreme Sensitivity of Adult Neurogenesis to Low Doses of X-Irradiation. *Cancer research*, *63*, 4021-4027.

[30] Tada, E., Parent, J., Lowenstein, D. & Fike, J. (2000). X-Irradiation Causes a Prolonged Reduction in Cell Proliferation in the Dentate Gyrus of Adult Rats. *Neuroscience*, *99*, 33-41.

[31] Monje, M. L., Mizumatsu, S., Fike, J. R. & Palmer, T. D. (2002). Irradiation Induces Neural Precursor-Cell Dysfunction. *Nature medicine*, *8*, 955-962.

[32] Sienkiewicz, Z., Haylock, R. & Saunders, R. (1994). Prenatal Irradiation and Spatial Memory in Mice: Investigation of Dose-Response Relationship. *International journal of radiation biology*, *65*, 611-618.

[33] Amaral, D. G., Scharfman, H. E. & Lavenex, P. (2007). The Dentate Gyrus: Fundamental Neuroanatomical Organization (Dentate Gyrus for Dummies). *Progress in brain research*, *163*, 3-790.

[34] Lopez-Rojas, J. & Kreutz, M. R. (2016). Mature Granule Cells of the Dentate Gyrus—Passive Bystanders or Principal Performers in Hippocampal Function? *Neuroscience & biobehavioral reviews*, *64*, 167-174.

[35] Parent, J. M., Tada, E., Fike, J. R. & Lowenstein, D. H. (1999). Inhibition of Dentate Granule Cell Neurogenesis with Brain Irradiation Does Not Prevent Seizure-Induced Mossy Fiber Synaptic Reorganization in the Rat. *Journal of neuroscience*, *19*, 4508-4519.

[36] Gueneau, G., Drouet, J. & Privat, A. (1979). Differential Radiosensitivity of Neurons and Neuroglia of the Hippocampus in the Adult Rabbit. *Acta neuropathological*, *48*, 199-209.

[37] Lacefield, C. O., Itskov, V., Reardon, T., Hen, R. & Gordon, J. A. (2012). Effects of Adult-Generated Granule Cells on Coordinated Network Activity in the Dentate Gyrus. *Hippocampus*, *22*, 106-116.

[38] Ivy, D. (2018). *Defining the Radioresponse of Mossy Cells.*

[39] Scharfman, H. E. (2016). The Enigmatic Mossy Cell of the Dentate Gyrus. *Nature reviews neuroscience*, *17*, 562.

[40] Bond, A. M., Ming, G. l. & Song, H. (2015). Adult Mammalian Neural Stem Cells and Neurogenesis: Five Decades Later. *Cell stem cell*, *17*, 385-395.

[41] Zaverucha-do-Valle, C., Gubert, F., Mesentier-Louro, L., Scemes, E., Pitossi, F., Santiago, M. F. & Mendez-Otero, R. (2013). Resident Neural Stem Cells. *Resident stem cells and regnerative therapy*, 69-88.

[42] Seri, B., Garcıa-Verdugo, J. M., McEwen, B. S. & Alvarez-Buylla, A. (2001). Astrocytes Give Rise to New Neurons in the Adult Mammalian Hippocampus. *Journal of neuroscience*, *21*, 7153-7160.

[43] Nagai, R., Tsunoda, S., Hori, Y. & Asada, H. (2000). Selective Vulnerability to Radiation in the Hippocampal Dentate Granule Cells. *Surgical neurology*, *53*, 503-507.

[44] Uberti, D., Piccioni, L., Cadei, M., Grigolato, P., Rotter, V. & Memo, M. (2001). P53 Is Dispensable for Apoptosis but Controls Neurogenesis of Mouse Dentate Gyrus Cells Following Γ-Irradiation. *Molecular brain research*, *93*, 81-89.

[45] Horrobin, D. F., Lonergan, P. E., Martin, D. S. & Lynch, M. A. (2002). Neuroprotective Effect of Eicosapentaenoic Acid in Hippocampus of Rats Exposed to Γ-Irradiation. *Journal of biological chemistry*, *277*, 20804-20811.

[46] Santarelli, L., Saxe, M., Gross, C., Surget, A., Battaglia, F., Dulawa, S., Weisstaub, N., Lee, J., Duman, R. & Arancio, O. (2003). Requirement of Hippocampal Neurogenesis for the Behavioral Effects of Antidepressants. *Science* (New York, N.Y.), *301*, 805-809.

[47] Couillard-Despres, S., Winner, B., Schaubeck, S., Aigner, R., Vroemen, M., Weidner, N., Bogdahn, U., Winkler, J., Kuhn, H. G. & Aigner, L. (2005). Doublecortin Expression Levels in Adult Brain Reflect Neurogenesis. *European journal of neuroscience*, *21*, 1-14.

[48] Jenrow, K. A., Brown, S. L., Liu, J., Kolozsvary, A., Lapanowski, K. & Kim, J. H. (2010). Ramipril Mitigates Radiation-Induced Impairment of Neurogenesis in the Rat Dentate Gyrus. *Radiation oncology*, *5*, 1-8.

[49] Katsura, M., Cyou-Nakamine, H., Zen, Q., Zen, Y., Nansai, H., Amagasa, S., Kanki, Y., Inoue, T., Kaneki, K. & Taguchi, A. (2016). Effects of Chronic Low-Dose Radiation on Human Neural Progenitor Cells. *Scientific reports*, *6*, 1-12.

[50] Casciati, A., Dobos, K., Antonelli, F., Benedek, A., Kempf, S. J., Bellés, M., Balogh, A., Tanori, M., Heredia, L. & Atkinson, M. J. (2016). Age-Related Effects of X-Ray Irradiation on Mouse Hippocampus. *Oncotarget*, *7*, 28040.

[51] Philipp, J., Le Gleut, R., Toerne, C. v., Subedi, P., Azimzadeh, O., Atkinson, M. J. & Tapio, S. (2020). Radiation Response of Human Cardiac Endothelial Cells Reveals a Central Role of the Cgas-Sting Pathway in the Development of Inflammation. *Proteomes*, *8*, 30.

[52] Rombouts, C., Aerts, A., Quintens, R., Baselet, B., El-Saghire, H., Harms-Ringdahl, M., Haghdoost, S., Janssen, A., Michaux, A. & Yentrapalli, R. (2014). Transcriptomic Profiling Suggests a Role for Igfbp5 in Premature Senescence of Endothelial Cells after Chronic Low Dose Rate Irradiation. *International journal of radiation biology*.

[53] Norton, S. & Kimler, B. F. (1990). Early Effects of Low Doses of Ionizing Radiation on the Fetal Cerebral Cortex in Rats. *Radiation research*, *124*, 235-241.

[54] Garman, R. H. (2011). Histology of the Central Nervous System. *Toxicologic pathology*, *39*, 22-35.

[55] Ung, M. C., Garrett, L., Dalke, C., Leitner, V., Dragosa, D., Hladik, D., Neff, F., Wagner, F., Zitzelsberger, H. & Miller, G. (2020). Dose-Dependent Long-Term Effects of a Single Radiation Event on Behaviour and Glial Cells. *International journal of radiation biology*, 1-42.

[56] Liu, J. L., Tian, D. S., Li, Z. W., Qu, W. S., Zhan, Y., Xie, M. J., Yu, Z. Y., Wang, W. & Wu, G. (2010). Tamoxifen Alleviates Irradiation-Induced Brain Injury by Attenuating Microglial Inflammatory Response *in Vitro* and *in Vivo*. *Brain research*, *1316*, 101-111.

[57] Ung, M. C., Garrett, L., Dalke, C., Leitner, V., Dragosa, D., Hladik, D., Neff, F., Wagner, F., Zitzelsberger, H. & Miller, G. (2021). Dose-Dependent Long-Term Effects of a Single Radiation Event on Behaviour and Glial Cells. *International journal of radiation biology*, *97*, 156-169.

[58] Jenrow, K. A., Brown, S. L., Lapanowski, K., Naei, H., Kolozsvary, A. & Kim, J. H. (2013). Selective Inhibition of Microglia-Mediated Neuroinflammation Mitigates Radiation-Induced Cognitive Impairment. *Radiation research*, *179*, 549-556.

[59] Hwang, S. Y., Jung, J. S., Kim, T. H., Lim, S. J., Oh, E. S., Kim, J. Y., Ji, K. A., Joe, E. H., Cho, K. H. & Han, I. O. (2006). Ionizing Radiation Induces Astrocyte Gliosis through Microglia Activation. *Neurobiology of disease*, *21*, 457-467.

[60] Neumann, S., Porritt, M. J., Osman, A. M. & Kuhn, H. G. (2020). Cranial Irradiation at Early Postnatal Age Impairs Stroke-Induced Neural Stem/Progenitor Cell Response in the Adult Brain. *Scientific reports*, *10*, 1-10.

[61] Chiang, C., McBride, W. & Withers, H. (1993). Radiation-Induced Astrocytic and Microglial Responses in Mouse Brain. *Radiotherapy and oncology*, *29*, 60-68.

[62] Turnquist, C., Beck, J. A., Horikawa, I., Obiorah, I. E., Von Muhlinen, N., Vojtesek, B., Lane, D. P., Grunseich, C., Chahine, J. J. & Ames, H. M. (2019). Radiation-Induced Astrocyte Senescence Is Rescued by Δ133p53. *Neuro-oncology*, *21*, 474-485.

[63] Han, X., Zhang, T., Liu, H., Mi, Y. & Gou, X. (2020). Astrocyte Senescence and Alzheimer's Disease: A Review. *Frontiers in aging neuroscience*, *12*, 148.

[64] Panagiotakos, G., Alshamy, G., Chan, B., Abrams, R., Greenberg, E., Saxena, A., Bradbury, M., Edgar, M., Gutin, P. & Tabar, V. (2007). Long-Term Impact of Radiation on the Stem Cell and Oligodendrocyte Precursors in the Brain. *PloS one*, *2*, e588.

[65] Sano, K., Morii, K., Sato, M., Mori, H. & Tanaka, R. (2000). Radiation-Induced Diffuse Brain Injury in the Neonatal Rat Model—Radiation-Induced Apoptosis of Oligodendrocytes—. *Neurologia medico-chirurgica*, *40*, 495-500.

[66] Sasaki, R., Matsumoto, A., Itoh, K., Kawabe, T., Ota, Y., Yamada, K., Maruta, T., Soejima, T. & Sugimura, K. (2000). Target Cells of Apoptosis in the Adult Murine Dentate Gyrus and O4

Immunoreactivity after Ionizing Radiation. *Neuroscience letters*, *279*, 57-60.

[67] Li, Y. Q., Jay, V. & Wong, C. S. (1996). Oligodendrocytes in the Adult Rat Spinal Cord Undergo Radiation-Induced Apoptosis. *Cancer research*, *56*, 5417-5422.

[68] Fu, Z., Zhao, Y., Zhang, K., Wang, J., Zhang, M. & Zhao, X. (2017). Age-Dependent Responses of Brain Myelin Integrity and Behavioral Performance to Radiation in Mice. *Radiation research*, *188*, 585-596.

[69] Vrdoljak, E., Bill, C., Stephens, L., Van Der Kogel, A., Ang, K. K. & Tofilon, P. (1992). Radiation-Induced Apoptosis of Oligodendrocytes *in Vitro*. *International journal of radiation biology*, *62*, 475-480.

[70] Licht, T. & Keshet, E. (2015). The Vascular Niche in Adult Neurogenesis. *Mechanisms of development*, *138*, 56-62.

[71] Shen, Q., Wang, Y., Kokovay, E., Lin, G., Chuang, S. M., Goderie, S. K., Roysam, B. & Temple, S. (2008). Adult Svz Stem Cells Lie in a Vascular Niche: A Quantitative Analysis of Niche Cell-Cell Interactions. *Cell stem cell*, *3*, 289-300.

[72] Karakatsani, A., Shah, B. & Ruiz de Almodovar, C. (2019). Blood Vessels as Regulators of Neural Stem Cell Properties. *Frontiers in molecular neuroscience*, *12*, 85.

[73] Culver, J. C., Vadakkan, T. J. & Dickinson, M. E. (2013). A Specialized Microvascular Domain in the Mouse Neural Stem Cell Niche. *PloS one*, *8*, e53546.

[74] Tavazoie, M., Van der Veken, L., Silva-Vargas, V., Louissaint, M., Colonna, L., Zaidi, B., Garcia-Verdugo, J. M. & Doetsch, F. (2008). A Specialized Vascular Niche for Adult Neural Stem Cells. *Cell stem cell*, *3*, 279-288.

[75] Warrington, J. P., Ashpole, N., Csiszar, A., Lee, Y. W., Ungvari, Z. & Sonntag, W. E. (2013). Whole Brain Radiation-Induced Vascular Cognitive Impairment: Mechanisms and Implications. *Journal of vascular research*, *50*, 445-457.

[76] Grabham, P. & Sharma, P. (2013). The Effects of Radiation on Angiogenesis. *Vascular cell*, *5*, 1-5.

[77] Boström, M., Hellström Erkenstam, N., Kaluza, D., Jakobsson, L., Kalm, M. & Blomgren, K. (2014). The Hippocampal Neurovascular Niche During Normal Development and after Irradiation to the Juvenile Mouse Brain. *International journal of radiation biology*, *90*, 778-789.

[78] Mao, X. W., Favre, C. J., Fike, J. R., Kubinova, L., Anderson, E., Campbell-Beachler, M., Jones, T., Smith, A., Rightnar, S. & Nelson, G. A. (2010). High-Let Radiation-Induced Response of Microvessels in the Hippocampus. *Radiation research*, *173*, 486-493.

[79] Berzaghi, R., Islam, A., Hellevik, T. & Martinez-Zubiaurre, I. (2021). Secretion Rates and Protein Composition of Extracellular Vesicles Released by Cancer-Associated Fibroblasts after Radiation. *Journal of radiation research*, *62*, 401-413.

[80] Rana, S., Kumar, R., Sultana, S. & Sharma, R. K. (2010). Radiation-Induced Biomarkers for the Detection and Assessment of Absorbed Radiation Doses. *Journal of pharmacy and bioallied sciences*, *2*, 189.

[81] Singh, V. K., Newman, V. L., Romaine, P. L., Hauer-Jensen, M. & Pollard, H. B. (2016). Use of Biomarkers for Assessing Radiation Injury and Efficacy of Countermeasures. *Expert review of molecular diagnostics*, *16*, 65-81.

[82] Wong, K., Siu, L., Ainsbury, E. & Moquet, J. (2013). Cytogenetic Biodosimetry: What It Is and How We Do It. *Hong Kong med J*, *19*, 168-173.

[83] Pawar, S. A., Shao, L., Chang, J., Wang, W., Pathak, R., Zhu, X., Wang, J., Hendrickson, H., Boerma, M. & Sterneck, E. (2014). C/Ebpδ Deficiency Sensitizes Mice to Ionizing Radiation-Induced Hematopoietic and Intestinal Injury. *PLoS one*, *9*, e94967.

[84] Burnett, A. F., Biju, P. G., Lui, H. & Hauer-Jensen, M. (2013). Oral Interleukin 11 as a Countermeasure to Lethal Total-Body Irradiation in a Murine Model. *Radiation research*, *180*, 595-602.

[85] Sultana, N., Sun, C., Katsube, T. & Wang, B. (2020). Biomarkers of Brain Damage Induced by Radiotherapy. *Dose-response, 18*, 1559325820938279.

[86] Fernström, E., Minta, K., Andreasson, U., Sandelius, Å., Wasling, P., Brinkmalm, A., Höglund, K., Blennow, K., Nyman, J. & Zetterberg, H. (2018). Cerebrospinal Fluid Markers of Extracellular Matrix Remodelling, Synaptic Plasticity and Neuroinflammation before and after Cranial Radiotherapy. *Journal of internal medicine 284*, 211-225.

[87] Singh, V. K., Santiago, P. T., Simas, M., Garcia, M., Fatanmi, O. O., Wise, S. Y. & Seed, T. M. (2018). Acute Radiation Syndrome: An Update on Biomarkers for Radiation Injury. *Journal of radiation and cancer research*, *9*, 132.

[88] Bertho, J. M., Roy, L., Souidi, M., Benderitter, M., Bey, E., Racine, R., Fagot, T. & Gourmelon, P. (2009). Initial Evaluation and Follow-up of Acute Radiation Syndrome in Two Patients from the Dakar Accident. *Biomarkers*, *14*, 94-102.

[89] Pedersen, N., Lok, E. & Wong, E. (2013). Decreased Cerebrospinal Fluid (Csf) Hypocretin 1 (Orexin a) Levels after Whole Brain Radiotherapy: A Candidate Biomarker for Radiation Encephalopathy (P02. 164). In: Editor, editor^editors. *Book Decreased Cerebrospinal Fluid (Csf) Hypocretin 1 (Orexin a) Levels after Whole Brain Radiotherapy: A Candidate Biomarker for Radiation Encephalopathy (P02. 164)*, AAN Enterprises.

In: The Dentate Gyrus
Editor: Feng-Ru Tang

ISBN: 978-1-68507-212-4

Chapter 5

PRE- AND POST-NATAL IRRADIATION-INDUCED NEUROPATHOLOGY IN THE DENTATE GYRUS

Feng-Ru Tang*, PhD, MD
Radiation Physiology Lab,
Singapore Nuclear Research and Safety Initiative,
National University of Singapore, Singapore

ABSTRACT

As one of the most radiosensitive regions in adult humans and animals, the dentate gyrus (DG) of the hippocampus has attracted intensive attention by radio-neuro-biologists. The effect of cranial or whole-body ionizing irradiation to rodents during prenatal or postnatal period, in particular, the postnatal irradiation has been evaluated extensively by neuropatholgical, molecular biological, neurophysiological and neurobehavioral studies. These animal experimental results suggest that acute or fractionated pre- or post-natal irradiation induces neuronal DNA damage, aging, apoptosis, and neuroinflammation. Irradiation significantly reduces neurogenesis, dendritic spinogenesis and synaptogenesis in DG leading to subsequent

* Corresponding Author's Email: tangfr@gmail.com.

cognitive impairment, depression, aging or other neurological and neuropsychological disorders. Furthermore, irradiation may also induce mature granule cell loss and gliosis in DG. Interestingly, acute irradiation of aged brain with low doses of radiation induces brain hormesis or neurogenesis. At molecular levels, inflammatory cytokines, chemokines, reactive oxygen species, neural growth factors, neurotransmitters, their receptors and signal transduction systems are involved in radiation-induced adverse effect on brain development and functions. Further study on low dose/dose rate radiation-induced epigenetic, non-coding RNA and omics changes may not only unravel the mechanisms of radiation-induced adverse brain effect or hormesis, but also provide clues for detection of radiation exposure and for diagnosis and therapeutic approaches to effectively prevent radiation-induced impairment of neurogenesis and cognition, aging, neurological and neuropsychological disorders. Using modern brain imaging techniques, investigation focusing on radiation-induced changes of critical brain development events and relevant molecules may reveal some novel biomarkers for early, non-invasive diagnosis of radiation-induced DG damage and subsequent disorders.

Keywords: Prenatal, postnatal radiation, dentate gyrus, pathology, cognition, molecular mechanisms

Introduction

In the adult human or animal brain, the dentate gyrus (DG) is one of the most radiosensitive regions due to the neurogenesis in the subgranular zone (SGZ). Radiosensitivity of DG is also dependent on the age, sex, strains and species of animals and cell types. The developing DG is in general more radiosensitive than mature DG due to much more cell divisions and neuronal proliferation in immature animals. The human brain is very radiosensitive in the first two years of age due to rapid brain development (weight reaches to 90-95% adult brain) including synaptogenesis, myelination and changes of neurotransmitter and receptor systems [1, 2]. For the mice, it has been reported that the postnatal day 10 (P10) represents the developmental stage most sensitive to neurotoxic insults including radiation exposure. Brain growth, gliogenesis, axonal and dendrite increase and oligodendrocyte maturation peak at this stage [2, 3]. Our recent studies suggest that P3 mice are more radiosensitive than P10 mice as irradiation at P3 induces much more extensive DNA damage in the entire brain at 1 day after irradiation [4] and significant volume reduction of different brain regions [5]. Therefore, information on the radiation effect on immature DG at different postnatal development stages and on mature or aged DG of the human or animals will be important for 1) estimation of the threshold of radiation dose/dose rate for inducing DG structural and functional abnormality or brain damage, 2) triage of victims after accidental radiation exposure or nuclear terrorism for different radio-neuro-protective treatment, 3) guiding radiotherapists to fine tuning radiation doses/does rates for individual patient in order to effectively treat or control brain tumor or diseases with minimized side effect on DG neurogenesis, Currently, radiation for pediatric brain tumors is usually delivered either to the primary tumor site (involved field) or to the entire craniospinal axis (for tumors with an underlying tendency to metastasize throughout the CNS [6] via external beam radiotherapy [7] according to the American Association of Neuroscience Nurses (AANN) Clinical Practice Guideline Series: Care of the Pediatric Patient with a Brain Tumor [8].

In this chapter, systematical review of animal experimental studies on DG effect of radiation exposure was done at different prenatal and postnatal days of the rodent life. The correlation of the postnatal mouse and human DG development was made in order to fill the knowledge gaps between the animal experimental studies and human research findings. The molecular mechanisms of radiation induced damages were also summarized. In the last part of the paper, we proposed further research directions.

Prenatal Ionizing Radiation-Induced DG Pathological Changes

The major prenatal developmental periods of the rodent include 1) the preimplantation period, i.e., prenatal days 0-5 days for mice, or 0-7 for rats, 2) the organogenesis period, i.e., prenatal days 6-13 for mice, or 8-15 for rats, and 3) the fetal period, i.e., prenatal days14-20 for mice, or 16-22 for rats [9]. Extensive experimental studies indicate that prenatal irradiation at different prenatal developmental periods may induce embryo resorption, death, brain gross malformations, significant reductions of the brain weight, size, cortical hypoplasias, dysplasia, callosal agenesis, and reactive gliosis depending on the animal developmental period, the dose/dose rate and sources of radiation exposure, animal genetic predisposition, and post-irradiation days examined for brain neuropathological changes. The first appearance of the primary radial glial scaffolding used by the early granule cells to migrate to the dentate anlage is at around day 14.5 of pregnancy in mice [10]. So far, few studies have been done to investigate prenatal radiation-induced DG pathological changes in postnatal immature or adult animals (Table 1). The low-dose prenatal radiation with 0.2Gy at an early organogenesis stage, i.e., day 5.5 of pregnancy (before DG genesis) induces impairment of neurogenesis at 3 and 12, but not 6 months of age in male mice. The significant changes in anxiety-like phenotypes, learning, and long-term memory are also observed at 3 and 12, but not 6 months of age, suggesting there is a transient recovery of neurogenesis around 6 months of age. In female mice, no significant difference in neurogenesis and behavioral functions is observed between the irradiated and control mice, suggesting a more radioresistant of DG in female than male mice [11]. During rat organogenesis period (pregnant 8-15 days), irradiation with 0.3Gy or more at day 15 of pregnancy (formation of the first proliferating matrix by DG precursors) induces aberrant mossy fiber terminals in the stratum oriens of the CA1-3 areas of hippocampus (infrapyramidal mossy fibers) [12], and irradiation with 1.5 Gy at day 15 of pregnancy induces disorganizations of DG granule cell layer [13]. During rat fetal period (pregnant 16-22 days), irradiation with 1 Gy at day 17 of pregnancy (formation of the secondary and tertiary proliferating matrix by DG migrating precursors) induces a significant reduction of proliferating cells in the hilus and SGZ, and mature neurons

Table 1. Prenatal ionizing irradiation—induced dentate gyrus (DG) neuropathological and neurobehavioral changes in immature and mature rodents

Animal strains	Radiation source	Age and Dose	Endpoint: (Animal age)	Neuronal or glial reactions and neurobehavioral changes	References
C57BL/6J mice	γ-ray (whole-body)	20 cGy (1.465 Gy/ min) at day 5.5 of pregnancy	3-, 6- and 12-month-old	Impairment of neurogenesis, anxiety-like phenotypes, learning, and long-term memory change at 3 and 12, but not 6 months of age in male mice.	11
Wistar rats	γ-ray (whole-body)	1.0 Gy at day 13, 15, 17 or 19 of pregnancy respectively	8- and 16- day-old	reduced astrocyte proliferation in DG, more obvious when irradiated on E19 than on E13.	15
Wistar rats	X-rays (whole-body)	0.3, 0.6, 1.2 or 1.8 Gy (180 kV), 0.25 Gy/min at day of 15 pregnancy	42-day-old	Aberrant mossy fiber terminals in the stratum oriens of the CA1-3 region (infrapyramidal mossy fibers) in rats exposed to 0.3 Gy or more.	12
Sprague-Dawley rats	X-rays (whole-body)	1.5 Gy (200 kVp, 20 mA) at day 15 of pregnancy	21-day-old	Stronly enhanced manganese-enhanced MRI (MEMRI) signals in the hilus and granular layer of DG, and disorganizations of the DG granule cell layer	13
Wistar rats	γ-ray (whole-body)	1Gy at day 17 of pregnancy	21- or 56-day-old	Significant reduction of proliferating cells in the hilus and subgranular zone, of mature neurons in the hilus and stratum granulosum and impairment of spatial memory	14

in the hilus and granule cell layer [14]. Irradiation with 1 Gy during both organogenesis (day 13 and 15) and fetal (day 17 and 19) periods of pregnancy reduces the intensity of astrocyte proliferation in DG. This reduction of astrocyte intensity is much stronger in brains irradiated on day19 than in those irradiated on day13 of pregnancy [15]. It suggests that astrocytes at the fetal period are more radiosensitive than the organogenesis period. Further study is needed to investigate how irradiation at various DG genesis period, i.e., formations of the first, second and tertiary proliferating matrixes, affects neurogenesis, gliogenesis or angiogenesis differently, why sex affects DG genesis before the formation of the first proliferating matrixes, and astrocytes are more radiosensitive at the late fetal (day 19) than earlier (day 13) pregnant period. Relevant molecular mechanisms are also need to be elucidated.

Postnatal Ionizing Radiation-Induced DG Pathological Changes

Irradiation of Immature Rodent Brain

The radiation effects vary when animals are exposed at different postnatal days due to the differences in DG neurogenesis and gliogenesis (Table 2). Experimental data indicate that at the day of the birth (postnatal day 0 or P0), X-ray irradiation of rats at 2Gy induces extensive DNA fragmentation and cell death (neurons, glial cells, immature cells) in DG hilar neurons and granule cells at 6h after irradiation by in-situ labeling of nuclear DNA fragmentation and Hu and vimentin immunohistochemistry respectively [16]. Gamma ray (γ-ray) irradiation of rat with 6Gy results in reduction of dentate granule cells and mossy fibers in the hilus and the stratum lucidum as early as 12 days after irradiation [17]. Selective irradiation of DG with 15Gy depletes neural stem/progenitor cells in SGZ. Irradiation of subventricular zone (SVZ) with 5, 10, and 15Gy significantly reduces neural stem/progenitor cells in SVZ in a dose-dependent manner, and down-regulates neural stem/progenitor cell associated proteins [18]. At P1, X-ray irradiation of rats with 2Gy increased the number of dying cells in DG granule cell layer and the hilus with the peak value at 6 h after irradiation. However, cell death is not induced in rats irradiated at P15 suggesting reduced radiosensitivity at the late time point of brain development [19]. Fractionated X-ray irradiation of the rat brain from P1 with 2, 4, 6 or 8 doses of 1.5-2 Gy progressively and permanently reduces the number of DG granule cells but not CA1 area of the hippocampus from the control levels by the different dosage schedules, suggesting a regional specific radiosensitivity [20, 21]. There is a marked increase in the specific activity of acetylcholinesterase (AChE) and choline acetyltransferase (CAT). A significantly potentiated spontaneous perseverative turning which is a behavioral correlate of lesions specific to the dentate granule cell layer of the hippocampus confirms neuropathological findings [2]. Fractionated irradiation of the rat brain from P2 to P15 with accumulated doses ranging from 4 to 12.5Gy also induces severe hippocampal granule cell hypoplasia and causes deficits in a memory-based discrimination [22, 23]. Acute irradiation with 5Gy at P3, P10 and P21 induces extensive γ-H2AX foci and apoptosis in the granule cell layer and the hilus of DG at 1 day after irradiation suggesting radiation-induced DNA damage, repairing and granule cell loss. γ-H2AX foci persist at 7, 120 days till 15 months after radiation exposure, these persistent DNA damage foci (PDDF) may be linked to brain aging and shorter life expectancy observed [4]. The brain volume of these animals is reduced significantly when examined with MRI at 13 months after irradiation [5]. Brain development in rodents from P1 to P3 is comparable to 23-32 weeks of gestation (preterm infant) in the human [2]. At this stage, the main developmental changes include predominance of mitotically active pre-oligodendrocytes [24-27], immune system development [28] and establishment of the blood-brain barrier [29-30]. It remains to be investigated whether high or low dose irradiation induces developmental changes in these three systems.

Table 2. Postnatal ionizing radiation–induced neuropathological changes in the dentate gyrus (DG) in immature rodents

Animal strains	Radiation source	Age and Dose	Endpoint: (age or post irradiation time)	Neuronal or glial reactions	References
Sprague-Dawley rats	X-rays	2Gy at P0 (taken as day of birth)	6h	Cell death in the hilus and granule cell layer of DG	16
Wistar rats	γ-rays (head)	6 Gy at P0	From P3 to P60	Reduction of granule cells and mossy fibers in the hilus and the stratum lucidum.	17
Sprague-Dawley rats	X-rays (SGZ)	15Gy at P0 and P28	P2, P30	A complete absence of DG after irradiation at P0, and elimination of BrdU+ proliferating cells in this neurogenic region after irradiation at P28	18
Sprague-Dawley rats	X-rays	2Gy at P1 or P15	3 to 48 h	Dying cells in the hilus and granule cell layer of DG at 6 and 24 h after irradiation	19
Wistar rats	X-rays (head)	2Gy at P1, P2, P3, followed by 1.5Gy at P5, P7, P9, P12, P15	From P23 to P135	Reduction of the developing granular neurons in DG and increased activity of acetylcholinesterase and choline acetyltransferase	20
Rats [Crl: CD(SD)BR]	X-rays (head)	2Gy at P1, 2, 1.5Gy at P5,7,9, 12, 14 and 16, with a total of 13Gy	P133	Significant depletion of dentate granule cells, perseveration in spontaneous exploration of the arms of a T-maze, retarded acquisition of a passive avoidance task, and increased horizontal locomotion	21
Purdue-Wistar rats	X-rays (head)	1.5-2 Gy at P2 with 2, 4, 6 or 8 doses. In 8x group, 2Gy was delivered at P2, P3 followed by 1.5Gy at P5,7,9, 11, 13 and 15. In 6x, 4x, or 2x group, 2Gy, the last exposure at P11, P7, P3 respectively.	P30, P60, P90 and P120 respectively	Progressively and permanently reduced DG granule cells from control levels by the different dosage schedules, i.e., 2x, 59% reduction; 4x, 77%; 6x, 83%; 8x, 84%.	22

Animal strains	Radiation source	Age and Dose	Endpoint: (age or post irradiation time)	Neuronal or glial reactions	References
Spraque-Dawley rats	X-rays	2Gy at P2, P3, 1.5Gy at P5,7,9,11, 13 and 15, with a total of 13Gy	P16-17, P60-65	Severe hippocampal granule cell hypoplasia and deficits in a memory-based discrimination.	23
Balb/c mice	γ-rays (whole body)	5Gy at P3, P10 and P21	24h, 7 and 120 days or 15M	DNA damage, apoptosis 24h after irradiation, reduced neurogenesis, and persistent DNA damage (γH2AX) foci 7, 120 days 15M after irradiation	4, 5
C57 BL /6 mice	X-rays (head)	6Gy at P9	36h and P93	Decreased neurogenesis at 36h and P93 after irradiation. Voluntary running rescued adult hippocampal neurogenesis after irradiation.	31
Wistar rat	X-rays (head)	6Gy at P9	24h or 63 days	A drastic reduction of neurogenesis at 1 day, of neurogenesis and radial glia-like stem cells in DG at 2 months after exposure	32
Rat	X-ray (right head)	16Gy at P7 or P14	2, 3, 6h, and 1, 3, 5 days	Apoptotic cells in DG at 1 day after irradiation	134
Wistar rat	X-rays (head)	6Gy at P9	16h	Reduced production of fibroblast growth factor 2 (Fgf2) from microglia leading to impairment of DG neurogenesis	33
Wistar rats	X-rays (head)	8 Gy at P9, P21	6h, 7days	Activated multiple inflammatory mechanisms 6 h after irradiation. Down-regulation of genes related to neurogenesis and cell cycle, up-regulation of glial fibrillary acidic protein (GFAP), hypertrophy, but not hyperplasia of astrocytes 7 days after irradiation. Loss of microglia in the young brain (P9 and P21).	34, 35
C57BL/6 mice	X-rays (head)	6Gy at P10	P70	Reduced neurogenesis in DG	36

Table 2. (Continued)

Animal strains	Radiation source	Age and Dose	Endpoint: (age or post irradiation time)	Neuronal or glial reactions	References
C57Bl/6J mice	X-rays (whole body or targeted dentate gyrus)	0.25, 0.5, 1 or 2 Gy at P10	P100	At the dose of 1 Gy, but not 2Gy, whole brain or targeted dorsal DG irradiation of P10 mice reduces adult hippocampal neurogenesis. A deficit in memory retrieval is identified after targeted dorsal DG exposure for the dose of 1 Gy, but not for 2 Gy	41
C57BL/6 mice	X-rays (head)	0.1, 2Gy at P10 and P70	1, 7 day(s), 1 and 6 month(s)	An increased GFAP-labelled radial glial-like cells (RGLs), apoptotic cells and decreased $PCNA^+$ cycling progenitors 1 day post-irradiation, increased $PCNA^+$ and $Sox2^+$ cells at 7 days after irradiation, reduced mature granule neurons at 1 and 6 month(s), reduced $PCNA^+$ cells 6 months after irradiation. Increased $Sox2^+$ cells, but decreased $PCNA^+$ cycling progenitor are observed 7 days after irradiation of P10 mice with 0.1Gy	40
C57BL/6J mice	X-rays (head)	8 Gy at P11	6 h or 49 days	Increased apoptosis in neural progenitor cells in SGZ of DG	37
Sprague-Dawley rats	X-rays (head)	6Gy or 12Gy at P10	49 days	Striking reduction of immature neurons after irradiation at 6 Gy, and 12 Gy respectively.	38
NMRI mice	γ-rays (whole body)	20mGy, 100mGy, 500mGy, 1 Gy at P10	P180 or P210	Reduced radial stem cells and progenitor cells after irradiation with 500mGy and 1Gy at P10, a dose-dependent decrease in mature granule cells in DG after irradiation with doses ranging from 100mGy to 1Gy	39
C57BL/6J mice	X-rays (head)	8Gy at P14	6h and 120 days	Reduced neurogenesis in SGZ, more obvious in the female	48

Animal strains	Radiation source	Age and Dose	Endpoint: (age or post irradiation time)	Neuronal or glial reactions	References
C57BL/6J mice	X-rays (head)	8Gy at P14	6h and 120 days	Induced apoptosis in the corpus callosum (CC) and reduced proliferating cells 6 h after irradiation and oligodendrocytes (Olig2(+) cells) 4 months after irradiation	49
C57BL/6J mice	X-rays (head)	8Gy at P14 (lipopolysaccharide was administered 24 h prior to cranial irradiation)	6h and 70 days	Lipopolysaccharide-induced inflammation aggravated irradiation-induced DG neurogenesis and growth	50
Wistar rats	γ-rays (head)	10Gy at P18	1, 2, 4, 8, and 24h	Enhancement of hypothalamic-pituitary-adrenal (HPA) axis activity and increase in relative glucocorticoid receptor / mineralocorticoid receptor ratio in hippocampus.	51
BALB/c	X-ray (whole body)	2Gy or 0.2Gyx10 at P21	P180	Impairment of cell proliferation and neurogenesis	52
BALB/c	γ-rays (whole body)	5Gy or 0.5Gyx10 at P26	90 days	Impairment of cell proliferation and neurogenesis	53
C57 BL/ 6J mice	X-rays (head)	3Gy or 10Gy at P28	140 days	Decreased neurogenesis	54
Sprague-Dawley rats	X-rays (head)	0.3Gy, 3Gy and 10Gy at preadolescent (P21), adolescent (P50), and postadolescent (P70)	90 days	Decreased neurogenesis in a dose-dependent pattern ranging from 0.3Gy to 10Gy	55
Sprague-Dawley rats	X-rays (head)	20Gy at P30	60 days	Impairment of DG neurogenesis	66

Irradiation with doses ranging from 100mGy to 12Gy at P9 or P10 significantly reduces hippocampal neurogenesis examined from 1 day to more than 3 months after irradiation [31-38]. Microglial cells exhibit decreased gene expression of growth factors involved in stem cell maintenance for a long period of time (9 weeks) after irradiation, which may be related to decreased neurogenesis in the hippocampus. Neurogenesis in the subventricular zone recovers with time [33]. At P9, irradiation with 8 Gy activates multiple inflammatory mechanisms in the acute phase 6 h after irradiation. In the subacute phase of 7 days after irradiation, genes related to neurogenesis and cell cycle are down-regulated, but glial fibrillary acidic protein (GFAP) is up-regulated. Hypertrophy, but not hyperplasia, of astrocytes occurs [32]. Loss of microglia in the brain (irradiated at P9 or P21) is also observed 7 days after irradiation [35]. At P10, which is assumed to represent the developmental stage most sensitive to neurotoxic insults [3], irradiation of mice with 6 Gy reduces animal body weight, hippocampal neurogenesis and impairs place learning. Irradiation with 500mGy and 1Gy also reduces cognitive performance 2 or 4 months and radial glia-like stem cells and progenitor cells 6 months after radiation exposure. The number of mature granule cells and of proliferating cells in the subgranular layer of DG is decreased after irradiation at a low dose of 100mGy [39]. Irradiation with 0.1Gy at P10 also reduces mitochondrial electron transport chain (ETC) complexes I 7 and 6 months after radiation exposure, depletes the proliferative compartment in the mouse DG at 6 months after irradiation [40]. Interestingly, whole brain or targeted dorsal DG irradiation of P10 mice with doses of 0.25, 0.5, 1 and 2Gy induces very different effects on DG neurogenesis and neurobehavioral changes. At the dose of 1Gy, but not 2Gy, whole brain or targeted dorsal DG irradiation of P10 mice reduces adult hippocampal neurogenesis. A deficit in memory retrieval is identified after targeted dorsal DG exposure for the dose of 1Gy, but not for 2Gy [41]. Brain development in rodents from P7 to P10 is comparable to 36-40 weeks of gestation (preterm infant) in the human [2]. During this period, there are peak brain growth spurt [42, 43] and gliogenesis [44, 45], increasing axonal and dendritic density [46, 47], pre-dominance of immature oligodendrocytes [24, 26, 27] and consolidation of the immune system [28]. Further study on radiation-induced axo- and dendro-architectonic changes of neurons, cytoarchitectonic changes of oligodendrocytes and astrocytes may unravel many previously unknown brain pathological changes.

From P11 to P14, while few studies have been done to evaluate low dose irradiation –induced brain pathological changes, high dose irradiation has been clearly shown to induce neuronal apoptosis and impairment of neurogenesis in SGZ of DG [27, 48]. Induced apoptosis, reduced proliferating cells 6 h after irradiation and oligodendrocytes (Olig2(+) cells) 4 months after irradiation are also observed in the corpus callosum (CC) [49]. Interestingly, reduced neurogenesis in SGZ and white matter is more obvious in the female than male at P14 [48, 49], suggesting a sex difference in reaction to irradiation. Lipopolysaccharide-induced inflammation aggravated injury of irradiation-induced hippocampal neurogenesis and the growth of DG, suggesting that brain inflammation exacerbates radiation-induced impairment of neurogenesis [50]. High dose irradiation with 10Gy during preadolescence (P18) enhances rat hypothalamic-pituitary-adrenal (HPA) axis activity and increased relative glucocorticoid receptor/mineralocorticoid receptor ratio in hippocampus [51]. At P21, X-ray irradiation with 2Gy induces impairment of DG neurogenesis although no cognitive impairment is demonstrated [52]. At P26, γ-ray irradiation with 5Gy induces not only impairment of DG neurogenesis, but also deficits in learning and memory in the contextual fear conditioning test. The memory for novel object recognition is also impaired [53]. During adolescence (P28), irradiation reduces postnatal neurogenesis and induces cognitive deficits and decreased locomotor activity in adulthood [54]. Decreased neurogenesis and impairment of associative memories occur at 3 months after irradiation at P21 (preadolescent), P50 (adolescent), and P70 (postadolescent). These changes are in a dose-dependent pattern ranging from 0.3Gy to 10Gy [55]. Brain development in rodents from P20 to P21 is comparable to 2-3-year-old children [2]. During this period, rapid brain development, synaptogenesis, myelination and changes of neuro-transmitter and receptor systems occur [2]. Systematical studies of the short and long-term effect of irradiation with a gradient low radiation dose/dose rate at early postnatal stages on neurological and neuropsychological changes in aged animals will undoubtedly shed light on better understanding the lifetime effect of radiation exposure in the early human life, especially neurological and neuropsychological disorders in the aged population.

Irradiation of Adult Rodent Brain

In adult rodent brain, acute or fractionated radiation exposures reduce DG neurogenesis [56-69] (Table 3). Radiation-induced cell death goes through apoptosis [59]. The impairment of neurogenesis is accompanied by marked alterations in the neurogenic microenvironment, including disruption of the microvascular angiogenesis and markedly increased activated microglia within the neurogenic zone. However, the production of new astrocytes or oligodendrocytes is not affected significantly [57, 59]. In the survival neurons, the number of dendritic branching, length, and area of the granule cells in DG are reduced. Significant reductions in synaptophysin expression at presynaptic sites in the hilus of DG and increases in postsynaptic density protein (PSD-95) along dendrites in the granule cell and molecular layers are observed [66].While irradiation at doses as low as 0.3Gy [55] or the radioadaptive dosing paradigm of 0.1Gy followed by 2Gy [69] reduces DG neurogenesis, irradiation with 0.3Gy to 1-year-old mice promotes hippocampal neurogenesis which is indicated by increased proliferation and neuronal differentiation of neural stem cells, cell survival, and reduced apoptotic death of neuronal stem cells [70]. It suggests that low dose irradiation of 1-year-old mice may induce brain hormesis or neurogenesis. This is supported by therapeutic approach using low to moderate doses of irradiation to control or treat aging related neurodegenerative diseases in Drosophila [71] and mouse [72-75] models and patients [76-79] with Alzheimer's disease (AD). The low-dose radiation therapy (LD-RT) may modulate amyloid load and neuroinflammation in AD, suppresses Aβ42-induced cell death through regulation of the protein kinase B (PKB, or AKT) and p38 mitogen-activated protein kinase (MAPK) signaling pathways, thus improve DG neurogenesis and in turn partially restored patient's cognition, memory, speech, movement, and appetite. With fractionated doses of 5Gy x4, increased neurodegenerative neurons in DG and CA1 subfield are observed at 30 and 100 days after irradiation. Decreased GFAP-immunoreactive astrocytes are only demonstrated at 100 days after irradiation [73]. Given current view that microglia and astrocytes are involved in learning and memory [80-82], it is concluded that radiation-induced loss of neurons, reduced number of dendritic branching, length, and area of the granule cells, astrocytes and microglial changes may result in learning and memory impairment. Interestingly, out-of-target irradiation (i.e., irradiation of the lower third of the mouse body, whilst the upper two thirds are shielded) also induces impairment of DG neurogenesis, so called abscopal effects [83].

Chronic low doses of galactic cosmic space radiation which contains highly charged, high-energy (HZE) particle such as ^{56}Fe beam also decreases hippocampal DG neurogenesis and disrupts hippocampal function in young adult rodents, raising the possibility of impaired astronaut cognition and risk of mission failure. ^{56}Fe beam irradiation with 2.0 Gy reduces the population of immature and proliferating neurons in DG and impairs the spatial memory of mice at later intervals [84] (Table 3). Acute ^{56}Fe beam exposure or five fractionated 20 cGy ^{56}Fe -particle exposure reduces adult-generated hippocampal neurons and stem cells 24 h or 3 months after irradiation [85]. Whole-body ^{28}Si-particle-iradiation with 0, 0.2 and 1 Gy of P69 C57BL/6J and Nestin-GFP mice induces dose-dependent reduction in DG cell proliferation and immature neurons at 24h after irradiation. ^{28}Si-radiation exposure damages neurogenesis, but to a lesser extent than ^{56}Fe beam radiation and that low-dose ^{28}Si exposure induces abnormalities in hippocampal function, disrupting fear memory but also inducing anxiety-like behavior.

Table 3. Postnatal ionizing radiation–induced neuropathological changes of the dentate gyrus in adult rodents

Animal strains	Radiation source	Age and Dose	Endpoint: (age or post irradiation time)	Neuronal or glial reactions	References
Fisher 344 rats	X-rays (head)	1Gy to 30Gy at P56 to P70	3h to 120 days	Apoptosis increases rapidly with radiation dose by 3-6h after irradiation, reaching a plateau with 3Gy, neurogenesis in SGZ decreases at 120 days after irradiation with ≥ 5Gy	56
Fisher 344 rats	X-rays (head)	2Gy or 10Gy on adult rats	60 days	A high dose irradiation at 10Gy induces significant depletion of dentate granule cells and alterations in the neurogenic microenvironment. The remaining neural precursors adopt glial fates.	57
Wistar rats	X-rays (hippocampus)	Fractionated 3Gy x 4 repeated 3 days later, with a total of 24Gy at P60	≥26 days	Fractionated irradiation prevents hippocampal neurogenesis, leading to poorer hippocampus-dependent place-recognition compared to the control.	58
C57BL/J6 mice	X-rays (head)	2, 5, or 10 Gy at P60	6 to 48h, and 60 days	Apoptosis peaks 12 h after irradiation. Proliferating SGZ cells are reduced by 93-96%; immature neurons are decreased from 40 to 60% in a dose-dependent pattern at 48h after irradiation. Impairment of neurogenesis also occurs at 2 months after irradiation	59
Sprague-Dawley rats	^{56}Fe -particles	2.5Gy at P60	30 days	Reduced granule cell proliferation and migration	60
Mongolian Gerbils	X-rays (head)	5Gy, 10 Gy or 5x2 Gy at P60	1, 2, 4, 8, 14, 30, 120, 270 days	Significant decline in the granule cell population 9 months later.	61

Animal strains	Radiation source	Age and Dose	Endpoint: (age or post irradiation time)	Neuronal or glial reactions	References
C57BL mice	Single, ^{56}Fe whole-body	2.0 Gy (0.88Gy/min) of 500 MeV/nucleon at 56 days	60 days	Impairment of neurogenesis and cell proliferation in DG	84
ICR mice	γ-rays (whole body)	500mGy, 2Gy, 4Gy at P60	6, 12, 24h, 3, 7, 14 days	Apoptosis in DG increases 6-12 h after irradiation at doses of 500mGy, 2 or 4 Gy. The number of Ki-67- and DCX-positive cells begins to decrease significantly 6 h postirradiation, reaching its lowest level 24 h after irradiation. The decrease is in a dose-dependent manner (0-4 Gy).	62
C57BL/6 mice	γ-rays (whole body)	5Gy, 1Gyx5, 0.5Gy x10 at P60	P180	Reduction of neurogenesis after both acute and fractionated radiation exposure, with more in acute than fractionated exposure.	63
Kunming mice	X-rays (head)	300mGy or 3Gy at the age of 12-month-old	7, 14 or 28 days	Low dose radiation (0.3Gy) increases neural stem cell proliferation neuronal differentiation, and neurogenesis, promots cell survival and reduces apoptotic death of neuronal stem cells	70
Thy1-EGFP transgene mice	γ-rays (head)	1Gy or 10Gy at P60	10 or 30 days	Significant reduction in the number of dendritic branching, length, and area of the granule cells in DG which is dose-responsive. There are also significant reductions in synaptophysin expression at presynaptic sites in the hilus, and significant increases in postsynaptic density protein (PSD-95) along dendrites in the granule cell and molecular layers.	65
Nestin-CreER^{T2}/R26R-YFP mice	^{56}Fe (whole-body)	Single (100cGy) or fractionated (20cGy x 5) at P64-P86.	24 h or 90 days	^{56}Fe -particle exposure reduces adult-generated DG neurons and stem cells	85

Table 3. (Continued)

Animal strains	Radiation source	Age and Dose	Endpoint: (age or post irradiation time)	Neuronal or glial reactions	References
C57BL/6 mice	γ-rays	100mGy, 2 Gy and 100 mGy + 2Gy at P60	30 days	Significant reductions (20–50%) in the number of newly generated cells 1 month after irradiation, an effect that is relatively dose-independent	69
Wistar rats	γ-rays (whole body)	5Gy x 4 at P210-P240	30 and 100 days	A significant increase of Fluoro-Jade C labelled degenerating neurons in DG	64
Nestin-GFP (NGFP) male	Single, ^{28}Si whole-body	1 Gy or 0.2 Gy (300 MeV/n, LET 67 KeV/μ) at a dose rate of 1.0 Gy/min at P69	24 h or 90 days	Dose-dependent reduction in DG cell proliferation and immature neurons at 24h after irradiation, and decreased survival of new neurons at 90 days male groups but not females	86
C57Bl/6J mice	Single, ^{56}Fe whole-body	10, 50, or 100 cGy, 10 cGy/min (600 MeV, 181 keV/μm) at 3-month-old	60 and 365 days	Impairment of neurogenesis at 2 months after irradiation, but a dramatic rebound 12 months after irradiation	88
Gottingen minipigs	γ-rays (^{60}Co)	1.79Gy, 0.485–0.502 Gy/min at 6.0 to 6.5-month-old	33–35 days	Initial astroglial reaction in the peri-dentate gyrus (peri-DG) area as assessed by HE staining and GFAP immunostaining	89
Thy1-EGFP transgene mice	^{4}He particles	0.3Gy of 400 MeV/n, 0.15–0.25 Gy/min) at 6-month-old	49-56 days	Significantly increased immunoreactivity of an activated microglial marker CD68, no changes in DG dendritic area and length	90

Furthermore, exposure to ^{28}Si decreases new neuron survival in long-term male groups but not females suggests that sex may be an important factor when performing brain health risk assessment for astronauts traveling in space [86]. Mice exposed to 100 cGy ^{12}C irradiation have a transient decrease (24 h after radiation) in the number of proliferating cells and immature neurons in DG, but restoration of proliferation and immature neurons occurs at 3 months post-^{12}C irradiation [87]. While ^{56}F beam irradiation with 10, 50, or 100 cGy, 10 cGy/min at 3-month-old induces impairment of neurogenesis, synaptic plasticity and learning at 2 months after irradiation, the deficit in spatial learning is absent at 6 months in irradiated mice, and synaptic potentiation is enhanced. Enhanced performance in spatial learning and facilitation of synaptic plasticity in irradiated mice persist 12 months postexposure, concomitant with a dramatic rebound in adult-born neurons [88]. In 6- to 6.5-month-old minipig model, acute irradiation with 1.79Gy induces initial astroglial reaction in the peri-dentate gyrus (peri-DG) area as assessed by hematoxylin and eosin (H&E) staining and GFAP immunostaining, but no pathological accumulation of insoluble intra- (e.g., phosphorylated-Tau or pTau neurofbrillary tangles-like lesions) or extra-cellular proteins (e.g., amyloid precursor protein or APP-positive lesions) [89]. ^{4}He particles irradiation (with 0.3Gy) of mice at 6-month-old significantly increases immunoreactivity of an activated microglial marker CD68, but no change in DG dendritic area and length is found [90]. Current studies suggest that different HZE particles may produce varied harmful effects, and low doses of HZE particles may affect brain neurogenesis and induce cognitive impairment. Further study with chronic exposure with combined different low dose HZE particles may provide more evidence to evaluate risk of deep space travel to astronaut brain neurogenesis and cognition.

RADIATION-INDUCED DG INFLAMMATION

Neuroinflammatory responses after clinical radiotherapy and radiosurgery have been well documented to be involved in brain injury, radiation somnolence syndrome, cognitive impairment and aging [27, 34, 35, 37, 91-102]. Radiotherapy may cause direct damage to endothelial and glial cells, particularly oligodendrocytes leading to vascular hyalinization and demyelination and subsequent brain inflammation, ischemia, and delayed radiation necrosis. Kalm et al. (2009) found transient activation of C–C motif chemokine ligand 2 (CCL2), growth-regulated oncogenes (GRO)/keratinocyte chemoattractant (KC) and IL-1alpha in the acute phase (6 h) after irradiation of P9 mice with 8Gy and activation of astrocytes in the subacute phase (7 days) after irradiation. Many cytokines such as interleukin (IL)-1α, IL-6, tumor necrosis factor (TNF)-α and chemokine networks, like the C-X-C motif chemokine ligand 12 (CXCL12)/C-X-C motif chemokine receptor 4 (CXCR4) axis, are up-regulated in the perinecrotic area [103, 104] (Table 4). Animal experimental study indicates that irradiation of immature mouse brain (P9) activates multiple inflammatory mechanisms such as up-regulation of CCL2, Gro/KC and IL-1-α at the acute stage 6 h after radiation exposure. CCL2 is expressed in astrocytes and microglia in DG and SVZ. Increased number and size of microglia with engulfment of cell debris is also observed [34, 35, 37]. Up-regulation of CCL2/monocyte chemoattractant protein-1 (MCP-1) after irradiation of the mouse hippocampus and prevention of reduced neurogenesis after deletion of CCL2 suggest that it may be a potential therapeutic target for prevention of impairment of neurogenesis and cognition following cranial radiation [69, 105]. Irradiation of immature mice also induces altered expression of numerous extracellular matrix (ECM)-related and coagulation-related genes for at least 1 month following irradiation. The changes are detectable within 24 h following cranial irradiation [106]. In young mature mice, irradiation also increases brain expression of proinflammatory molecules such as TNF-α, IL-β, intercellular adhesion molecule-1 (ICAM-1), α1-antichymotrypsin, IL-lα and GFAP mRNA as early as 2h after the exposure [107]. Increase in total activated microglia per hippocampus in both the granule cell layer and the hilus at 2 months after irradiation with 10Gy suggests a dramatic chronic inflammatory response in the adult brain [51]. This is supported by increases in the levels of nuclear factor kappa B (NF-κB) and GFAP 75 days after low dose radiation exposure ranging from 50 mGy to 1 Gy [108]. While comparative study indicates that irradiation induces more proinflammatory response in adult brain than the juvenile [109], there is a significant age-dependent decrease in proinflammatory response from 4 to 24 h after irradiation of rats at the age of 4, 16, and 24 months, thereby suggesting the suppression of pro-inflammatory responses in aged animals [110].

Radiation-induced proinflammatory response is regionally specific [111]. For instance, TNF-α levels are significantly elevated in cortex compared to hippocampus, whereas IL-1β levels are elevated in hippocampus compared to cortical samples. Irradiation effect on microglia is also heterogeneous between white and gray matter and among regions of gray matter, indicating that there are regional regulators of the neural response to brain irradiation. The CA3 region of the hippocampus appears to be differentially sensitive to effects of aging and irradiation [112]. Therefore, radiation-induced inflammatory responses may be related not only to animal ages, species or strains, but also to brain regions and radiation doses. Proinflammatory response may lead to significant reductions in neurogenesis as inflammatory blockade restores hippocampal neurogenesis and impairment of cognition [113]. Pre-treatment of adult C57BL/6 with Fingolimod (FTY720), inhibits microglia activation 24 h after X-ray exposure in DG, while astrocyte activation is unaffected and no lymphocyte infiltrations are found. It protects radiation-induced damage of neuronal precursor cells [114]. Carbon monoxide releasing molecule-3 could effectively improve the inflammatory response induced by activation of the microglia, reduce neuronal apoptosis, promote neural regeneration, and improve the learning and memory performance of mice after radiation [115].

Table 4. Postnatal ionizing radiation-induced inflammation in the hippocampus

Animal strains	Radiation source	Age and Dose	Endpoint: (age or Post irradiation time)	Parameter or biomarker changes	References
NMRI mice	γ-rays (whole body)	20mGy, 100mGy, 500mGy, 1 Gy at P10	P180 or P210	Astrogliosis, activation of insulin-growth factor/insulin signalling and increased level of microglial cytokine tumor necrosis factor-α (TNFα)	39
C3Hf/Sed/Kam mice	X-rays (midbrain)	2, 7, 12, 17, 25Gy at P58-P70	15min, 30 min, 1, 2, 4, 8, 18, 24 h.	Increased TNF-α, IL-β, ICAM-1, α1-antichymotrypsin, and to a lesser extent IL-lα and GFAP mRNA	105
Sprague-Dawley rats	^{16}O-particle	50, 500 mGy and 1Gy at P60	36 h or 75 days	The loss of autophagy function shortly after exposure and increased nuclear factor kappa B (NF-κB) and GFAP 75 days after exposure.	106
CCL2−/− and BALB/c	X-rays (head)	10 Gy at P60-P90	7, 30, 60 days	Absence of CCL2 signalling after irradiation allows partial recovery of neurogenesis in the second month after irradiation.	107
C57BL/6 and Balb/c mice	X-rays (head)	X-rays (head)	24h and 30 days	Persistent proinflammatory profile of microglia for at least 1 month following irradiation, with altered expression of numerous extracellular matrix (ECM)-related and coagulation-related genes. The microglia transcriptome changes are similar to those in aging.	108
Wistar rats	X-rays (head)	6Gy at P9 and P180	6h, 7, 28 days	More proinflammatory response in adult brain than the juvenile	109

Animal strains	Radiation source	Age and Dose	Endpoint: (age or Post irradiation time)	Parameter or biomarker changes	References
F344xBN rats	γ-rays (head)	10Gy at the age of 4-, 16-, and 24- month-old	4, 8, and 24h	A significant age-dependent decrease in TNF-α expression at 8 and 24h after irradiation and a similar age-related attenuation in IL-1beta, ICAM-1, VCAM-1, monocyte chemoattractant protein-1 (MCP-1) and MMP-9 expression 4 and 8h post-irradiation.	110
F344xBN rats	γ-rays (head)	10Gy at the age of 4- month-old	4, 8, and 24h	Irradiation induces regionally specific pro-inflammatory environments through activation of AP-1, NF-κB, cAMP-response element binding protein (CREB) and over expression of TNF-α, IL-1β, and MCP-1 in rat brain and may contribute to unique pathways for the radiation-induced impairments in tissue function.	111
Fischer 344 x Brown Norway F1 hybrid rat	γ-rays (head)	10Gy at 8-, 18- or 28- month-old	7 or 70 days	Irradiation induces heterogeneous microglia responses between white- and gray-matter and among regions of gray matter such as CA3 and CA1 areas. Gray matter and CA3 area show a greater response than white matter and CA1 area respectively.	112

Nuclear factor kappa-light-chain-enhancer of activated B (NF-κB) expression increased in whole and nuclear fractions 4 hours after cranial radiation therapy (CRT), inhibition of NF-κB activation using an NF-κB essential modulator binding domain (NBD) peptide mitigates CRT-induced neuroinflammation and improves behavioral outcomes [116]. Selective autophagy related 7 (Atg7) knockout (KO) reduced the number of radiation-induced activated microglia, preventing radiotherapy-induced neural stem and progenitor cell death and its associated long-term side effects [117]. Further study is needed to evaluate the long-term effect of low dose/dose rate radiation-induced brain inflammatory responses and damage.

Radiation-Induced Cognitive Deficits

Radiation-induced DG neuropathological changes may result in cognitive impairment in the human or animals (Table 5). Clinical data have indicated the involvement of neuroinflammatory responses in brain injury, radiation somnolence syndrome, cognitive impairment and aging [98-102, 118-120]. Extensive animal experimental data support clinical findings. Acute exposure to a single intermediate dose of ionizing radiation to P3, P10 or P19 mice causes functional defects at adult age in mice exposed to the two earlier time points (P3 and P10) while no neurobehavioral alteration is observed in those exposed at P19. Furthermore, the effect on those exposed at P10 is dose-response related and to be long-lasting or persistent as these significant defects are evident in both 2- and 4-month-old mice [121]. Acute irradiation (at radiation doses ranging from 1 to 20Gy) of immature mice at P10 [36], P12 [37], P14 [48], P 21 [122], P30 [69] induces hippocampus-dependent memory deficit and increased anxiety levels when animals are tested at mature age. Interestingly, increased anxiety levels are more severe in female than male, and impairment of place learning occurs in female but not male [48]. In amyloid precursor protein (APP) 23 transgenic mice, acute irradiation with 1, 2, 4 Gy at the age of P35 accelerates Alzheimer's disease-related neurological deficits [123]. Acute (at dose of ≥2Gy) [63] or fractionated (a total of 20 to 45Gy) [59, 118, 124-126] irradiation of young or aging adult rodents also induces significant memory deficits. ^{56}Fe irradiation impacts hippocampus-dependent contextual freezing 3 months following irradiation. The upper blade blade might be more important for contextual freezing and the lower blade for cued freezing [127].

Molecular Mechanism of Radiation-Induced DG Pathophysiological Changes and Cognitive Impairment

Oxidative stress is one of the major mechanisms implicated in radiation-induced hippocampal pathophysiological changes as reactive oxygen species (ROS) increase significantly after irradiation which may damage DG neurons and prevent neurogenesis. The use of the antioxidant such as lipoic acid (LA) or N-acetylcysteine (NAC) is able to reduce ROS levels which in turn to effectively prevent radiation-induced oxidative neuronal loss and promote DG functional recovery [128-133]. Both acute and chronic inflammatory responses are involved in pathophysiological changes of DG and cognition impairment (Table 3). This is further supported by evidence showing the protective effect of anti-inflammatory treatment such as anti-TNF on the brain's microvascular network, or deletion of CCR2 on hippocampal neurogenesis [64, 82, 132]. Changes of signaling pathways related to synaptic actin remodeling such as the Rac1-Cofilin, Rac1 and LIMK1, and synaptic proteins MAP-2 and PSD-95after neonatal radiation exposure with 1Gy result in abnormal synaptic plasticity leading to cognitive impairment [37]. Down-regulation of phosphorylated cAMP-response element binding protein (CREB) and brain-derived neurotrophic factor (BDNF) protein levels, and the levels of mRNAs encoding common BDNF transcripts, and exons IIC, III, IV, VII, VIII, and IXA in the hippocampus may also be associated with synaptogenesis and subsequent memory deficits after cranial irradiation [106].

Table 5. Postnatal ionizing radiation-induced cognitive deficits

Animal strains	Radiation source	Age and Dose	Endpoint: (age or post irradiation time)	Neurobehavioral changes	References
Naval Medical Research Institute (NMRI) and C57bl/6 mice	γ-rays (whole body)	0.02, 0.1, 0.5 and 1Gy at P3, P10 or P19	P60 and P120	Altered adult spontaneous behavior and impaired habituation atrer irradiation with 0.5 or 1Gy, but not 0.020 or 0.1Gy on P10 mice	121
C57Bl/6J mice	X-rays (whole body or targeted dentate gyrus)	0.25, 0.5, 1 or 2 Gy at P10	P100	Deficit in memory retrieval after targeted dorsal DG exposure with 1 Gy, but not for 2 Gy.	41
C57BL/J6 mice	X-rays (head)	2, 5, 10Gy at P21	48h, 30, 90day	Hippocampal-dependent memory deficits	122
BALB/c	γ-rays (whole body)	5Gy or 0.5Gyx10 at P26	90 days	Deficits in learning and memory in the contextual fear conditioning test, Impairment of memory for novel object recognition	53
C57BL/J6 mice	γ-rays (head)	4Gy x 5	1 and 5 month(s)	Persistent and progressive hippocampus-dependent learning deficits	118
Sprague-Dawley rats	X-rays (head)	20Gy at P30	60 days	Cognitive deficits	66
NMRI mice	γ-rays (whole body)	20mGy, 100mGy, 500mGy, 1 Gy at P10	P180 or P210	Significant alterations in spontaneous behaviour at 2 and 4 months following a single 0.5 or 1.0 Gy exposure.	39
Amyloid precursor protein (APP) transgenic mice	^{56}Fe-particle	1, 2, 4 Gy at P35	7, 28, 49, 84, 112-154 days	Acceleration of Alzheimer's disease-related neurological deficits	123
Fischer 344 x Brown Norway rats	X-rays (head)	40 Gy, 8 fractions over 4 weeks, at the age of 12-month-old	26-30- month-old	Impairments in the reversal Morris water maze performance, in spatial learning and memory	124

Animal strains	Radiation source	Age and Dose	Endpoint: (age or post irradiation time)	Neurobehavioral changes	References
C57BL/6 mice	γ-rays (head)	36Gy (4.5Gy/fraction, 2x/wk for 4wk) at P77-P84	90 days	A transient deficit in contextual learning, disruption of working memory, and progressive impairment of spatial learning which is completely reversed by systemic hypoxia	137
C57Bl6/J mice	^{56}Fe (whole body)	600 MeV, 0.5 or 1 Gy at P 56	30min after cognitive test from 3 months after irradiation	Changes in hippocampus-dependent contextual freezing and the percentage of Arc-positive cells in the upper and lower blades of granule cell layer 3 months following irradiation.	129
C57BL/6 mice	γ-rays (head)	1 and 10Gy at P56	30 and 90 days after irradiation	Significant depression-like behaviors after irradiation at 10Gy	67
C57Bl/6J mice	Single, ^{56}Fe whole-body	10, 50, or 100 cGy, 10 cGy/min (600 MeV, 181 keV/μm) at 3-month-old	60 and 365 days	Impairment of learning at 2 months after irradiation, By six months, no defcits in spatial learning, synaptic potentiation and spatial learning are enhanced which persists 12 months after irradiation	88
C57BL mice	Single, ^{56}Fe whole-body	2.0 Gy (0.88Gy/ min) 500 MeV/ nucleon at 56 days	60 days	Impaired spatial memory	84

Radiation-induced increased oxidative stress, neuroinflammation and loss of autophagy by significant inhibition of autophagy function in the hippocampus as measured by accumulation of ubiquitin inclusion bodies such as P62/SQSTM1, autophagosome marker microtubule-associated protein 1 beta light chain 3 (MAP1B-LC3), beclin1 and proteins such as mammalian target of rapamycin (mTOR) may be involved in the aging process [85]. The delay of myelination may be related to radiation-induced apoptosis and depletion of oligodendrocytes [134]. Irradiation increases the expression of metabotrophic glutamate receptor 1, and triggers the altered neuronal differentiation in undifferentiated neural stem cells or stem-like cells through PI3K-STAT3-mGluR1 and PI3K-p53 signaling in the mouse primary neural stem cells and C17.2 mouse neural stem-like cells, suggesting that the altered neuronal differentiation may be related to the impairment of DG neurogenesis and cognition [135]. Activation of cytokines has been associated with abscopal (or out-of-target) radiation effect and macrophage activation, followed by a storm of cytokines including IL-1a, IL-1b, IL-6, TNF-α and TGF-β, accompanied the induction of abscopal radiation effects [136-138]. The out-of-target radiation effect may also be related to the alterations in diacylglycerol (DAG)/Inositol trisphosphate/calcium (IP3) and tumor growth factor (TGF-β) signaling pathways as well as in the expression of proteins involved in the regulation of long-term neuronal synaptic plasticity and synapse organization [83]. On the other hand, low dose irradiation-induced increased neurogenesis or hormesis may be related to increment of Wnt1, Wnt3a, Wnt5a, and β-catenin expression in neural stem cells [70].

FUTURE RESEARCH DIRECTIONS

Animal experimental data indicates that ionizing radiation induces impairment of hippocampal neurogenesis, neuronal loss, abnormal gliogenesis, neuroinflammatory responses, capillary loss or microvascular rarefaction, and subsequent cognitive impairment and aging. The molecular response of the mouse brain within a few hours after low-dose irradiation (100mGy) may involve molecular networks and pathways associated with cognitive functions, advanced aging, Alzheimer's disease and diverse neuropsychiatric disorders. Irradiation-induced changes are age, sex, cell, animal strain/species, radiation component, dose/dose rate, and endpoint specific. Further studies in the following areas are still needed: 1) differentiation of the effect of radiation exposure before or during the formation of first, secondary and tertiary DG proliferative matrixes, for instance, why irradiation before generation of DG progenitor cells, i.e., during the organogenesis period of pregnancy affects only neurogenesis but not gliogenesis or angiogenesis in DG; 2) evaluation of long-term effect of low dose (≤100mGy)/dose rate (≤6mGy/h) irradiation on hippocampal neurogenesis, gliogenesis, endotheliogenesis, inflammation, neural plasticity, and subsequent cognitive impairment and aging. Using modern sophisticated technology to study cyto-, axo- and dendro-architectonic changes of neurons, neural plasticity, reactive responses of microglia, astrocytes, and oligodendrocytes, many previously unknown brain pathological changes may be unraveled; 3) establishment of the relationships among irradiation, changes of hippocampal ion channels and gap junction proteins, cognition and aging as it has been known that hippocampal ion channels and gap junction proteins are required for proper hippocampal neurogenesis and cognitive functions; 4) investigation of low and high dose/dose rate irradiation-induced changes of different omics and non-coding RNA (ncRNA) in the hippocampus and blood. Results from these studies may not only provide clues for detection or diagnosis of radiation exposures, but also shed light on understanding the mechanism of radiation-induced biopositive and bionegetive effect; non-invasive monitoring blood omics and non-coding RNA (ncRNA) levels or brain imaging at different stages of animal life, and correlation of their changes to brain pathological or animal behavioral changes will undoubtedly shed light on development of bio- or image-markers for diagnosis of neurological and neuropsychological disorders at early stages after radiation exposures; 5) Revelation of radiation-induced changes of critical brain development events in the early life of the animals. Changes of critical brain development events after irradiation may cause fundamental hippocampal functional changes leading to cognitive impairment and aging which may affect the quality of the rest of human life.

ACKNOWLEDGMENT

This work was sponsored by the National Research Foundation of Singapore.

REFERENCES

[1] Padovani, L., André, N., Constine, L. S., Muracciole, X. 2012. Neurocognitive function after radiotherapy for paediatric brain tumours. *Nat. Rev. Neurol.* 8, 578-88.

[2] Semple, B. D., Blomgren, K., Gimlin, K., Ferriero, D. M., Noble-Haeusslein, L. J. 2013. Brain development in rodents and humans: Identifying benchmarks of maturation and vulnerability to injury across species. *Prog. Neurobiol.* 106-107, 1-16.

[3] Eriksson, P. 1997. Developmental neurotoxicity of environmental agents in the neonate. *NeuroToxicology*. 18, 719–26.

[4] Tang, F. R., Liu, L., Wang, H., Ho, K. J. N., Sethi, G. 2021. Spatiotemporal dynamics of γH2AX in the mouse brain after acute irradiation at different postnatal days with special reference to the dentate gyrus of the hippocampus. *Aging* Jun 23;13. doi: 10.18632/aging.203202. Online ahead of print.

[5] Ren, B. X., Huen, I., Wu, Z. J., Wang, H., Duan, M., Guenther, I., Bhanu Prakash, K. N., Tang, F. R. 2021. Early postnatal irradiation-induced age-dependent changes in adult mouse brain: MRI based characterization. *BMC Neuroscience* 22(1), 28.

[6] Robertson, P. L. 2006. Advances in treatment of pediatric brain tumors. *NeuroRx*. 3, 276–91.

[7] Chalabi, J., & Patel, S. 2009. Radiation therapy in children. *Int. Anesthesiol. Clin.* 47, 45–53.

[8] American Association of Neuroscience Nurses (AANN). *Care of the Pediatric Patient with a Brain Tumor.* Chicago: American Association of Neuroscience Nurses (AANN); 2014. P. 25.

[9] Streffer, C., & Molls, M. 1987. Cultures of preimplantation mouse embryos: A model for radiological studies. *Adv. Radiat. Biology* 13, 169-213.

[10] Stanfield, B. B., Cowan, W. M. 1979. The development of the hippocampus and dentate gyrus in normal and reeler mice. *J. Comp. Neurol.* 185(3), 423-59.

[11] Ganapathi, R., & Manda, K. 2017. Later life changes in hippocampal neurogenesis and behavioral functions after low-dose prenatal irradiation at early organogenesis stage. *Int. J. Radiat. Oncol. Biol. Phys.* 98(1), 63-74.

[12] Miki, T., Sawada, K., Sun, X. Z., Hisano, S., Takeuchi, Y., Fukui, Y. 1999. Abnormal distribution of hippocampal mossy fibers in rats exposed to X-irradiation in utero. *Brain Res. Dev. Brain Res.* 112(2), 275-80.

[13] Saito, S., Sawada, K., Aoki, I. 2018. Prenatal irradiation-induced hippocampal abnormalities in rats evaluated using manganese-enhanced MRI. *Front. Neural. Circuits.* 12,112.

[14] Pipová Kokošová, N., Kisková, T., Vilhanová, K., Štafuriková, A., Jendželovský, R., Račeková, E., Šmajda, B. 2020. Melatonin mitigates hippocampal and cognitive impairments caused by prenatal irradiation. *Eur. J. Neurosci.* 52(6), 3575-3594.

[15] Janeczko, K., Setkowicz, Z., Fraczek, M., Kochowska, J. 1999. Effects of prenatal gamma-irradiation on postnatal astrogliogenesis in the hippocampal formation of rat. *Brain Res.* 816(2), 628-32.

[16] Ferrer, I., Macaya, A., Blanco, R., Olivé, M., Cinós, C., Munell, F., Planas, A. M. 1995. Evidence of internucleosomal DNA

fragmentation and identification of dying cells in X-ray-induced cell death in the developing brain. *Int. J. Dev. Neurosci.* 13, 21-8.

[17] Gaiarsa, J. L., Beaudoin, M., Ben-Ari, Y. 1992. Effect of neonatal degranulation on the morphological development of rat CA3 pyramidal neurons: inductive role of mossy fibers on the formation of thorny excrescences. *J. Com. Neurol.* 321, 612-25.

[18] McGinn, M. J., Sun, D., Colello, R. J. 2008. Utilizing X-irradiation to selectively eliminate neural stem/progenitor cells from neurogenic regions of the mammalian brain. *J. Neurosci. Methods* 170, 9-15.

[19] Ferrer. I., Serrano, T., Alcantara, S., Tortosa, A., Graus, F. 1993. X-ray-induced cell death in the developing hippocampal complex involves neurons and requires protein synthesis. *J. Neuropath. Exp. Neurol.* 52, 370-8.

[20] Ben-Barak, J. 1981. The development of the cholinergic system in rat hippocampus following postnatal x-irradiation. *Brain Res.* 226, 171-86.

[21] Mickley, G. A., Ferguson, J. L., Nemeth, T. J., Mulvihill, M. A., Alderks, C. E. 1989. Spontaneous perseverative turning in rats with radiation-induced hippocampal damage. *Behav. Neurosci.* 103, 722-30.

[22] Bayer, S. A., & Altman, J. 1975. Radiation-induced interference with postnatal hippocampal cytogenesis in rats and its long-term effects on the acquisition of neurons and glia. *J. Comp. Neurol.* 163, 1-19.

[23] Diaz-Granados, J. L., Greene, P. L., Amsel, A. 1992. Memory-based learning in preweanling and adult rats after infantile x-irradiation-induced hippocampal granule cell hypoplasia. *Behav. Neurosci.* 106, 940-6.

[24] Craig, A., Luo, N. L., Beardsley, D. J., Wingate-Pearse, N., Walker, D. W., Hohimer, A. R., Back, S. A. 2003. Quantitative analysis of perinatal rodent oligodendrocyte lineage progression and its correlation with human. *Exp. Neurol.* 181, 231–40.

[25] Lodygensky, G. A., Vasung, L., Sizonenko, S. V., Huppi, P. S. 2010. Neuroimaging of cortical development and brain connectivity in human newborns and animal models. *J. Anat.* 217, 418–28.

[26] Dean, J. M., Moravec, M. D., Grafe, M., Abend, N., Ren, J., Gong, X., Volpe, J. J., Jensen, F. E., Hohimer, A. R., Back, S. A. 2011. Strain-specific differences in perinatal rodent oligodendrocyte lineage progression and its correlation with human. *Dev. Neurosci.* 33, 251-60.

[27] Dean, J. M., Riddle, A., Maire, J., Hansen, K. D., Preston, M., Barnes, A. P., Sherman, L. S., Bach, S. A. 2011. An organotypic slice culture model of chronic white matter injury with maturation arrest of oligodendrocyte progenitors. *Mol. Neurodegener.* 6, 46.

[28] Holsapple, M. P., West, L. J., Landreth, K. S. 2003. Species comparison of anatomical and functional immune system development. *Birth Defects Res. B Dev. Reprod. Toxicol.* 68, 321–34.

[29] Engelhardt, B. 2003. Development of the blood-brain barrier. *Cell Tissue Res.* 314, 119–29.

[30] Daneman, R., Zhou, L., Kebede, A. A., Barres, B. A. 2010. Pericytes are required for blood-brain barrier integrity during embryogenesis. *Nature* 468, 562-6.

[31] Naylor, A. S., Bull, C., Nilsson, M. K., Zhu, C., Björk-Eriksson, T., Eriksson, P. S., Blomgren, K., Kuhn, H. G. 2008. Voluntary running rescues adult hippocampal neurogenesis after irradiation of the young mouse brain. *Proc. Natl. Acad. Sci. USA* 105, 14632-7.

[32] Hellström, N. A., Björk-Eriksson, T., Blomgren, K., Kuhn, H. G. 2009. Differential recovery of neural stem cells in the subventricular zone and dentate gyrus after ionizing radiation. *Stem Cells* 27, 634-41.

[33] Hellström, N. A., Lindberg, O. R., Ståhlberg, A., Swanpalmer, J., Pekny, M., Blomgren, K., Kuhn, H. G. 2011. Unique gene

expression patterns indicate microglial contribution to neural stem cell recovery following irradiation. *Mol. Cell Neurosci.* 46, 710-9.

[34] Kalm, M., Fukuda, A., Fukuda, H., Ohrfelt, A., Lannering, B., Björk-Eriksson, T., Blennow, K., Márky, I., Blomgren, K. 2009. Transient inflammation in neurogenic regions after irradiation of the developing brain. *Radiat. Res.* 171, 66-76.

[35] Kalm, M., Lannering, B., Björk-Eriksson, T., Blomgren, K. 2009. Irradiation-induced loss of microglia in the young brain. *J. Neuroimmunol.* 206, 70-5.

[36] Barlind, A., Karlsson, N., Björk-Eriksson, T., Isgaard, J., Blomgren, K. 2010. Decreased cytogenesis in the granule cell layer of the hippocampus and impaired place learning after irradiation of the young mouse brain evaluated using the IntelliCage platform. *Exp. Brain Res.* 201, 781-7.

[37] Huo, K., Sun, Y., Li, H., Du, X., Wang, X., Karlsson, N., Zhu, C. L., Blomgren, K. 2012. Lithium reduced neural progenitor apoptosis in the hippocampus and ameliorated functional deficits after irradiation to the immature mouse brain. *Mol. Cell. Neurosci.* 51, 32-42.

[38] Kremer, T., Jagasia, R., Herrmann, A., Matile, H., Borroni, E., Francis, F., Kuhn, H. G., Czech, C. 2013. Analysis of adult neurogenesis: evidence for a prominent "non-neurogenic" DCX-protein pool in rodent brain. *PLoS One* 2013; 8: e59269.

[39] Kempf, S. J., Casciati, A., Buratovic, S., Janik, D., von Toerne, C., Ueffing, M., Neff, F., Moertl, S., Stenerlöw, B., Saran, A., Atkinson, M. J., Eriksson, P. 2014. The cognitive defects of neonatally irradiated mice are 2016.accompanied by changed synaptic plasticity, adult neurogenesis and neuroinflammation. *Mol. Neurodegener.* 9, 57.

[40] Casciati, A., Dobos, K., Antonelli, F., Benedek, A., Kempf, S. J., Bellés, M., Balogh, A., Tanori, M., Heredia, L., Atkinson, M. J., von Toerne, C., Azimzadeh, O., Saran, A., Sáfrány, G., Benotmane, M. A., Linares-Vidal, M. V., Tapio, S., Lumniczky,

K., Pazzaglia, S. 2016. Age-related effects of X-ray irradiation on mouse hippocampus. *Oncotarget* 7(19), 28040-58.

[41] Serrano, C., Dos Santos, M., Kereselidze, D., Beugnies, L., Lestaevel, P., Poirier, R., Durand, C. 2021. Targeted dorsal dentate gyrus or whole brain irradiation in juvenile mice differently affects spatial memory and adult hippocampal neurogenesis. *Biology* (Basel). 10(3),192.

[42] Dobbing, J., & Sands, J. 1979. Comparative aspects of the brain growth spurt. *Early Hum. Dev.* 3, 79–83.

[43] Bockhorst, K. H., Narayana, P. A., Liu, R., Ahobila-Vijjula, P., Ramu, J., Kamel, M., Wosik, J., Bockhorst, T., Hahn, K., Hasan, K. M., Perez-Polo, J. R. 2008. Early postnatal development of rat brain: in vivo diffusion tensor imaging. *J. Neurosci. Res.* 86, 1520–8.

[44] Catalani, A., Sabbatini, M., Consoli, C., Cinque, C., Tomassoni, D., Azmitia, E., Angelucci, L., & Amenta, F. 2002. Glial fibrillary acidic protein immunoreactive astrocytes in developing rat hippocampus. *Mech. Ageing Dev.* 123, 481–90.

[45] Kriegstein, A., & Alvarez-Buylla, A. 2009. The glial nature of embryonic and adult neural stem cells. *Ann. Rev. Neurosci.* 32, 149–84.

[46] Cowan, W. M. 1979. The development of the brain. *Sci. Am.* 241, 113–33.

[47] Baloch S., Verma R., Huang H., Khurd P., Clark S., Yarowsky P., Abel, T., Mori, S., Davatzikos, C. 2009. Quantification of brain maturation and growth patterns in C57BL/6J mice via computational neuroanatomy of diffusion tensor images. *Cereb. Cortex* 19, 675–87.

[48] Roughton, K., Kalm, M., Blomgren, K. 2012. Sex-dependent differences in behavior and hippocampal neurogenesis after irradiation to the young mouse brain. *Eur. J. Neurosci*. 36, 2763-72.

[49] Roughton, K., Andreasson, U., Blomgren, K., Kalm, M. 2013. Lipopolysaccharide-induced inflammation aggravates irradiation-

induced injury to the young mouse brain. *Dev. Neurosci.* 35, 406-15.

[50] Roughton, K., Boström, M., Kalm, M., Blomgren, K. 2013. Irradiation to the young mouse brain impaired white matter growth more in females than in males. *Cell Death Dis.* 4, e897.

[51] Velickovic, N., Djordjevic, A., Drakulic, D., Stanojevic, I., Secerov, B., Horvat, A. 2009. Cranial irradiation modulates hypothalamic-pituitary-adrenal axis activity and corticosteroid receptor expression in the hippocampus of juvenile rat. *Gen. Physiol. Biophys.* 28, 219-27.

[52] Peng, S., Yang, B., Duan, M. Y., Liu, Z. W., Wang, W. F., Zhang, X. Z., Ren, B. X., Tang, F. R. 2019. The Disparity of impairment of neurogenesis and cognition after acute or fractionated radiation exposure in adolescent BALB/c mice. *Dose Response* 17(1),1559325818822574.

[53] Tang, F. R., Loke, W. K., Wong. P. Y., Khoo, B. C. 2017. Radioprotective effect of ursolic acid in radiation-induced impairment of neurogenesis, learning and memory in adolescent BALB/c mouse. *Physiol. Behav.* 175, 37-46.

[54] Hayashi, F., Takashima, N., Murayama, A., Inokuchi, K. 2008. Decreased postnatal neurogenesis in the hippocampus combined with stress experience during adolescence is accompanied by an enhanced incidence of behavioral pathologies in adult mice. *Mol. Brain* 1, 22.

[55] Achanta, P., Fuss, M., Martinez, J. L. Jr. 2009. Ionizing radiation impairs the formation of trace fear memories and reduces hippocampal neurogenesis. *Behav. Neurosci.* 123,1036-45.

[56] Tada, E., Parent, J. M., Lowenstein, D. H., Fike, J. R. 2000. X-irradiation causes a prolonged reduction in cell proliferation in the dentate gyrus of adult rats. *Neurosci.* 99, 33-41.

[57] Monje, M. L., Mizumatsu, S., Fike, J. R., Palmer, T. D. 2002. Irradiation induces neural precursor-cell dysfunction. *Nat. Med.* 8, 955-62.

[58] Madsen, T. M., Kristjansen, P. E., Bolwig, T. G., Wörtwein, G. 2003. Arrested neuronal proliferation and impaired hippocampal function following fractionated brain irradiation in the adult rat. *Neurosci.* 119, 635-42.

[59] Mizumatsu, S., Monje, M. L., Morhardt, D. R., Rola, R., Palmer, T. D., Fike, J. R. 2003. Extreme sensitivity of adult neurogenesis to low doses of X-irradiation. *Cancer Res.* 63, 4021-7.

[60] Casadesus, G., Shukitt-Hale, B., Stellwagen, H. M., Smith, M. A., Rabin, B. M., Joseph, J. A. 2005. Hippocampal neurogenesis and PSA-NCAM expression following exposure to 56Fe particles mimics that seen during aging in rats. *Exp. Gerontol.* 40, 249-54.

[61] Fan, Y., Liu, Z., Weinstein, P. R., Fike, J. R., Liu, J. 2007. Environmental enrichment enhances neurogenesis and improves functional outcome after cranial irradiation. *Eur. J. Neurosci.* 25, 38-46.

[62] Kim, J. S., Lee, H. J., Kim, J. C., Kang, S. S., Bae, C. S., Shin, T., Jin, J. K., Kim, S. H., Wang, H., Moon, C. 2008. Transient impairment of hippocampus-dependent learning and memory in relatively low-dose of acute radiation syndrome is associated with inhibition of hippocampal neurogenesis. *J. Radiat. Res.* 49, 517-26.

[63] Park, M. K., Kim, S., Jung, U., Kim, I., Kim, J. K., Roh, C. 2012. Effect of acute and fractionated irradiation on hippocampal neurogenesis. *Molecules* 17, 9462-8.

[64] Bálentová, S., Hajtmanová, E., Filova, B., Borbelyova, V., Lehotský, J. 2015. Effect of fractionated irradiation on the hippocampus in an experimental model. *Klin. Onkol.* 28, 191-9.

[65] Parihar, V. K., Limoli, C. L. 2013. Cranial irradiation compromises neuronal architecture in the hippocampus. *Proc. Natl. Acad. Sci. USA* 110, 12822-7.

[66] Ji. J. F., Ji, S. J., Sun, R., Li, K., Zhang, Y., Zhang, L. Y., Tien, Y. 2014. Forced running exercise attenuates hippocampal neurogenesis impairment and the neurocognitive deficits induced

by whole-brain irradiation via the BDNF-mediated pathway. *Biochem. Biophys. Res. Commun.* 443, 646-51.

[67] Son, Y., Yang, M., Kim, J. S., Kim, J., Kim, S. H., Kim, J. C., Shin, T., Wang, H. B., Jo, S. K., Jung, U., Moon, C. J. 2014. Hippocampal dysfunction during the chronic phase following a single exposure to cranial irradiation. *Exp. Neurol.* 254, 134-44.

[68] Son, Y., Yang, M., Wang, H. B., Moon, C. J. 2015. Hippocampal dysfunctions caused by cranial irradiation: a review of the experimental evidence. *Brain Behav. Immun.* 45, 287-96.

[69] Acharya M. M., Patel N. H., Craver B. M., Tran K. K., Giedzinski E., Tseng B. P., Parihar, V. K., Limoli, C. L. 2015. Consequences of low dose ionizing radiation exposure on the hippocampal microenvironment. *PLoS One* 10, e0128316.

[70] Wei L. C., Ding Y. X., Liu Y. H., Duan L., Bai Y., Shi M., Chen, L. W. 2012. Low-dose radiation stimulates Wnt/β-catenin signaling, neural stem cell proliferation and neurogenesis of the mouse hippocampus in vitro and in vivo. *Curr. Alzheimer Res.* 9, 278-89.

[71] Hwang, S., Jeong, H., Hong, E. H., Joo, H. M., Cho, K. S., Nam, S. Y. 2019. Low-dose ionizing radiation alleviates Aβ42-induced cell death via regulating AKT and p38 pathways in Drosophila Alzheimer's disease models. *Biol. Open* 8(2), bio036657.

[72] Khandelwal, M., Manglani, K., Gupta, S., Tiku, A. B. 2020. Gamma radiation improves AD pathogenesis in APP/PS1 mouse model by potentiating insulin sensitivity. *Heliyon.* 6(7), e04499.

[73] Kim, S., Nam, Y., Kim, C., Lee, H., Hong, S., Kim, H. S., Shin, S. J., Park, Y. H., Mai, H. N., Oh, S. M., Kim, K. S., Yoo, D. H., Chung, W. K., Chung, H., Moon, M. 2020. Neuroprotective and anti-inflammatory effects of low-moderate dose ionizing radiation in models of Alzheimer's disease. *Int. J. Mol. Sci.* 21(10), 3678.

[74] Wilson, G. D., Wilson, T. G., Hanna, A., Fontanesi, G., Kulchycki, J., Buelow, K., Pruetz, B. L., Michael, D. B., Chinnaiyan, P., Maddens, M. E., Martinez, A. A., Fontanesi, J. 2020. Low dose

brain irradiation reduces Amyloid-β and Tau in 3xTg-AD mice. *J. Alzheimers Dis.* 75(1), 15-21.

[75] Ceyzériat, K., Zilli, T., Fall, A. B., Millet, P., Koutsouvelis, N., Dipasquale, G., Frisoni, G. B., Tournier, B. B., Garibotto, V. 2021. Treatment by low-dose brain radiation therapy improves memory performances without changes of the amyloid load in the TgF344-AD rat model. *Neurobiol. Aging* 103,117-127.

[76] Cuttler, J. M., Moore, E. R., Hosfeld, V. D., Nadolski, D. L. 2016. Treatment of Alzheimer disease with CT scans: A case report. *Dose Response.* 14(2):1559325816640073.

[77] Ceyzériat, K., Tournier, B. B., Millet, P., Frisoni, G. B., Garibotto, V., Zilli, T. 2020. Low-dose radiation therapy: A new treatment strategy for Alzheimer's disease? *J. Alzheimers Dis.* 74(2), 411-419.

[78] Chung, M., Rhee, H. Y., Chung, W. K. 2021. Clinical approach of low-dose whole-brain ionizing radiation treatment in Alzheimer's disease dementia patients. *J Alzheimers Dis.* 2021;80(3):941-947. doi: 10.3233/JAD-210042. *Erratum in J. Alzheimers Dis.* 81(3), 1343.

[79] Cuttler, J. M., Abdellah, E., Goldberg, Y., Al-Shamaa, S., Symons, S. P., Black, S. E., Freedman, M. 2021. Low doses of ionizing radiation as a treatment for Alzheimer's disease: A pilot s tudy. *J. Alzheimers Dis.* 80(3), 1119-1128.

[80] Moraga-Amaro, R., Jerez-Baraona, J. M., Simon, F., Stehberg, J. 2014. Role of astrocytes in memory and psychiatric disorders. *J. Physiol. Paris* 108, 240-51.

[81] Szu, J. I., & Binder, D. K. 2016. The role of astrocytic aquaporin-4 in synaptic plasticity and learning and memory. *Front. Integr. Neurosci.* 10, 8.

[82] Walker, F. R., & Yirmiya, R. 2016. Microglia, physiology and behavior: A brief commentary. *Brain Behav. Immun.* 55, 1-5.

[83] Pazzaglia, S., Tanno, B., Antonelli, F., Giardullo, P., Babini, G., Subedi, P., Azimzadeh, O., Khan, Z. N., Oleksenko, K., Metzger, F., Toerne, C. V., Traynor, D., Medipally, D., Meade, A. D.,

Kadhim, M., Lyng, F. M., Tapio, S., Saran, A., Mancuso, M. 2021. Out-of-field hippocampus from partial-body irradiated mice displays changes in multi-omics profile and defects in neurogenesis. *Int. J. Mol. Sci.* 22(8), 4290.

[84] Manda, K., Ueno, M., Anzai, K. 2008. Space radiation-induced inhibition of neurogenesis in the hippocampal dentate gyrus and memory impairment in mice: ameliorative potential of the melatonin metabolite, AFMK. *J. Pineal Res.* 45(4), 430-8.

[85] Rivera, P. D., Shih, H. Y., Leblanc, J. A., Cole, M. G., Amaral, W. Z., Mukherjee, S., Zhang, S., Lucero, M. J., Decarolis, N. A., Chen, B. P., Eisch, A. J. 2013. Acute and fractionated exposure to high-LET (56)Fe HZE-particle radiation both result in similar long-term deficits in adult hippocampal neurogenesis. *Radiat. Res.* 180(6), 658-67.

[86] Whoolery, C. W., Walker, A. K., Richardson, D. R., Lucero, M. J., Reynolds, R. P., Beddow, D. H., Clark, K. L., Shih, H. Y., LeBlanc, J. A., Cole, M. G., Amaral, W. Z., Mukherjee, S., Zhang, S., Ahn, F., Bulin, S. E., DeCarolis, N. A., Rivera, P. D., Chen, B. P. C., Yun, S., Eisch, A. J. 2017. Whole-body exposure to ^{28}Si-radiation dose-dependently disrupts dentate gyrus neurogenesis and proliferation in the short term and new neuron survival and contextual fear conditioning in the long term. *Radiat. Res.* 188(5), 532-551.

[87] Zanni, G., Deutsch, H. M., Rivera, P. D., Shih, H. Y., LeBlanc, J. A., Amaral, W. Z., Lucero, M. J., Redfield, R. L., DeSalle, M. J., Chen, B. P. C., Whoolery, C. W., Reynolds, R. P., Yun, S., Eisch, A. J. 2018. Whole-body ^{12}C irradiation transiently decreases mouse hippocampal dentate gyrus proliferation and immature neuron number, but does not change new neuron survival rate. *Int. J. Mol. Sci.* 19(10), 3078.

[88] Miry, O., Zhang, X. L., Vose, L. R., Gopaul, K. R., Subah, G., Moncaster, J. A., Wojnarowicz, M. W., Fisher, A. M., Tagge, C. A., Goldstein, L. E., Stanton, P. K. 2021. Life-long brain

compensatory responses to galactic cosmic radiation exposure. *Sci. Rep.* 11(1), 4292.

[89] Iacono, D., Murphy, E. K., Avantsa, S. S., Perl, D. P., Day, R. M., Iacono, D., Murphy, E. K., Avantsa, S. S., Perl, D. P., Day, R. M. 2021. Reduction of pTau and APP levels in mammalian brain after low-dose radiation. *Sci. Rep.* 11(1), 2215.

[90] Allen, B. D., Syage, A. R., Maroso, M., Baddour, A. A. D., Luong, V., Minasyan, H., Giedzinski, E., West, B. L., Soltesz, I., Limoli, C. L., Baulch, J. E., Acharya, M. M. 2020. Mitigation of helium irradiation-induced brain injury by microglia depletion. *J. Neuroinflammation* 17(1), 159.

[91] Wong-Goodrich, S. J., Pfau, M. L., Flores, C. T., Fraser, J. A., Williams, C. L., Jones, L. W. 2010. Voluntary running prevents progressive memory decline and increases adult hippocampal neurogenesis and growth factor expression after whole-brain irradiation. *Cancer Res.* 70(22), 9329-38.

[92] Conner, K. R., Forbes, M. E., Lee, W. H., Lee, Y. W., Riddle, D. R., 2011. AT1 receptor antagonism does not influence early radiation-induced changes in microglial activation or neurogenesis in the normal rat brain. *Radiat. Res.* 176(1), 71-83.

[93] Schindler, M. K., Bourland, J. D., Forbes, M. E., Hua, K., Riddle, D. R. 2011. Neurobiological responses to stereotactic focal irradiation of the adult rodent hippocampus. *J. Neurol. Sci.* 306(1-2), 129-37.

[94] Jenrow, K. A., Brown, S. L., Lapanowski, K., Naei, H., Kolozsvary, A., Kim, J. H. 2013. Selective inhibition of microglia-mediated neuroinflammation mitigates radiation-induced cognitive impairment. *Radiat. Res.* 179(5), 549-56.

[95] Parthsarathy, V., & Hölscher, C. 2013. The type 2 diabetes drug liraglutide reduces chronic inflammation induced by irradiation in the mouse brain. *Eur. J. Pharmacol.* 700(1-3), 42-50.

[96] Tomé, W. A., Gökhan, Ş., Gulinello, M. E., Brodin, N. P., Heard, J., Mehler, M. F., Guha, C. 2016. Hippocampal-dependent neurocognitive impairment following cranial irradiation observed

in pre-clinical models: current knowledge and possible future directions. *Br. J. Radiol.* 89(1057), 20150762.

[97] Cheng, Z., Zheng, Y. Z., Li, Y. Q., Wong, C. S. 2017. Cellular senescence in mouse hippocampus after irradiation and the role of p53 and p21. *J. Neuropathol. Exp. Neurol.* 76(4), 260-269.

[98] Kureshi, S. A., Hofman, F. M., Schneider, J. H., Chin, L. S., Apuzzo, M. L., Hinton, D. R. 1994. Cytokine expression in radiation-induced delayed cerebral injury. *Neurosurgery* 35, 822-9.

[99] Ballesteros-Zebadúa, P., Chavarria, A., Celis, M. A., Paz, C., Franco-Pérez, J. 2012. Radiation-induced neuroinflammation and radiation somnolence syndrome. *CNS Neurol. Disord. Drug Targets* 11, 937-49.

[100] Daams, M., Schuitema, I., van Dijk, B. W., van Dulmen-den Broeder, E., Veerman, A. J., van den Bos, V., Sude Sonneville, L. M. 2012. Long-term effects of cranial irradiation and intrathecal chemotherapy in treatment of childhood leukemia: a MEG study of power spectrum and correlated cognitive dysfunction. *BMC Neurol.* 12, 84.

[101] Greene-Schloesser, D., Moore, E., Robbins, M. E. 2013. Molecular pathways: radiation-induced cognitive impairment. *Clin. Cancer Res.* 19, 2294-300.

[102] Ness, K. K., Armstrong, G. T., Kundu, M., Wilson, C. L., Tchkonia, T., Kirkland, J. L. 2015. Frailty in childhood cancer survivors. *Cancer* 121, 1540-7.

[103] Yoritsune, E., Furuse, M., Kuwabara, H., Miyata, T., Nonoguchi, N., Kawabata, S., Hayasaki, H., Kuroiwa, T., Ono, K., Shibayama, Y., Miyatake, S. 2014. Inflammation as well as angiogenesis may participate in the pathophysiology of brain radiation necrosis. *J. Radiat. Res.* 55, 803-11.

[104] Furuse, M., Nonoguchi, N., Kawabata, S., Miyatake, S., Kuroiwa, T. 2015. Delayed brain radiation necrosis: pathological review and new molecular targets for treatment. *Med. Mol. Morphol.* 48, 183-90.

[105] Hong, J. H., Chiang, C. S., Campbell, I. L., Sun, J. R., Withers, H. R., McBride, W. H. 1995. Induction of acute phase gene expression by brain irradiation. *Int. J. Radiat. Oncol. Biol. Phys.* 33, 619-26.

[106] Poulose, S. M., Bielinski, D. F., Carrihill-Knoll, K., Rabin, B. M., Shukitt-Hale, B. 2011. Exposure to 16O-particle radiation causes aging-like decrements in rats through increased oxidative stress, inflammation and loss of autophagy. *Radiat. Res.* 176, 761-9.

[107] Lee, S. W., Haditsch, U., Cord, B. J., Guzman, R., Kim, S. J., Boettcher, C., Priller, J., Ormerod, B. K., Palmer, T. D. 2013. Absence of CCL2 is sufficient to restore hippocampal neurogenesis following cranial irradiation. *Brain Behav. Immun.* 30, 33-44.

[108] Li, M. D., Burns, T. C., Kumar, S., Morgan, A. A., Sloan, S. A., Palmer, T. D. 2015. Aging-like changes in the transcriptome of irradiated microglia. *Glia* 63, 754-67.

[109] Blomstrand, M., Kalm, M., Grandér, R., Björk-Eriksson, T., Blomgren, K. 2014. Different reactions to irradiation in the juvenile and adult hippocampus. *Int. J. Radiat. Biol.* 90, 807-15.

[110] Lee, W. H., Sonntag, W. E., Lee, Y. W. 2010. Aging attenuates radiation-induced expression of pro-inflammatory mediators in rat brain. *Neurosci. Lett.* 476, 89-93.

[111] Lee, W. H., Sonntag, W. E., Mitschelen, M., Yan, H., Lee, Y. W. 2010. Irradiation induces regionally specific alterations in pro-inflammatory environments in rat brain. *Int. J. Radiat. Biol.* 86, 132-44.

[112] Hua, K., Schindler, M. K., McQuail, J. A., Forbes, M. E., Riddle, D. R. 2012. Regionally distinct responses of microglia and glial progenitor cells to whole brain irradiation in adult and aging rats. *PLoS One* 7, e52728.

[113] Monje, M. L., & Palmer, T. 2003. Radiation injury and neurogenesis. *Curr. Opin. Neurol.* 16,129-34.

[114] Metzdorf, J., Hobloss, Z., Schlevogt, S., Ayzenberg, I., Stahlke, S., Pedreiturria, X., Haupeltshofer, S., Gold, R., Tönges, L., Kleiter, I.

2019. Fingolimod for irradiation-induced neurodegeneration. *Front. Neurosci.* 13, 699.

[115] Lu, K., Wu, W. J., Zhang, C., Zhu, Y. L., Zhong, J. Q., Li, J. 2020. CORM-3 regulates microglia activity, prevents neuronal injury, and improves memory function during radiation-induced brain injury. *Curr. Neurovasc. Res.* 17(4), 464-470.

[116] Beamish, C. A., Zawaski, J. A., Inoue, T., Sarkar, P., Grosshans, D. R., Sabek, O. M., Gaber, M. W. 2021. NF-kappa B blockade by NEMO binding domain peptide ameliorates inflammation and neurobehavioral sequelae after cranial radiation therapy in juvenile mice. *Int. J. Radiat. Oncol. Biol. Phys.* 109(5),1508-1520.

[117] Wang, Y., Zhou, K., Li, T., Xu, Y., Xie, C., Sun, Y., Zhang, Y., Rodriguez, J., Blomgren, K., Zhu, C. 2017. Inhibition of autophagy prevents irradiation-induced neural stem and progenitor cell death in the juvenile mouse brain. *Cell Death Dis.* 8(3), e2694.

[118] Rao, A. A., Ye, H., Decker, P. A., Howe, C. L., Wetmore, C. 2011. Therapeutic doses of cranial irradiation induce hippocampus-dependent cognitive deficits in young mice. *J. Neurooncol.* 105, 191-8.

[119] Armstrong, G. T., Reddick, W. E., Petersen, R. C., Santucci, A., Zhang, N., Srivastava, D., Ogg, R. J., Hillenbrand, C. M., Sabin, N., Krasin, M. J., Kun, L., Pui, C. H., Hudson, M. M., Robison, L. L., Krull, K. R. 2013. Evaluation of memory impairment in aging adult survivors of childhood acute lymphoblastic leukemia treated with cranial radiotherapy. *J. Natl. Cancer. Inst.* 105, 899-907.

[120] Son, Y., Yang, M., Kang, S., Lee, S., Kim, J., Kim, J., Park, S., Kim, J. S., Jo, S. K., Jung, U., Shin, T., Kim, S. H., Wang, H., Moon, C. 2015. Cranial irradiation regulates CREB-BDNF signaling and variant BDNF transcript levels in the mouse hippocampus. *Neurobiol. Learn. Mem.* 121,12-9.

[121] Eriksson, P., Buratovic, S., Fredriksson, A., Stenerlöw, B., Sundell-Bergman, S. 2016. Neonatal exposure to whole body ionizing radiation induces adult neurobehavioural defects: Critical

period, dose-response effects and strain and sex comparison. *Behav. Brain Res.* 304, 11-9.

[122] Rola, R., Raber, J., Rizk, A., Otsuka, S., VandenBerg, S. R., Morhardt, D. R., Fike, J. R. 2004. Radiation-induced impairment of hippocampal neurogenesis is associated with cognitive deficits in young mice. *Exp. Neurol.* 188, 316-30.

[123] Vlkolinsky, R., Titova, E., Krucker, T., Chi, B. B., Staufenbiel, M., Nelson, G. A., Obenaus, A. 2010. Exposure to 56Fe-particle radiation accelerates electrophysiological alterations in the hippocampus of APP23 transgenic mice. *Radiat. Res.* 173, 342-52.

[124] Shi, L., Olson, J., D'Agostino, R. Jr., Linville, C., Nicolle, M. M., Robbins, M. E., Wheeler, K. T., Brunso-Bechtold, J. K. 2011. Aging masks detection of radiation-induced brain injury. *Brain Res.* 1385, 307-16.

[125] Schindler, M. K., Forbes, M. E., Robbins, M. E., Riddle, D. R. 2008. Aging-dependent changes in the radiation response of the adult rat brain. *Int. J. Radiat. Oncol. Biol. Phys.* 70, 826-34.

[126] Seltser, R., & Sartwell, P. E. 1965. The influence of occupational exposure to radiation on the mortality of American radiobiologists and other medical specialists. *Am. J. Epidemiol.* 81, 2-22.

[127] Kholodova, N. B., Zhavoronkova, L. A., Ryzhov, B. N., Kuznetsova, G. D. 2007. Premature aging of an organism and characteristics of its manifestation in remote period after low dose irradiation (in Russian). *Adv. Gerontol.* 20, 48-55.

[128] Richardson, R. B. 2009. Ionizing radiation and aging: rejuvenating an old idea. *Aging* (Albany NY) 1, 887-902.

[129] Raber, J., Allen, A. R., Rosi, S., Sharma, S., Dayger, C., Davis, M. J., Fike, J. R. 2013. Effects of whole body (56)Fe radiation on contextual freezing and Arc-positive cells in the dentate gyrus. *Behav. Brain Res.* 246,162-7.

[130] Li, J., Meng, Z., Zhang, G., Xing, Y., Feng, L., Fan, S., Fan, F., Buren, B., Liu, Q. 2015. N-acetylcysteine relieves oxidative stress and protects hippocampus of rat from radiation-induced apoptosis by inhibiting caspase-3. *Biomed. Pharmacother.* 70, 1-6.

[131] Riley, P. A. 1994. Free radicals in biology: oxidative stress and the effects of ionizing radiation. *Int. J. Radiat. Biol.* 65, 27-33.

[132] Limoli, C. L., Giedzinski, E., Baure, J., Rola, R., Fike, J. R. 2007. Redox changes induced in hippocampal precursor cells by heavy ion irradiation. *Radiat. Environ. Biophys.* 46, 167-72.

[133] Huang, T. T., Leu, D., Zou, Y. 2015. Oxidative stress and redox regulation on hippocampal-dependent cognitive functions. *Arch. Biochem. Biophys* 576, 2-7.

[134] Sano, K., Morii, K., Sato, M., Mori, H., Tanaka, R. 2000. Radiation-induced diffuse brain injury in the neonatal rat model--radiation-induced apoptosis of oligodendrocytes. *Neurol. Med. Chir.* (Tokyo). 40, 495-9.

[135] Eom, H. S., Park, H. R., Jo, S. K., Kim, Y. S., Moon, C., Kim, S. H., Jung, U. 2016. Radiation induces altered neuronal differentiation by mGluR1 through PI3K-STAT3 signaling in C17.2 mouse neural stem-like cells. *PLos One* 11, e0147538.

[136] Pouget, J. P., Georgakilas, A. G., Ravanat, J. L. 2018. Targeted and off-target (bystander and abscopal) effects of radiation therapy: Redox mechanisms and risk/benefit analysis. *Antioxid. Redox Signal.* 29, 1447–1487.

[137] Van der Meeren, A., Monti, P., Vandamme, M., Squiban, C., Wysocki, J., Griffiths, N. 2005. Abdominal radiation exposure elicits inflammatory responses and abscopal effects in the lungs of mice. *Radiat. Res.* 163, 144–152.

[138] Rastogi, S., Coates, P. J., Lorimore, S. A., Wright, E. G. 2012. Bystander-type effects mediated by long-lived inflammatory signaling in irradiated bone marrow. *Radiat. Res.* 177, 244–250.

In: The Dentate Gyrus
Editor: Feng-Ru Tang
ISBN: 978-1-68507-212-4

Chapter 6

NEUROGENESIS IN THE ADULT DENTATE GYRUS AND EPILEPTOGENESIS

Qun Liu and Bo-Xu Ren*
Medical School, Yangtze University,
Jingzhou, People's Republic of China

ABSTRACT

Neurogenesis in the adult brain may replace lost neurons and mitigate patients' suffering. On the other hand, aberrant neurogenesis may produce more harm than benefit to patients with neurological and neuropsychological diseases. In the neurogenic regions of the dentate gyrus from animal models and patients with temporal lobe epilepsy (TLE), increased newly generated neurons in the subgranular zone (SGZ) at early stages after brain insults have been speculated to be involved in epileptogenesis. However, this argument is not supported by other research findings showing that 1) spontaneously recurrent seizures occur before newly generated neurons are integrated into hippocampal neural pathways, 2) hippocampal neurogenesis is decreased at chronic stages, 3) decreased neurogenesis is involved in epileptogenesis. Therefore, the hypothesis of increased neurogenesis in

* Corresponding Author's Email: boxuren188@163.com.

epileptogenesis may need to be re-evaluated. Here we systemically reviewed brain neurogenesis in the dentate gyrus and relevant molecules in the regulation of neurogenesis in SGZ. We then updated researchers and epileptologists on current progresses on pathophysiological changes of neurogenesis at different stages of TLE in animal models and in patients with TLE. The relationships among neurogenesis, epileptogenesis and cognitive impairment and molecules mechanism involved in neurogenesis were also discussed. In the last part of this paper, we proposed future research directions.

Keywords: neurogenesis, temporal lobe epilepsy, epileptogenesis, molecular mechanisms, dentate gyrus, cognition

INTRODUCTION

Neurogenesis occurs in the hippocampal subgranular zone (SGZ) of the dentate gyrus (DG) and in the subventricular zone (SVZ) of the lateral ventricle in the adult mammalian brain [1-7]. In chronic neurological disorders, such as temporal lobe epilepsy, stroke, ischemia, depression, Alzheimer's disease, Huntington's disease, and Parkinson's disease, both increased and reduced brain neurogeneses have been reported depending on the types and developmental stages of disorders. For increased neurogenesis at early stages of temporal lobe epilepsy (TLE), the fate of newly generated neurons at the chronic stages of TLE is still in debate as the survivability of newly generated neurons in the sclerotic hippocampus remains unknown. In other words, long-term study is still needed to demonstrate whether newly generated neurons could survive in pathological DG niche, be integrated into local neural circuits, and become functional. At chronic stages of TLE, the demonstration of reduced neurogenesis suggests that the characteristic neuropathological changes of epileptic hippocampus including gliosis, sclerosis, axon reorganization, and atrophy may significantly change neurogenic niche. The functional link between reduced neurogenesis and epileptogenesis further suggests that increased neurogenesis may not be related to epileptogenesis. This is supported by anatomical evidence showing that spontaneously recurrent seizures occur before newly generated neurons are integrated into abnormal hippocampal neural pathways.

In this paper, we systemically reviewed neurogenesis and the related molecular mechanisms in normal and epileptic mammalian brain. The relationship among increased or reduced neurogenesis, epileptogenesis and cognitive changes were discussed.

REGULATION OF NEUROGENESIS IN SGZ OF THE DENTATE GYRUS IN THE ADULT MAMMALIAN BRAIN

In the hippocampus, neurogenesis occurs in SGZ of the dentate gyrus. Precursor cells in this niche, including vascular endothelial cells, (quiescent) stem cells, and astrocytes [8, 9], are supported by a basal lamina that provides the obligatory extracellular matrix and produces new neurons in the mammal (Figure1) [9-11]. Neurogenesis in SGZ is regulated by different growth factors and signaling pathways, including fibroblast growth factor2 (FGF2) and fibroblast growth factor receptor (FGFR1) axis, brain-derived neurotrophic factor (BDNF), endothelial-derived growth factor (VEGF), insulin-like growth factor 1 (IGF-1), epidermal growth factor (EFG), Wnt signaling, and Notch signaling [12-20]. Wnt promotes activation of quiescent stem cells and enhances neuronal differentiation. Bone morphogenetic protein receptor type IA (BMPR-1A) maintains stem cells in a quiescent state, Notch maintains the NSC pool by preventing exit from quiescence, and the T-box transcription factor Tbr2 is essential for the proliferation and differentiation of immediate progenitor cells. Homeobox factor Prox1 and bHLH transcription factor NeuroD1 are expressed by granule neuron precursor cells and promote their differentiation.

The nuclear orphan receptor TlX, Cyclin D2 (CcnD2), and Achaete-scute homolog 1 (Ascl1) are essential for the proliferation of adult NSCs [21]. By destabilizing Ascl1 protein, E3-ubiquitin ligase HECT, UBA and WWE domain–containing 1 (Huwe1) maintain neural stem cells in a static state and prevent the accumulation of Cyclin Ds [22]. Inhibitor of DNA binding protein Id4, a direct downstream target of Notch2, prevents DG NSCs from cell-cycle entry to maintain NSCs quiescence [23]. One possible reason is that Id4 and other Id proteins promote the degradation of Ascl1 in NSC [24]. In addition, transcription factors such as hairy and enhancer of split (Hes), forkhead O-box (FoxO), and repressor element 1-silencing transcription (REST) are involved in regulating quiescence and proliferation of NSCs in adult DG [25]. GABAergic transmission can regulate the proliferation and differentiation of neural progenitor cells.

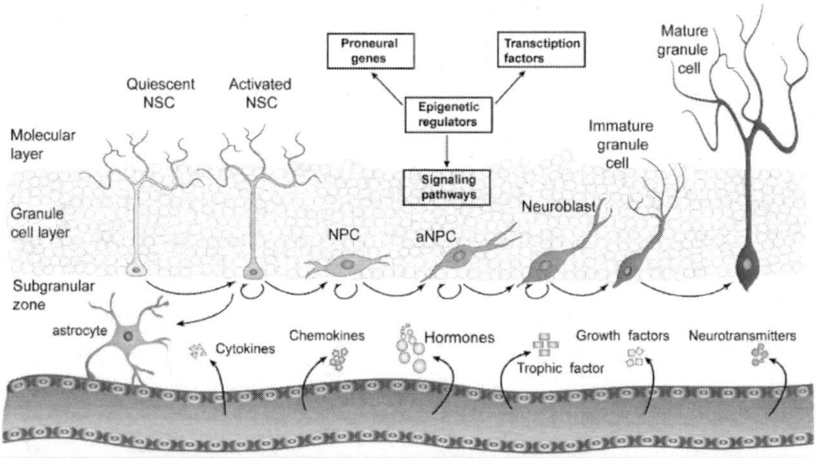

	Quiescense	Activation/ Proliferation	Fate Specification	Differation	Maturation
Signals	Notch, BMP, GABA	Canonical Wnt, FGF-2, EGF, VEGF, IGF-1, Shh, Glutamate, eCB	Canonical Wnt, IGF-1, FGF-2	BDNF, FGF-2, Wnt/PCP, IGF-1, GABA, Glutamate, Reelin	Glutamate, IGF-1, NRG2
Transctiption Factors	Hes, FoXO, REST, Id4	Ascl1, Sox2, TLX, CcnD2, Sox11	NeuroD1, Tbr2, Prox1	Prox1, NeuroD1, CREB	CREB
Epigenetic Regulators	Huwe1	Ezh2, FMRP, Gadd45b	FMRP, Ezh2, Mbd1	Gadd45b, FMRP, MeCP2	HDAC2, MeCP2
		Let-7b, miR-9, miR-184, miR-137, miR-34a, miR-153, miR-25, miR-19-92 cluster	miR-9, miR-124, miR-184	miR-132, miR-153, miR-211	miR-22, miR-137, miR-132, miR-134, miR-211, miR-34a

Figure 1. Schematic illustration of dentate gyrus neurogenic niche, the different processes underlying neurogenesis, and its regulation. Neurogenic niche, consisting of multiple cell types, allow NSC transform into the mature neuron. The transition is regulated by numerous factors, including signaling pathways, transcription factors, and epigenetic regulators.

BDNF and stromal cell-derived factor-1 (SDF-1)/CXC chemokine receptor 4 (CXCR4) signaling may regulate SGZ neurogenesis by decreasing and enhancing GABAergic transmission, respectively [26, 27]. In both SGZ and SVZ of adult mice, sonic hedgehog (Shh) stimulates adult neural progenitors to reenter the cell cycle and generate new neurons [28]. Ras-related GTPase, Rit, is a critical player in the survival of immature hippocampal neurons within SGZ following brain injury [29]. For endocannabinoid (eCB) signaling, long-term activation of CB1 cannabinoid receptor by arachidonyl-2-chloroethylamide (ACEA) promotes neural proliferation [30]. Compared to the CB1, CB2 in regulating adult neurogenesis showed a more complex effect. Although the proliferation of neural progenitor cells is suppressed in the SGZ of two-month-old mice with CB2 knockout and CB2 often plays a role in promoting neurogenesis in brain injury [31, 32], a recent study in 4-month-old mice showed that the cannabinoid receptor CB2 deficiency did not affect neural progenitor cell proliferation [33]. Sox2 is expressed in adult neural stem cells in SVZ and SGZ, and regulates survivin expression. Reduced Sox2 in neural stem cells may affect neurogenesis and induce apoptosis [34]. Similarly, Deletion of transcription factor Sox11 in adult NPC blunted proliferation in SGZ, suggesting that Sox11 was essential for hippocampal neurogenesis [35]. Of glutamate and receptor system, neurogenesis in SGZ may be regulated by N-methyl-D-aspartate (NMDA) receptors (NR1 and NR2B) present in precursor cells and in differentiating granule neurons [36]. Recently, it was shown that metabotropic glutamate receptor 5 (mGluR5) regulated the proliferation and differentiation of neuronal progenitors in SGZ [37]. The reduction of newly generated neurons in the adult SVZ and SGZ in an anosmic model suggested that olfactory sensory input might play roles in regulating adult neurogenesis [38]. In adult mouse SGZ, Ghrelin [39] and enhancer of zeste homolog2 (Ezh2) [40] could also stimulate proliferation and differentiation of neural progenitors. NSCs short of methyl-CpG-binding domain 1 (Mbd1) in the adult DG fail to differentiate into immature neurons and present an upregulation of astrocyte transcripts [41]. The highly expressed methyl-CpG-binding protein 2 (MeCP2) during DG neuronal maturation is necessary for dendritic growth and the integration of newborn neurons [42]. Other intrinsic and extrinsic factors that regulate adult neurogenesis at different stages in SGZ include genetic background [43], epigenetic regulators [44, 45], aging [46-48], various neurotransmitters [49], environmental stimuli [50-52], physical exercise [53-57], hippocampus-dependent learning [58-60], physical and psychosocial stress, depression [61, 62], hormone or activation of the hypothalamic-pituitary-adrenal axis [46], psychotropic drugs [59-63], and alcohol intoxication [64]. The experimental data from the current publications suggest that SGZ neurogenesis may be regulated by similar molecules and mechanisms. Predictably, TLE-induced changes of these molecules may affect neurogenesis in SGZ. Further study may be needed to establish whether any molecules are specifically involved in SGZ neurogenesis and/or gliogenesis.

Neurogenesis in SGZ in the Animal Models of TLE

Hippocampal neuronal loss, sclerosis, and axon reorganization are characteristic neuropathological changes in patients with temporal lobe epilepsy. While most of the granule cells survive repeated seizures [65], loss of some granule cells does occur in patients with intractable TLE [66, 67]. Based on pathological changes in DG, including granule cell dispersion, ectopic localization, axon reorganization, and neurogenesis observed in TLE patients [65, 66, 68-70], and animal models [71-89], it has been hypothesized that newly generated aberrant granule cells may be integrated into hippocampal neural pathways, and play an important role in the occurrence of spontaneously recurrent seizure. In fact, experimental data did support seizure-induced increased neurogenesis at early stages after seizure induction by pilocarpine [81-83, 86, 87], kainic acid [78, 89], pentylenetrazol [88], kindling [77, 79, 80, 84], electroconvulsive shock [85] and in pediatric patients with TLE [90]. Neuronal fate-mapping studies also revealed that more than half of the newborn dentate granule cells (DGCs) showed severe morphological abnormalities [91], including ectopic granule cells, formation of abnormal basal dendrites, and abnormal mossy fiber sprouting (MFS) into the inner molecular layer. These pathological changes have been observed as an essential structural basis for the integration of new abnormal granulosa cells into the hippocampal neural circuits [92-95].

In contrast to the increased neurogenesis at the time of the initial seizure induction, neurogenesis returned to the baseline by 7 [84], 27 days [76], or about two months [93] after SE and dropped substantially below the baseline level by five months [96] or one year [76] after SE. The decreased DG neurogenesis has also been confirmed by other studies in animal models of TLE [97, 98]. In the mouse pilocarpine model, we showed a significant reduction of calretinin-labeled newly generated neurons in SGZ at two months after pilocarpine-induced status epilepticus [98]. One possible explanation is that pathological changes in chronic TLE may significantly change brain neurogenetic niche, leading to reduced neurogenesis in SGZ. This change may also be linked to a dramatic decline in the neuronal fate-choice decision of newly generated cells [99].

NEUROGENESIS IN SGZ IN PATIENTS WITH TLE

In pediatric patients with TLE, either increased [90] or decreased [99] neurogenesis has been observed in DG. In adult TLE patients, increased neurogenesis is demonstrated in SGZ [100] and the hippocampal fissure [101]. However, careful analysis of data from adult patients suggests that the increase in neurogenesis may be due to age difference rather than seizure onset because the average age of epilepsy patients was much younger than the control group [102, 103]. No difference in neurogenesis-associated proteins in the hippocampus between TLE patients and the control group also suggests that neurogenesis may not be involved in the occurrence of spontaneously recurrent seizures or epileptogenesis [104]. Furthermore, a recent neuropathological study indicates that decreased neurogenesis in SGZ may result in mesial temporal sclerosis (MTS) and alterations of dentate gyrus granule cells [105]. It cannot be ignored that the pathological tissue from TLE patients is usually collected in the late stage of the disease. The analysis for surgical specimens may not allow us to obtain the early characteristics of neurogenesis in the epilepsy process. Therefore, there is a limitation of studies in samples from patients with TLE and it has to be very careful when we link epileptogenesis to neurogenesis in patients with TLE. Further study with better experimental designs is still needed to clarify whether increased or decreased neurogenesis occurs in patients with TLE. Factors such as age, sex, etiology, history of anti-epileptic drug usage, frequency of seizure occurrence, brain pathology of patients, and age-matched control have to be taken into consideration before the experiment is done.

Molecular Mechanisms of Neurogenesis in Epilepsy

Neurogenesis may be induced by brain damage after seizures. This is supported by in vitro study which shows that brain cell proliferation occurs after seizure-induced damage [106]. However, an in vivo experiment indicates that it is the seizure event and not hippocampal neuronal death that provokes neurogenesis, i.e., neurogenesis is independent of cell death [107], but coupled to neuronal activity. The most severe SE state may induce the most extensive neurogenesis, but the survival rate of new neurons may be the lowest at the late stages of the disease [108, 109]. As mentioned above, brain neurogenesis is regulated by various molecules including growth factors, neurotransmitters, cytokines, chemokines and their receptor systems, ion channels, EPOR, and immediate early genes. TLE-induced expression changes of these molecules may not only induce brain pathophysiological changes but also neurogenesis changes [76, 84, 106-109]. Experimental data suggest that seizure-induced upregulations of BDNF, FGF-2, and VEGF are capable of enhancing neurogenesis [110-118]. Neurotransmitters and/or neuromodulators, their receptors and related signal transduction molecules including cannabinoid system [30], GABA [119], acetylcholine, galanin type 2 receptors [120], glutamate, 5-hydroxy-tryptamine (5HT)-1A, neuropeptides, nitric oxide, opioid system, serotonin [121-124], and neuropeptide Y (NPY) via its Y1 receptor [125] or Sonic hedgehog (Shh) signaling [126], paracrine signaling molecules, bone morphogenic proteins and Sonic hedgehog; transcriptional regulators, such as cAMP response element-binding (CREB) and neuronal PAS domain protein 3; protein kinase B (Akt); stress and aging may also be involved in progenitor proliferation and neurogenesis [127]. The cysteine protease cystatin C, which is expressed on astrocytes and microglia after SE [123, 124], and hippocampal inflammation, which is commonly observed after injury, can considerably suppress dentate neurogenesis [128-131]. On the other hand, reduced production of growth factors such as FGF-2, IGF-1, BDNF, and glial cell line-derived neurotrophic factor (GDNF) may result in decreased neurogenesis [96, 132]. GDNF exhibits neurogenic effects [133, 134] and anti-convulsive properties [135]. Decreased GDNF may contribute to both reduced neurogenesis and increased frequency of epileptic attacks. Furthermore, elevated Dickkopf-1, an inhibitor of Wnt in mesial temporal lobe epilepsy (mTLE) may contribute to decreased DG neurogenesis in epilepsy as Wnt/β-catenin signaling pathway mediates TLE neurogenesis [136]. In pentylenetetrazol (PTZ) kindling model, increased neurogenesis in SGZ may be modulated by the upregulation of bone morphogenetic proteins-4 (BMP4) [137]. Ephrin-A5/EphA4 interaction plays an essential role in the suppression of neurogenesis, microvessel remodeling, and spontaneous recurrent seizures (SRS), and Ephrin-A5/EphA4 complex has been considered as a potential therapeutic target for the treatment of TLE [138]. Ephrin-B3 is involved in the regulation of Reelin signaling pathway and reduces aberrant hippocampal neurogenesis during seizures induced by pilocarpine [11]. Gadd45b is a member of the growth arrest and DNA damage protein 45 family [139]. In the adult mouse models of electroconvulsive shock and pilocarpine-induced TLE, Gadd45b induces DNA demethylation in promoter regions of BDNF and IGF-1 genes, increases the expression of BDNF and IGF-1, and thus promotes the proliferation of NPCs in DG, along with dendritic and axonal growth of neurons [140, 141]. Fragile X family of RNA-binding proteins, including fragile X mental retardation protein (FMRP), fragile X related protein 1 (FXR1P), and FXR2P, all regulate the proliferation of NSCs [142-146]. Moreover, FMRP is required for the differentiation of adult NPCs [143, 147]. Another RNA-binding protein Pumilio accelerates the degradation of its target RNA to regulate an extensive mRNA network [148]. Both in vivo and in vitro studies have demonstrated that the loss of pumilio 1 (Pum1) and Pum2 leads to impaired neurogenesis in DG, manifested by reduced proliferation and differentiation of NSCs and increased apoptosis [149]. Pum2 expression is downregulated in humans and mice with TLE [150]. Inactivation or downregulation of Pum2 may show a propensity for TLE by altering the expression of voltaged-gated sodium channels (NAV) and GABA receptor subunit alpha-2 [151, 152]. It has become clear that histone deacetylases (HDACs) may also play an important role in neurogenesis [153]. Pharmacological inhibition of HDACs reduced aberrant neurogenesis and allowed mice to avoid seizure-induced cognitive impairment in the kainic acid-induced intrahippocampal epilepsy model [154]. Due to the multiple functions of each molecule mentioned above and shared signal transduction pathways among them, therapeutic approaches should be carefully designed as targeting particular molecule to promote neurogenesis may, at the same time, exacerbate epileptic activity leading to neuronal death or induce neuropsychological problems.

Table 1. miRNAs that regulate neurogenesis involved in epileptogenesis

miRNA	Epilepsy model	Expression	Target	Effect	Reference
Let-7b	kainic acid rat model	down	STAT3	regulates glial cell activation, inflammatory response and epileptic seizure	[163]
miR-20a	pentylenetetrazole mouse model	up	RGMa	regulates synaptic plasticity, axon growth and epileptogenesis	[168]
miR-25	kainic acid rat model	down	OXSR1	attenuates neuronal apoptosis and epileptiform discharges	[173]
miR-184	kainic acid mouse model	up	unclear	attenuates neuronal apoptosis	[175]
miR-124	pilocarpine rat model and pentylenetetrazole mouse model	down	CREB	alleviates seizure severity and prolongs onset latency	[181]
	kainic acid rat model	down	NRSF	promotes microglia activation and inflammatory cytokines	[182]
miR-153	temporal cortex of TLE patients	up	HIF-1a		[185, 186]
miR-211	pilocarpine mouse model	down	TGFBR2	regulates neuronal excitability	[192]
miR-34a	lithium-pilocarpine rat model	up	unclear	promotes neuronal apoptosis	[199]
	kainic acid mouse model	up	unclear	promotes neuronal apoptosis	[203]
	mg^{2+}-free neuronal model	up	Notch	regulates epileptiform discharges and neuronal apoptosis	[204]
miR-132	lithium-pilocarpine rat model and mg^{2+}-free neuronal model	up	p250GAP	regulates frequency of spontaneous seizures, epileptiform discharges and neuronal morphology	[211, 212]
	kainic acid mouse model	up	unclear	regulates neuronal death	[213]
	electrics stimulation model and human primary astrocytes	up	unclear	promotes expression of pro-epileptogenic factor in astrocytes	[217]
miR-134	kainic acid mouse model	up	unclear	alters epileptogenesis, hippocampal toxicity and dendritic spine density	[218, 219]
	kainic acid mouse model	up	limk1	increase the frequency of SRS	[229]

Table 1. (Continued)

miRNA	Epilepsy model	Expression	Target	Effect	Reference
	kainic acid mouse model	up	tubby-like protein1	regulates neuronal excitotoxicity	[233]
	kainic acid rat model	up	CREB	promotes spontaneous seizures and neuronal death	[232]
	pilocarpine mouse model	up	unclear	alters development of SE and dendritic spine volume	[222]
	lithium-pilocarpine rat model and mg^{2+}-free neuronal model	up	limk1		[221]
	lithium-pilocarpine rat model	up	unclear	regulates neuronal death, learning and memory ability of rat	[231]
	pentylenetetrazole mouse model and perforant pathway stimulation rat model	up	unclear	promotes seizure onset and spontaneous seizures	[223]
miR-137	kainic acid mouse model	up	unclear	changes composition of NSC pool	[180]
	pilocarpine mouse model and pentylenetetrazol mouse model	down	unclear	increase seizures severity and SRS latency	[234]
miR-22	kainic acid mouse model	up	P2X7R	regulates epileptogenesis, changes morphogenesis of newborn NSC, and reduces neuroinflammation and spontaneous seizures	[242-244]

MicroRNAs as Regulators of Neurogenesis in the Adult DG and Targets for Treatment of Epilepsy

As crucial post-transcriptional regulators, microRNAs (miR) are widely involved in the regulation of epilepsy (Table 1) and neurogenesis (Figure 1). MiR-9 is highly expressed in neurogenic regions of the adult brain. Overexpression of miR-9 inhibits the TLX, resulting in the inhibition of the proliferation of neural stem cells and premature differentiation of neurons [155]. MiR-9 also regulates the expression of several key genes involved in neuronal differentiation, such as REST, CREB, and FoxO1 [156]. Work in NSCs from telencephalon of adult zebrafish has shown that with the help of shuttle protein TNRC6, miR-9 translocation to the nucleus from cytoplasm enhances Notch signal and makes NSCs in a quiescent state [157]. MiR-9 nuclear localization is also observed parallel to the activation of NSCs in adult mouse DG [157]. In view of the upregulation of miR-9 in the hippocampus during chronic TLE, it has been suggested that miR-9 may be involved in the decrease of hippocampal neurogenesis at this stage [158]. It should be noted that miR-9 regulates FoxO1 to decrease the Notch signal, and maintain the self-renewal of NSCs in SVZ of adult mice [159]. Let-7b inhibits the proliferation of NSCs from adult mice and promotes neuronal differentiation by targeting TLX [160]. It decreases at 2, 7, and even 50 days after pilocarpine-induced SE [161]. Decreased let-7b is also recognized in the hippocampus of TLE patients [162]. let-7b reduces the number of proliferating glial cells and suppresses the inflammatory response in the hippocampus of TLE by targeting STAT3 and its overexpression reduces the frequency and severity of seizures [163]. Long noncoding RNA H19, which is highly upregulated during the epileptic latency, may function as a competitive endogenous RNA to sponge let-7b. Overexpressed H19 could competitively bind to let-7b to contributes to hippocampal glial cell activation and neuronal apoptosis in TLE rats [163, 164].

MiR-17-92 cluster, composed of miR-17, miR-18a, miR-19a, miR-20a, miR-19b-1, and miR-92a [165], is highly expressed in the hippocampus of adult mice [166]. MiR-17-92 cluster targets kinase Sgk1, a downstream effector of glucocorticoid receptor signaling, to maintain the NSCs proliferation [166]. Mice with the genetic knockout of the miR-17-92 cluster exhibit a reduction of neurogenesis in DG, whereas overexpression enhances neurogenesis [167]. Ablation of the miR-17-92 cluster significantly restrains the proliferation of NSCs and neuroblasts in DG and impairs the hippocampal-dependent learning and memory ability of mice compared to wild-type mice. It is further indicated that enigma homolog 1 (ENH1) and phosphatase and tensin homolog (PTEN) may also be downstream effectors of the miR-17-92 cluster [167]. MiR-20a is a member of the miR-17-92 cluster and upregulated in the epilepsy model [168]. As a downstream target of miR-20a, repulsive guidance molecule a (RGMa) inhibits neuronal axon growth and regulates synaptic plasticity by inhibiting Rho GTPase family member A (RhoA) [168, 169]. Silencing miR-20a prevents PTZ-induced epileptogenesis through RGMa-RhoA pathway-mediated synaptic plasticity and axon growth. Moreover, although RGMa inhibits MSF in epileptogenesis, silencing miR-20a does not change MFS in the hippocampus of rats with epilepsy [168]. Unlike miR-20a, the miR-92a level is decreased in the hippocampus of mesial TLE (mTLE) patients [162]. MiR-92a controls the expression of GluA1, a subunit of AMPA receptors to regulates homeostatic synaptic scaling [170]. Furthermore, this miRNA is also a vital regulator of neuronal excitability through inhibition of some A-type voltage-gated potassium channel family members [171]. However, the specific role of miR-92a in neurogenesis in epilepsy needs to be elucidated.

MiR-106b-25 cluster is involved in adult NSCs proliferation and is predicted to interact with the insulin/IGF-foxo3 pathway [172]. MiR-25, the most important member of the miR-106b-25 cluster, promotes the proliferation of adult NSCs [173]. Along with the downregulation of miR-25-3p in the hippocampus of kainic acid-treated rats, the expression of oxidative-stress responsive 1 (OXSR1) is upregulated. MiR-25-3p attenuates apoptosis and spontaneous recurrent epileptiform discharges of primary neurons from the rat hippocampus by restricting the expression of OXSR1 [173].

MiR-184, together with its upstream Mbd1 and downstream target Numblike, forms a delicate regulatory network to maintain the balance between proliferation and differentiation of NSC in adult DG [174]. This miRNA is identified as an upregulated antiapoptotic factor in the hippocampus of epileptic mice [175]. MiR-184 inhibition significantly increased seizure-induced neuronal death in the hippocampal CA1 subfield without affecting seizure susceptibility. MiR-124, an extremely abundant miRNA in the brain, is a key factor in determining the fate of neuron and glial cells. MiR-124 could inhibit Sox9 to maintain neuronal differentiation in SVZ in adult mice [176, 177]. Knockdown of miR-124 in the SVZ confers astrocytic characteristics on neuroblasts, whereas overexpression of miR-124 promotes neuronal differentiation, culminating in depletion of the adult NSC pool with loss of neurogenesis [178]. A study of embryonic stem cell neurogenesis in mice has shown reduced STAT3 phosphorylation by miR-124, which drives neuroblasts to progress to neuronal development rather than in glial cells [179]. Therefore, miR-124 downregulation in epilepsy patients, mice, rats may be an underlying mechanism for the unbalanced number of glial cells and neurons after SE [180]. Indeed, the therapeutic efficacy varies when targeting miR-124 to treat SE. Preemptive intrahippocampal supplementation with miR-124 mimics suppresses CREB1 expression and attenuates the epileptic effect [181]. Analogous to miR-9, miR-124 can interact with NRSF/REST to drive neuronal differentiation of NSCs [156, 182]. However, although miR-124 could suppress the expression of NRSF that promotes epileptogenesis [182, 183], increased miR-124 does not affect the seizure frequency and severity after kainic acid-induced spontaneous seizures in rats. Intrahippocampal administration of synthetic miR-124, on the other hand, enhances microglial activation and inflammatory factors [182]. Thus, neuroinflammation may antagonize the seizure reduction resulting from NRSF downregulation.

MiR-153 regulates the Notch signaling pathway by simultaneously targeting both Jagged1 and Hey2, thereby inhibiting gliogenesis and promoting neurogenesis [184]. Overexpression of miR-153 attenuates aging-related cognitive impairments by enhancing hippocampus-dependent neurogenesis. Analysis of surgical specimens from the temporal cortex of TLE patients attests that miR-153 expression is reduced [185, 186]. Thus, it is speculated that increased miR-153 may ameliorate cognitive impairment caused by reduced DG neurogenesis in TLE. Many studies indicate that overexpressed hypoxia-inducible factor-1α (HIF-1α) may be a risk factor for multidrug resistance in epilepsy [186-188]. HIF-1α is a direct target of miR-153, and decreased miR-153 in the TLE promotes HIF-1α expression [185, 186].

Knockdown of miR-211 significantly reduced neurons undergoing differentiation and maturation in DG of adult rats [189]. Studies on primary cortical neuron culture also show that miR-211-5p ameliorates aberrant neurite outgrowth and branching through targeting NUAK1, an AMPK-related kinase [190]. The expression of miR-211 is downregulated in pilocarpine-induced epilepsy models [191, 192]. Dynamic expression of miR-211 in the mouse forebrain enhances spontaneous seizures and neuronal excitability [192]. This change in excitability thresholds may be mediated by miR-211 through regulation of transforming growth factor-beta receptor type 2 (TGFBR2) signaling and cholinergic synapse pathways, as well as expression of another excitatory miRNA, miR-134.

MiR-34a targets multiple genes expression to regulate differentiation and maturation of NPCs isolated from embryonic brain, including SIRT1 [193], Numblike [194], syntaxin 1a [195], synaptotagmin 1 [195, 196], autophagy-related protein 9a [196], DCX [197], and cyclin D1 [198]. Overexpression of miR-34a utilizing recombinant adenoviral vectors in the adult rat DG promotes precursor cell proliferation and maturation, and rats also consequently exhibit better task-dependent learning and memory abilities [197]. In addition, elevated miR-34a restricts dendritic growth and alters the morphology of dendritic spines [194, 195, 197]. MiR-34a, identified as a pro-apoptotic miRNA regulated by P53, is upregulated in epileptic models [199, 200]. However, miRNA profiles for the neocortex and hippocampus from patients with mTLE showed the downregulation of miR-34a [201, 202]. Targeting miR-34a after SE reduces the level of activated caspase-3 and resists apoptosis in hippocampal neurons [199, 203]. Overexpression of miR-34a also inhibits apoptosis and suppresses epileptiform discharges in rat hippocampal neurons treated with Mg^{2+}-free medium, which the Notch signal may mediate [204]. However, intrahippocampal injection of miR-34a antagomirs before SE does not show a neuroprotective effect, although it reduces the upregulation of miR-34a in CA3 and CA1 in epileptic mouse hippocampus [203]. Given these controversial results and the different expression patterns of miR-34a in epileptic animals and humans, more detailed studies to clarify the role of miR-34a in the treatment of epilepsy are necessary.

MiR-132 expression is induced by CREB downstream of neuronal activity [205, 206]. Accumulating evidence suggests that miR-132 targets p250GAP to regulate dendritic growth, dendritic spine formation, and integration of newborn neurons in the adult DG [207-210]. MiR-132 inhibition in adult mouse or rat models of epilepsy presents anti-epileptogenic effects, as evidenced by the decreased frequency of spontaneous seizures in the chronic stage, the reduced abnormal dendritic spine formation, and the suppression of neuronal death in the hippocampal CA3 subfield [211-213]. The role of miR-132 in enhancing the differentiation of hippocampal neurons has been verified from animal to cell level [214]. MiR-132 overexpression in NSCs in the adult DG promotes the differentiation of NSCs. However, recent studies show that miR-132 inhibits neuronal differentiation and promotes glial cell differentiation and neurite growth [215, 216]. As mentioned earlier, MeCP2 is highly expressed and functions during neuronal maturation. Indeed, MeCP2 is the downstream target of miR-132. MiR-132 overexpression decreases MeCP2 in NSCs, which enhances glial differentiation [216]. As one of the most commonly upregulated miRNAs in animal models of epilepsy, miR-132 has recently been found to be increased in reactive glial cells in the human epileptogenic hippocampus

[217]. More importantly, human primary astrocytes transfected with miR-132 showed reduced expression of pro-epileptogenic cyclooxygenase-2 (COX-2), interleukin-1β (IL-1β), transforming growth factor-β2 (TGF-β2), C-C motif chemokine ligand 2 (CCl2), and metalloproteinases 3 (MMP3). Thus, targeting astrocytes miR-132 might ameliorate epilepsy severity by inhibiting the generation of pro-inflammatory and extracellular matrix factors.

Expression of miR-134 is elevated in a variety of experimental epilepsy models [218-223], which is also confirmed in the transcriptional analysis of hippocampal tissue and cerebral cortex obtained from TLE patients [219, 220, 223]. The anti-epileptic effect of inhibiting miR-134 expression has been established in many models in which seizures are triggered through different mechanisms. Dendritic spines are major contact points for excitatory synaptic transmission in the brain, and dendritic reorganization may influence seizures [224]. The activity-dependent miR-134 is enriched in dendrites under the mediation of BDNF [225], where it modulates synaptic homeostasis in the hippocampus by targeting CREB [226], promotes dendritogenesis by targeting pum2 and LIM domain kinase 1 (limk1) [227, 228], and increases the size of the dendritic spine by targeting limk. Reducing limk1 level in vivo increases the frequency of SRS in miR-134 antagomirs treated SE mice, implying partial abrogation of the anti-seizure phenotype of miR-134 antagomirs [229]. Thus, silencing miR-134 suppresses seizures in part by decreasing the density of the pyramidal neuron spine and increasing the spine volume in the hippocampus [219, 222]. There are also different experimental models to support neuroprotective effects from inhibition of miR-134. Inhibiting miR-134 with lentivirus in cultured hippocampal neurons relieves SE-like electrographic activity and decreases SE-induced neuronal death significantly [230]. Intracranial injection of miR-134 antagomirs rescues neuronal death in CA3 and CA1 areas of the hippocampus and reduces the expression of apoptosis-related Bim proteins and cytoplasmic cytochrome C after SE [218, 219, 231, 232]. Moreover, miR-134 antagomirs also ameliorate oxidative stress [231] and endoplasmic reticulum stress [232], reduce MFS [232] and astrogliosis [219], and may increase vulnerability to excitotoxicity [233] in the hippocampus of the Sprague-Dawley rat epilepsy model. In short, current data suggest that the inhibition of miR-134 may prevent epileptogenesis.

MiR-137 is abundant in the CNS, especially in the molecular layer of DG [234]. MiR-137 promotes the proliferation of adult NSCs by acting synergistically with epigenetic regulators, including lysine specific demethylase 1 (LSD1), MeCP2, and Ezh2, and negatively regulates dendritic branching and phenotype maturation during neuronal differentiation [156, 235]. The expression pattern of miR-137 is yet inconclusive in the DG of the TLE animal model. During the acute phase of kainic acid-induced SE in mice, the expression of miR-137 is increased [236, 237]. Inhibition of miR-137 using miR-137 antimicrorna oligonucleotides (miR-137 AMOs) partially corrects the aberrant composition of the NSC pool in DG and suppresses the excessive proliferation of reactive neuroblasts [180]. The simultaneous application of miR-124 Amos enhances this neuroprotective effect against TLE [180]. However, miR-137 is down-regulated in the long term after pilocarpine or electrically induced SE [234, 238, 239]. Overexpression of miR-137 inhibits neuronal excitability by regulating presynaptic neurotransmission, which in turn prolongs the latency of SE in pilocarpine-induced TLE mice and reduces the severity of epilepsy [234].

MiR-22 lengthens the cell cycle and regulates cell migration during neurogenesis [240, 241]. In the mouse model with unilateral microinjection of kainic acid into the amygdala, miR-22 is elevated in the DG along with abnormal neurogenesis in the bilateral hippocampus [242]. Inhibition of miR-22 exacerbates this abnormal neurogenesis, which is not limited to the increase in the number of newborn neurons but also involves the changes in the migration pathways of newborn neurons, reduction in the complexity of the dendritic tree, and increase in the volume and density of dendritic spines. Notably, the modulation of neuroinflammation by miR-22 is dramatically involved in the pathology of TLE. MiR-22 restrains the development of bilateral hippocampal epileptic foci by suppressing purinergic P2X7 receptors (P2X7R) [243] and TLE mice with gene ablation of miR-22 present more severe SE [244]. However, RNA-Seq reveals extensive downregulation of inflammatory signaling pathways by miR-22 deletion, contrary to the pathogenicity of neuroinflammation [244]. Therefore, it should be cautious when using miR-22 and its downstream pathways as therapeutic targets for the treatment of epilepsy.

NEUROGENESIS, EPILEPTOGENESIS AND COGNITION IN EPILEPSY

Extensive experimental studies suggest that newly generated aberrant or ectopic granule cells may be involved in epileptogenesis. Seizure-induced DGCs in epileptogenesis form recurrent excitatory circuits with neighboring granule cells through axonal sprouting or abnormal basal dendrite formation. Research over the last decades has emphasized that this pathological change may lead to hyperexcitability of the dentate gyrus [245-249]. Similarly, using rabies virus-mediated retrograde tracing technology, Zhu et al. recently found that newborn DGCs participated in the formation of excitatory synaptic connections and repetitive excitatory circuits with other DGCs [94]. Granule cells ectopically migrating into the hilus are characterized by hyperexcitability in rodent models and tissue resected from patients with TLE and discharge spontaneous bursts of action potentials which are synchronized with CA3 pyramidal cell population discharges leading to epileptic activity [83, 250, 251]. Finally, by selectively deleting phosphatase and tensin homolog in newborn DGCs of the mouse, Pun et al. induced abnormal morphology of newborn DGCs similar to those in epilepsy, which is sufficient to lead to SRS in an intact mouse [252].

Compared with the above morphological and electrophysiological studies, the application of chemogenetic methods in living epilepsy models allows specific manipulation of neuronal activity without altering circuit anatomy [253]. An initial study using this approach strongly supported the vital role of newborn DGCS in the formation and function of hippocampal excitatory circuits [94]. Selective silencing of newborn DGCs significantly reduced the frequency of epileptic spikes and SRS, whereas activating newborn DGCs produced precisely the reverse effect. Similarly, combining chemogenetic approaches with mono-synaptic tracers, Lybrand et al. showed that aberrant neurogenesis caused hippocampal circuit remodeling exacerbating epilepsy in mice [95]. Silencing aberrant newborn DGCs reduced SRS and histopathological features of epilepsy, including abnormal dendritic morphology and ectopic DGCs. Furthermore, similar bidirectional manipulation of epileptic-related newborn granule cells also revealed that cognition impairment is closely associated with abnormal newborn granule cells [254].

However, the relationship between neurogenesis and epileptogenesis is still in controversy. Conceivably, if newborn granule cells do contribute to epileptogenesis, eliminating these cells or blocking granule cell production should be protective. In fact, by blocking neurogenesis with pharmacological methods or ionizing radiation, earlier studies have demonstrated conflicting results [125, 255-260]. The inhibition of neurogenesis does not lead to complete seizures remission or pathological improvement; a considerable proportion of the findings suggest a harmless or even protective effect of newborn granule cells on hippocampal network function. Since pharmacological inhibition has certain off-target effects and ionizing radiation has the potential to induce neuroinflammation, conditionally induced transgenic mouse models with temporal and cellular specificity have been employed in subsequent studies [261, 262]. Ablation of newborn granule cells just before or following pilocarpine-induced SE significantly reduces SRS frequency and improves cognition. A recent study reported that prolonging the elimination of aberrant neurogenesis to 4 weeks following SE reduced SRS formation by 65% [263]. However, by reducing neurogenesis with deleting the transcription factor NeuroD1 in NSC, Brulet et al. did not observe a reduction in pilocarpine-induced SRS compared with control mice [264]. The factor that spontaneously recurrent seizures occur much earlier before newly generated neurons being integrated into the brain neural circuits indicates that epileptogenesis may be independent of neurogenesis [265-268]. This is supported by other observations which show reduced neurogenesis in animal models and patients with TLE [97-99, 105]. Furthermore, drastic pathological changes in the hippocampus, including gliosis, sclerosis, synaptic reorganization, increased total wall thickness of microvessels, and inflammation at the late stages of TLE may significantly change the neurogenic niches, leading to the impairment of neurogenesis [269]. It may explain why consistent atrophy instead of hypertrophy of the hippocampus occurs in animal models and patients with TLE, in particular, at the advanced stages of the disease. Other functional and pathological changes of granular cells also suggest that reduced neurogenesis may play an important role in epileptogenesis [270-276].

In a normal hippocampus, newly generated neurons in DG are integrated into the hippocampal circuitry and play important roles in learning and memory [277]. Neuroanatomical studies showed that these neurons sent axons to the CA3 area, and meanwhile, they received inputs mainly from the entorhinal cortex [278-280]. Functional studies indicated that newly generated neurons exhibited similar electrophysiological characteristics to the existing granule cells [281], responded to hippocampus-dependent learning tasks [282], and survived for prolonged periods [283]. When dividing cells in DG were experimentally eliminated, an animal had reduced learning ability [284]. Environmental enrichment could induce neurogenesis [50]. It is understandable that characteristic neuropathological changes of the hippocampus may lead to the impairment of cognition. This is supported by data from patients with TLE [59, 285-293] and from various animal models of TLE [294-303]. In animal models, cognitive deficits differ among animal strains and ages, and worsen as a function of the cumulative number of seizures. It is likely to progress even if seizures are controlled. The hippocampal-dependent cognitive deficits may also be linked to diminished dentate neurogenesis [304-306]. A failure of neurogenesis in the adult DG has also been associated with depression [307]. In patients with TLE, it remains to be determined whether a therapeutic approach by promoting brain neurogenesis could significantly improve learning and memory.

FUTURE RESEARCH DIRECTIONS IN TEMPORAL LOBE EPILEPSY

Extensive neurophathological changes of the brain from patients and animal models of TLE suggest that systemic study of pan-brain reorganized neural circuits or connectome may be a cornerstone for understanding the neurobiological mechanism of epileptogenesis [4, 308]. By tracing the fate of newly generated neurons, the synaptic connections these neurons established with surviving neurons in pathological brain regions, the electrical connections or gap junctions between newly generated neurons and glial cells, combined with the functional study of the roles of the newly established neural circuits in epileptogenesis, we may provide new evidence to support neurogenesis in epileptogenesis. Given that numerous signaling pathways have been involved in physiological neurogenesis, further studies may be needed to clarify which and how each of these pathways directly or indirectly mediates epileptogenesis. The results from these studies will provide valuable clues for the development of clinical treatments for epilepsy by targeting these molecular pathways.

Epileptogenesis is associated with a wide range of brain changes, including but not limited to aberrant neurogenesis, loss of granule cells, activated glial cells, and inflammatory responses. Abnormal neurogenesis may be one of the many inducers of epileptogenesis. Targeting only this single pathological change may be difficult to achieve practical efficacy on epileptogenesis. Therefore, it is urgent to focus on the role of other pathological alterations in epileptogenesis and seizure susceptibility. Astrocytes modulate neuronal activityand synaptic transmission by gliotransmission and they probably set the tone for neuronal activity and determine the sphere of influenced neurons since neuro-glial interaction exists. Astrocytes give rise to new neurons in the adult mammalian hippocampus [309], induce neurogenesis from adult neural stem cells [310], and may even serve as adult neural stem cells [311]. Therefore, further investigation of astrocytes in neurogenesis and epileptogenesis, in particular, induction of astrocyte-like neural stem cells to differentiate into neurons, will undoubtedly shed light on understanding the mechanism of neurogenesis in epileptogenesis and for designing cell therapy to control TLE. Acquired channelopathy (A-type potassium ion channels) is likely to amplify neuronal activity and may contribute to the initiation and/or propagation of seizures in TLE [312]; whether channelopathy occurs in newly generated neurons to initiate SRS may be another interesting area to explore. Cascades of inflammation cause hyperexcitability or seizures, leading to neuronal death, which in turn activates microglia and astrocytes. These glial cells produce pro-inflammatory cytokines and chemokine, which induces leukocyte-endothelium interactions and subsequent leukocyte recruitment in the brain parenchyma. Pro-inflammatory cytokines and chemokine have now been considered to play important roles in epileptogenesis as inhibition of brain inflammation could attenuate SRS [313]. Further investigation of the roles of the pro-inflammatory and anti-inflammatory cytokines and chemokines in neurogenesis and epileptogenesis may provide clues to develop new anti-inflammatory approaches to promote neurogenesis and prevent epileptogenesis. The number of progenitor cells in SVZ is much more than those in SGZ. With the neuronal loss in different brain regions in TLE and mogration of newly generated neurons from SVZ to pathological foci, focusing on the synaptic connections and pathophysiological changes of newly generated neurons from SVZ may provide novel clues for understanding the mechanism of epileptogenesis and for prevention of epileptogenesis by promoting newly generated neurons to migrate to pathological foci. Current studies have identified multiple differentially expressed miRNAs in animal models and patients with epilepsy. These miRNAs play important roles in seizure susceptibility and seizure-associated pathological changes such as abnormal neurogenesis, neuroinflammation, and apoptosis. Since targeting miRNAs has reduced TLE-related neuropathological changes and epileptic activitires in the animal models, further study in patients with TLE may shed light on targeting miRNAs to effectively control intractable TLE.

REFERENCES

[1] Altman, J. 1962. Are new neurons formed in the brains of adult mammals? *Science.* 135(3509), 1127-8.

[2] Eriksson, P.S., Perfilieva, E., Bjork-Eriksson, T., Alborn, A.M., Nordborg, C., Peterson, D.A., Gage, F.H. 1998. Neurogenesis in the adult human hippocampus. *Nat Med.* 4(11), 1313-7.

[3] Hastings, N.B., & Gould, E. 1999. Rapid extension of axons into the CA3 region by adult-generated granule cells. *J Comp Neurol.* 413(1), 146-54.

[4] Seri, B., Garcia-Verdugo, J.M., McEwen, B.S., Alvarez-Buylla, A. 2001. Astrocytes give rise to new neurons in the adult mammalian hippocampus. *J Neurosci.* 21(18), 7153-60.

[5] Ge, S., Goh, E.L., Sailor, K.A., Kitabatake, Y., Ming, G.L., Song, H. 2006. GABA regulates synaptic integration of newly generated neurons in the adult brain. *Nature.* 439(7076), 589-93.

[6] Ramirez-Amaya, V., Marrone, D.F., Gage, F.H., Worley, P.F., Barnes, C.A. 2006. Integration of new neurons into functional neural networks. *J Neurosci.* 26(47), 12237-41.

[7] Rikani, A.A., Choudhry, Z., Choudhry, A.M., Zenonos, G., Tariq, S., Mobassarah, N.J. 2013. Spatially regulated adult neurogenesis. *Ann Neurosci.* 20(2), 67-70.

[8] Ma, D.K., Ming, G.L., Song, H. 2005. Glial influences on neural stem cell development: cellular niches for adult neurogenesis. *Curr Opin Neurobiol.* 15(5), 514-20.

[9] Palmer, T.D., Willhoite, A.R., Gage, F.H. 2000. Vascular niche for adult hippocampal neurogenesis. *J Comp Neurol.* 425(4), 479-94.

[10] Falk, S., & Gotz, M. 2017. Glial control of neurogenesis. *Curr Opin Neurobiol.* 47, 188-195.

[11] Liu, T.T., Li, Y., Shu, Y., Xiao, B., Feng, L. 2018. Ephrinb3 modulates hippocampal neurogenesis and the reelin signaling pathway in a pilocarpineinduced model of epilepsy. *Int J Mol Med.* 41(6), 3457-3467.

[12] Li, X., Barkho, B.Z., Luo, Y., Smrt, R.D., Santistevan, N.J., Liu, C., Kuwabara, T., Gage, F.H., Zhao, X. 2008. Epigenetic regulation of the stem cell mitogen Fgf-2 by Mbd1 in adult neural stem/progenitor cells. *J Biol Chem.* 283(41), 27644-27652.

[13] Arredondo, S.B., Valenzuela-Bezanilla, D., Mardones, M.D., Varela-Nallar, L. 2020. Role of Wnt Signaling in Adult Hippocampal Neurogenesis in Health and Disease. *Front Cell Dev Biol.* 8, 860.

[14] Ferreira, F.F., Ribeiro, F.F., Rodrigues, R.S., Sebastiao, A.M., Xapelli, S. 2018. Brain-Derived Neurotrophic Factor (BDNF) Role in Cannabinoid-Mediated Neurogenesis. *Front Cell Neurosci.* 12, 441.

[15] Fournier, N.M., Lee, B., Banasr, M., Elsayed, M., Duman, R.S. 2012. Vascular endothelial growth factor regulates adult hippocampal cell proliferation through MEK/ERK- and PI3K/Akt-dependent signaling. *Neuropharmacology.* 63(4), 642-52.

[16] Han, J., Calvo, C.F., Kang, T.H., Baker, K.L., Park, J.H., Parras, C., Levittas, M., Birba, U., Pibouin-Fragner, L., Fragner, P., Bilguvar, K., Duman, R.S., Nurmi, H., Alitalo, K., Eichmann, A.C., Thomas, J.L. 2015. Vascular endothelial growth factor receptor 3 controls neural stem cell activation in mice and humans. *Cell Rep.* 10(7), 1158-72.

[17] Nieto-Estevez, V., Oueslati-Morales, C.O., Li, L., Pickel, J., Morales, A.V., Vicario-Abejon, C. 2016. Brain Insulin-Like Growth Factor-I Directs the Transition from Stem Cells to Mature Neurons During Postnatal/Adult Hippocampal Neurogenesis. *Stem Cells.* 34(8), 2194-209.

[18] Zhou, Y., Bond, A.M., Shade, J.E., Zhu, Y., Davis, C.O., Wang, X., Su, Y., Yoon, K.J., Phan, A.T., Chen, W.J., Oh, J.H., Marsh-Armstrong, N., Atabai, K., Ming, G.L., Song, H. 2018. Autocrine Mfge8 Signaling Prevents Developmental Exhaustion of the Adult Neural Stem Cell Pool. *Cell Stem Cell.* 23(3), 444-452 e4.

[19] Lie, D.C., Colamarino, S.A., Song, H.J., Desire, L., Mira, H., Consiglio, A., Lein, E.S., Jessberger, S., Lansford, H., Dearie, A.R., Gage, F.H. 2005. Wnt signalling regulates adult hippocampal neurogenesis. *Nature.* 437(7063), 1370-5.

[20] Androutsellis-Theotokis, A., Leker, R.R., Soldner, F., Hoeppner, D.J., Ravin, R., Poser, S.W., Rueger, M.A., Bae, S.K., Kittappa, R., McKay, R.D. 2006. Notch signalling regulates stem cell numbers in vitro and in vivo. *Nature.* 442(7104), 823-6.

[21] Frontiers Production, O. 2015. Erratum on: Neurogenesis in the embryonic and adult brain: same regulators, different roles. *Front Cell Neurosci.* 9, 160.

[22] Urban, N., van den Berg, D.L., Forget, A., Andersen, J., Demmers, J.A., Hunt, C., Ayrault, O., Guillemot, F. 2016. Return to quiescence of mouse neural stem cells by degradation of a proactivation protein. *Science.* 353(6296), 292-5.

[23] Zhang, R., Boareto, M., Engler, A., Louvi, A., Giachino, C., Iber, D., Taylor, V. 2019. Id4 Downstream of Notch2 Maintains Neural Stem Cell Quiescence in the Adult Hippocampus. *Cell Rep.* 28(6), 1485-1498 e6.

[24] Blomfield, I.M., Rocamonde, B., Masdeu, M.D.M., Mulugeta, E., Vaga, S., van den Berg, D.L., Huillard, E., Guillemot, F., Urban, N. 2019. *Id4 promotes the elimination of the pro-activation factor Ascl1 to maintain quiescence of adult hippocampal stem cells.* Elife. 8.

[25] Goncalves, J.T., Schafer, S.T., Gage, F.H. 2016. Adult Neurogenesis in the Hippocampus: From Stem Cells to Behavior. *Cell.* 167(4), 897-914.

[26] Bhattacharyya, B.J., Banisadr, G., Jung, H., Ren, D., Cronshaw, D.G., Zou, Y., Miller, R.J. 2008. The chemokine stromal cell-

derived factor-1 regulates GABAergic inputs to neural progenitors in the postnatal dentate gyrus. *J Neurosci.* 28(26), 6720-30.

[27] Waterhouse, E.G., An, J.J., Orefice, L.L., Baydyuk, M., Liao, G.Y., Zheng, K., Lu, B., Xu, B. 2012. BDNF promotes differentiation and maturation of adult-born neurons through GABAergic transmission. *J Neurosci.* 32(41), 14318-30.

[28] Jiao, J., & Chen, D.F. 2008. Induction of neurogenesis in nonconventional neurogenic regions of the adult central nervous system by niche astrocyte-produced signals. *Stem Cells.* 26(5), 1221-30.

[29] Cai, W., Carlson, S.W., Brelsfoard, J.M., Mannon, C.E., Moncman, C.L., Saatman, K.E., Andres, D.A. 2012. Rit GTPase signaling promotes immature hippocampal neuronal survival. *J Neurosci.* 32(29), 9887-97.

[30] Andres-Mach, M., Zagaja, M., Haratym-Maj, A., Rola, R., Maj, M., Haratym, J., Dudra-Jastrzebska, M., Luszczki, J.J. 2017. A Long-Term Treatment with Arachidonyl-2'-Chloroethylamide Combined with Valproate Increases Neurogenesis in a Mouse Pilocarpine Model of Epilepsy. *Int J Mol Sci.* 18(5).

[31] Palazuelos, J., Ortega, Z., Diaz-Alonso, J., Guzman, M., Galve-Roperh, I. 2012. CB2 cannabinoid receptors promote neural progenitor cell proliferation via mTORC1 signaling. *J Biol Chem.* 287(2), 1198-209.

[32] Oddi, S., Scipioni, L., Maccarrone, M. 2020. Endocannabinoid system and adult neurogenesis: a focused review. *Curr Opin Pharmacol.* 50, 25-32.

[33] Mensching, L., Djogo, N., Keller, C., Rading, S., Karsak, M. 2019. Stable Adult Hippocampal Neurogenesis in Cannabinoid Receptor CB2 Deficient Mice. *Int J Mol Sci.* 20(15).

[34] Thiel, G. 2013. How Sox2 maintains neural stem cell identity. *Biochem J.* 450(3), e1-2.

[35] Wang, Y., Lin, L., Lai, H., Parada, L.F., Lei, L. 2013. Transcription factor Sox11 is essential for both embryonic and adult neurogenesis. *Dev Dyn.* 242(6), 638-53.

[36] Nacher, J., Varea, E., Miguel Blasco-Ibanez, J., Gomez-Climent, M.A., Castillo-Gomez, E., Crespo, C., Martinez-Guijarro, F.J., McEwen, B.S. 2007. N-methyl-d-aspartate receptor expression during adult neurogenesis in the rat dentate gyrus. *Neuroscience.* 144(3), 855-64.

[37] Xiao, X.L., Ma, D.L., Wu, J., Tang, F.R. 2013. Metabotropic glutamate receptor 5 (mGluR5) regulates proliferation and differentiation of neuronal progenitors in the developmental hippocampus. *Brain Res.* 1493, 1-12.

[38] Andersen, J., Urban, N., Achimastou, A., Ito, A., Simic, M., Ullom, K., Martynoga, B., Lebel, M., Goritz, C., Frisen, J., Nakafuku, M., Guillemot, F. 2014. A transcriptional mechanism integrating inputs from extracellular signals to activate hippocampal stem cells. *Neuron.* 83(5), 1085-97.

[39] Li, E., Kim, Y., Kim, S., Sato, T., Kojima, M., Park, S. 2014. Ghrelin stimulates proliferation, migration and differentiation of neural progenitors from the subventricular zone in the adult mice. *Exp Neurol.* 252, 75-84.

[40] Zhang, J., Ji, F., Liu, Y., Lei, X., Li, H., Ji, G., Yuan, Z., Jiao, J. 2014. Ezh2 regulates adult hippocampal neurogenesis and memory. *J Neurosci.* 34(15), 5184-99.

[41] Jobe, E.M., Gao, Y., Eisinger, B.E., Mladucky, J.K., Giuliani, C.C., Kelnhofer, L.E., Zhao, X. 2017. Methyl-CpG-Binding Protein MBD1 Regulates Neuronal Lineage Commitment through Maintaining Adult Neural Stem Cell Identity. *J Neurosci.* 37(3), 523-536.

[42] Sun, Y., Gao, Y., Tidei, J.J., Shen, M., Hoang, J.T., Wagner, D.F., Zhao, X. 2019. Loss of MeCP2 in immature neurons leads to impaired network integration. *Hum Mol Genet.* 28(2), 245-257.

[43] Kempermann, G., & Gage, F.H. 2002. Genetic influence on phenotypic differentiation in adult hippocampal neurogenesis. *Brain Res Dev Brain Res.* 134(1-2), 1-12.

[44] Hagg, T. 2005. Molecular regulation of adult CNS neurogenesis: an integrated view. *Trends Neurosci.* 28(11), 589-95.

[45] Faigle, R., & Song, H. 2013. Signaling mechanisms regulating adult neural stem cells and neurogenesis. *Biochim Biophys Acta.* 1830(2), 2435-48.

[46] Cameron, H.A., & Gould, E. 1994. Adult neurogenesis is regulated by adrenal steroids in the dentate gyrus. *Neuroscience.* 61(2), 203-9.

[47] Kuhn, H.G., Dickinson-Anson, H., Gage, F.H. 1996. Neurogenesis in the dentate gyrus of the adult rat: age-related decrease of neuronal progenitor proliferation. *J Neurosci.* 16(6), 2027-33.

[48] Cameron, H.A., & McKay, R.D. 1999. Restoring production of hippocampal neurons in old age. *Nat Neurosci.* 2(10), 894-7.

[49] Kempermann, G. 2002. Regulation of adult hippocampal neurogenesis - implications for novel theories of major depression. *Bipolar Disord.* 4(1), 17-33.

[50] Kempermann, G., Kuhn, H.G., Gage, F.H. 1997. More hippocampal neurons in adult mice living in an enriched environment. *Nature.* 386(6624), 493-5.

[51] Nilsson, M., Perfilieva, E., Johansson, U., Orwar, O., Eriksson, P.S. 1999. Enriched environment increases neurogenesis in the adult rat dentate gyrus and improves spatial memory. *J Neurobiol.* 39(4), 569-78.

[52] Brown, J., Cooper-Kuhn, C.M., Kempermann, G., Van Praag, H., Winkler, J., Gage, F.H., Kuhn, H.G. 2003. Enriched environment and physical activity stimulate hippocampal but not olfactory bulb neurogenesis. *Eur J Neurosci.* 17(10), 2042-6.

[53] van Praag, H., Christie, B.R., Sejnowski, T.J., Gage, F.H. 1999. Running enhances neurogenesis, learning, and long-term potentiation in mice. *Proc Natl Acad Sci U S A.* 96(23), 13427-31.

[54] van Praag, H., Kempermann, G., Gage, F.H. 1999. Running increases cell proliferation and neurogenesis in the adult mouse dentate gyrus. *Nat Neurosci.* 2(3), 266-70.

[55] Fabel, K., Fabel, K., Tam, B., Kaufer, D., Baiker, A., Simmons, N., Kuo, C.J., Palmer, T.D. 2003. VEGF is necessary for exercise-

induced adult hippocampal neurogenesis. *Eur J Neurosci.* 18(10), 2803-12.

[56] Cao, L., Jiao, X., Zuzga, D.S., Liu, Y., Fong, D.M., Young, D., During, M.J. 2004. VEGF links hippocampal activity with neurogenesis, learning and memory. *Nat Genet.* 36(8), 827-35.

[57] Pereira, A.C., Huddleston, D.E., Brickman, A.M., Sosunov, A.A., Hen, R., McKhann, G.M., Sloan, R., Gage, F.H., Brown, T.R., Small, S.A. 2007. An in vivo correlate of exercise-induced neurogenesis in the adult dentate gyrus. *Proc Natl Acad Sci U S A.* 104(13), 5638-43.

[58] Gould, E., Beylin, A., Tanapat, P., Reeves, A., Shors, T.J. 1999. Learning enhances adult neurogenesis in the hippocampal formation. *Nat Neurosci.* 2(3), 260-5.

[59] Rausch, R. 2002. Epilepsy surgery within the temporal lobe and its short-term and long-term effects on memory. *Curr Opin Neurol.* 15(2), 185-9.

[60] Leuner, B., Mendolia-Loffredo, S., Kozorovitskiy, Y., Samburg, D., Gould, E., Shors, T.J. 2004. Learning enhances the survival of new neurons beyond the time when the hippocampus is required for memory. *J Neurosci.* 24(34), 7477-81.

[61] Fuchs, E., & Gould, E. 2000. Mini-review: in vivo neurogenesis in the adult brain: regulation and functional implications. *Eur J Neurosci.* 12(7), 2211-4.

[62] Duman, R.S., Malberg, J., Nakagawa, S. 2001. Regulation of adult neurogenesis by psychotropic drugs and stress. *J Pharmacol Exp Ther.* 299(2), 401-7.

[63] Eisch, A.J., Barrot, M., Schad, C.A., Self, D.W., Nestler, E.J. 2000. Opiates inhibit neurogenesis in the adult rat hippocampus. *Proc Natl Acad Sci U S A.* 97(13), 7579-84.

[64] Di Rocco, G., Baldari, S., Pani, G., Toietta, G. 2019. Stem cells under the influence of alcohol: effects of ethanol consumption on stem/progenitor cells. *Cell Mol Life Sci.* 76(2), 231-244.

[65] Houser, C.R., Swartz, B.E., Walsh, G.O., Delgado-Escueta, A.V. 1992. Granule cell disorganization in the dentate gyrus: possible

alterations of neuronal migration in human temporal lobe epilepsy. *Epilepsy Res Suppl.* 9, 41-8; discussion 48-9.

[66] Houser, C.R. 1990. Granule cell dispersion in the dentate gyrus of humans with temporal lobe epilepsy. *Brain Res.* 535(2), 195-204.

[67] O'Connor, W.M., Masukawa, L., Freese, A., Sperling, M.R., French, J.A., O'Connor, M.J. 1996. Hippocampal cell distributions in temporal lobe epilepsy: a comparison between patients with and without an early risk factor. *Epilepsia.* 37(5), 440-9.

[68] de Lanerolle, N.C., Kim, J.H., Robbins, R.J., Spencer, D.D. 1989. Hippocampal interneuron loss and plasticity in human temporal lobe epilepsy. *Brain Res.* 495(2), 387-95.

[69] Sutula, T., Cascino, G., Cavazos, J., Parada, I., Ramirez, L. 1989. Mossy fiber synaptic reorganization in the epileptic human temporal lobe. *Ann Neurol.* 26(3), 321-30.

[70] Babb, T.L., Kupfer, W.R., Pretorius, J.K., Crandall, P.H., Levesque, M.F. 1991. Synaptic reorganization by mossy fibers in human epileptic fascia dentata. *Neuroscience.* 42(2), 351-63.

[71] Represa, A., & Ben-Ari, Y. 1992. Kindling is associated with the formation of novel mossy fibre synapses in the CA3 region. *Exp Brain Res.* 92(1), 69-78.

[72] Isokawa, M., Levesque, M.F., Babb, T.L., Engel, J., Jr. 1993. Single mossy fiber axonal systems of human dentate granule cells studied in hippocampal slices from patients with temporal lobe epilepsy. *J Neurosci.* 13(4), 1511-22.

[73] Franck, J.E., Pokorny, J., Kunkel, D.D., Schwartzkroin, P.A. 1995. Physiologic and morphologic characteristics of granule cell circuitry in human epileptic hippocampus. *Epilepsia.* 36(6), 543-58.

[74] Okazaki, M.M., Evenson, D.A., Nadler, J.V. 1995. Hippocampal mossy fiber sprouting and synapse formation after status epilepticus in rats: visualization after retrograde transport of biocytin. *J Comp Neurol.* 352(4), 515-34.

[75] Van der Zee, C.E., Rashid, K., Le, K., Moore, K.A., Stanisz, J., Diamond, J., Racine, R.J., Fahnestock, M. 1995. Intraventricular

administration of antibodies to nerve growth factor retards kindling and blocks mossy fiber sprouting in adult rats. *J Neurosci.* 15(7 Pt 2), 5316-23.

[76] Parent, J.M., Yu, T.W., Leibowitz, R.T., Geschwind, D.H., Sloviter, R.S., Lowenstein, D.H. 1997. Dentate granule cell neurogenesis is increased by seizures and contributes to aberrant network reorganization in the adult rat hippocampus. *J Neurosci.* 17(10), 3727-38.

[77] Bengzon, J., Kokaia, Z., Elmer, E., Nanobashvili, A., Kokaia, M., Lindvall, O. 1997. Apoptosis and proliferation of dentate gyrus neurons after single and intermittent limbic seizures. *Proc Natl Acad Sci U S A.* 94(19), 10432-7.

[78] Gray, W.P., & Sundstrom, L.E. 1998. Kainic acid increases the proliferation of granule cell progenitors in the dentate gyrus of the adult rat. *Brain Res.* 790(1-2), 52-9.

[79] Parent, J.M., Janumpalli, S., McNamara, J.O., Lowenstein, D.H. 1998. Increased dentate granule cell neurogenesis following amygdala kindling in the adult rat. *Neurosci Lett.* 247(1), 9-12.

[80] Scott, B.W., Wang, S., Burnham, W.M., De Boni, U., Wojtowicz, J.M. 1998. Kindling-induced neurogenesis in the dentate gyrus of the rat. *Neurosci Lett.* 248(2), 73-6.

[81] Parent, J.M., Tada, E., Fike, J.R., Lowenstein, D.H. 1999. Inhibition of dentate granule cell neurogenesis with brain irradiation does not prevent seizure-induced mossy fiber synaptic reorganization in the rat. *J Neurosci.* 19(11), 4508-19.

[82] Covolan, L., Ribeiro, L.T., Longo, B.M., Mello, L.E. 2000. Cell damage and neurogenesis in the dentate granule cell layer of adult rats after pilocarpine- or kainate-induced status epilepticus. *Hippocampus.* 10(2), 169-80.

[83] Scharfman, H.E., Goodman, J.H., Sollas, A.L. 2000. Granule-like neurons at the hilar/CA3 border after status epilepticus and their synchrony with area CA3 pyramidal cells: functional implications of seizure-induced neurogenesis. *J Neurosci.* 20(16), 6144-58.

[84] Nakagawa, E., Aimi, Y., Yasuhara, O., Tooyama, I., Shimada, M., McGeer, P.L., Kimura, H. 2000. Enhancement of progenitor cell division in the dentate gyrus triggered by initial limbic seizures in rat models of epilepsy. *Epilepsia.* 41(1), 10-8.

[85] Scott, B.W., Wojtowicz, J.M., Burnham, W.M. 2000. Neurogenesis in the dentate gyrus of the rat following electroconvulsive shock seizures. *Exp Neurol.* 165(2), 231-6.

[86] Auvergne, R., Lere, C., El Bahh, B., Arthaud, S., Lespinet, V., Rougier, A., Le Gal La Salle, G. 2002. Delayed kindling epileptogenesis and increased neurogenesis in adult rats housed in an enriched environment. *Brain Res.* 954(2), 277-85.

[87] Faverjon, S., Silveira, D.C., Fu, D.D., Cha, B.H., Akman, C., Hu, Y., Holmes, G.L. 2002. Beneficial effects of enriched environment following status epilepticus in immature rats. *Neurology.* 59(9), 1356-64.

[88] Jiang, W., Wan, Q., Zhang, Z.J., Wang, W.D., Huang, Y.G., Rao, Z.R., Zhang, X. 2003. Dentate granule cell neurogenesis after seizures induced by pentylenetrazol in rats. *Brain Res.* 977(2), 141-8.

[89] Kralic, J.E., Ledergerber, D.A., Fritschy, J.M. 2005. Disruption of the neurogenic potential of the dentate gyrus in a mouse model of temporal lobe epilepsy with focal seizures. *Eur J Neurosci.* 22(8), 1916-27.

[90] Blumcke, I., Schewe, J.C., Normann, S., Brustle, O., Schramm, J., Elger, C.E., Wiestler, O.D. 2001. Increase of nestin-immunoreactive neural precursor cells in the dentate gyrus of pediatric patients with early-onset temporal lobe epilepsy. *Hippocampus.* 11(3), 311-21.

[91] Hester, M.S., & Danzer, S.C. 2014. Hippocampal granule cell pathology in epilepsy - a possible structural basis for comorbidities of epilepsy? *Epilepsy Behav.* 38, 105-16.

[92] Ribak, C.E., Tran, P.H., Spigelman, I., Okazaki, M.M., Nadler, J.V. 2000. Status epilepticus-induced hilar basal dendrites on

rodent granule cells contribute to recurrent excitatory circuitry. *J Comp Neurol.* 428(2), 240-53.

[93] Jessberger, S., Zhao, C., Toni, N., Clemenson, G.D., Jr., Li, Y., Gage, F.H. 2007. Seizure-associated, aberrant neurogenesis in adult rats characterized with retrovirus-mediated cell labeling. *J Neurosci.* 27(35), 9400-7.

[94] Zhou, Q.G., Nemes, A.D., Lee, D., Ro, E.J., Zhang, J., Nowacki, A.S., Dymecki, S.M., Najm, I.M., Suh, H. 2019. Chemogenetic silencing of hippocampal neurons suppresses epileptic neural circuits. *J Clin Invest.* 129(1), 310-323.

[95] Lybrand, Z.R., Goswami, S., Zhu, J., Jarzabek, V., Merlock, N., Aktar, M., Smith, C., Zhang, L., Varma, P., Cho, K.O., Ge, S., Hsieh, J. 2021. A critical period of neuronal activity results in aberrant neurogenesis rewiring hippocampal circuitry in a mouse model of epilepsy. *Nat Commun.* 12(1), 1423.

[96] Hattiangady, B., Rao, M.S., Shetty, A.K. 2004. Chronic temporal lobe epilepsy is associated with severely declined dentate neurogenesis in the adult hippocampus. *Neurobiol Dis.* 17(3), 473-90.

[97] Heinrich, C., Nitta, N., Flubacher, A., Muller, M., Fahrner, A., Kirsch, M., Freiman, T., Suzuki, F., Depaulis, A., Frotscher, M., Haas, C.A. 2006. Reelin deficiency and displacement of mature neurons, but not neurogenesis, underlie the formation of granule cell dispersion in the epileptic hippocampus. *J Neurosci.* 26(17), 4701-13.

[98] Tang, F.R., Chia, S.C., Jiang, F.L., Ma, D.L., Chen, P.M., Tang, Y.C. 2006. Calcium binding protein containing neurons in the gliotic mouse hippocampus with special reference to their afferents from the medial septum and the entorhinal cortex. *Neuroscience.* 140(4), 1467-79.

[99] Mathern, G.W., Leiphart, J.L., De Vera, A., Adelson, P.D., Seki, T., Neder, L., Leite, J.P. 2002. Seizures decrease postnatal neurogenesis and granule cell development in the human fascia dentata. *Epilepsia.* 43 Suppl 5, 68-73.

[100] Thom, M., Martinian, L., Williams, G., Stoeber, K., Sisodiya, S.M. 2005. Cell proliferation and granule cell dispersion in human hippocampal sclerosis. *J Neuropathol Exp Neurol.* 64(3), 194-201.

[101] Crespel, A., Rigau, V., Coubes, P., Rousset, M.C., de Bock, F., Okano, H., Baldy-Moulinier, M., Bockaert, J., Lerner-Natoli, M. 2005. Increased number of neural progenitors in human temporal lobe epilepsy. *Neurobiol Dis.* 19(3), 436-50.

[102] Liu, Y.W., Curtis, M.A., Gibbons, H.M., Mee, E.W., Bergin, P.S., Teoh, H.H., Connor, B., Dragunow, M., Faull, R.L. 2008. Doublecortin expression in the normal and epileptic adult human brain. *Eur J Neurosci.* 28(11), 2254-65.

[103] Fahrner, A., Kann, G., Flubacher, A., Heinrich, C., Freiman, T.M., Zentner, J., Frotscher, M., Haas, C.A. 2007. Granule cell dispersion is not accompanied by enhanced neurogenesis in temporal lobe epilepsy patients. *Exp Neurol.* 203(2), 320-32.

[104] Engel, T., Schindler, C.K., Sanz-Rodriguez, A., Conroy, R.M., Meller, R., Simon, R.P., Henshall, D.C. 2011. Expression of neurogenesis genes in human temporal lobe epilepsy with hippocampal sclerosis. *Int J Physiol Pathophysiol Pharmacol.* 3(1), 38-47.

[105] Marucci, G., Giulioni, M., Rubboli, G., Paradisi, M., Fernandez, M., Del Vecchio, G., Pozzati, E. 2013. Neurogenesis in temporal lobe epilepsy: relationship between histological findings and changes in dentate gyrus proliferative properties. *Clin Neurol Neurosurg.* 115(2), 187-91.

[106] Sadgrove, M.P., Chad, J.E., Gray, W.P. 2005. Kainic acid induces rapid cell death followed by transiently reduced cell proliferation in the immature granule cell layer of rat organotypic hippocampal slice cultures. *Brain Res.* 1035(2), 111-9.

[107] Smith, P.D., McLean, K.J., Murphy, M.A., Turnley, A.M., Cook, M.J. 2005. Seizures, not hippocampal neuronal death, provoke neurogenesis in a mouse rapid electrical amygdala kindling model of seizures. *Neuroscience.* 136(2), 405-15.

[108] Mohapel, P., Ekdahl, C.T., Lindvall, O. 2004. Status epilepticus severity influences the long-term outcome of neurogenesis in the adult dentate gyrus. *Neurobiol Dis.* 15(2), 196-205.

[109] Deisseroth, K., Singla, S., Toda, H., Monje, M., Palmer, T.D., Malenka, R.C. 2004. Excitation-neurogenesis coupling in adult neural stem/progenitor cells. *Neuron.* 42(4), 535-52.

[110] Cheng, C.M., Cohen, M., Tseng, V., Bondy, C.A. 2001. Endogenous IGF1 enhances cell survival in the postnatal dentate gyrus. *J Neurosci Res.* 64(4), 341-7.

[111] Jin, K., Mao, X.O., Sun, Y., Xie, L., Jin, L., Nishi, E., Klagsbrun, M., Greenberg, D.A. 2002. Heparin-binding epidermal growth factor-like growth factor: hypoxia-inducible expression in vitro and stimulation of neurogenesis in vitro and in vivo. *J Neurosci.* 22(13), 5365-73.

[112] Jin, K., Zhu, Y., Sun, Y., Mao, X.O., Xie, L., Greenberg, D.A. 2002. Vascular endothelial growth factor (VEGF) stimulates neurogenesis in vitro and in vivo. *Proc Natl Acad Sci U S A.* 99(18), 11946-50.

[113] Lee, J., Duan, W., Mattson, M.P. 2002. Evidence that brain-derived neurotrophic factor is required for basal neurogenesis and mediates, in part, the enhancement of neurogenesis by dietary restriction in the hippocampus of adult mice. *J Neurochem.* 82(6), 1367-75.

[114] Lichtenwalner, R.J., Forbes, M.E., Bennett, S.A., Lynch, C.D., Sonntag, W.E., Riddle, D.R. 2001. Intracerebroventricular infusion of insulin-like growth factor-I ameliorates the age-related decline in hippocampal neurogenesis. *Neuroscience.* 107(4), 603-13.

[115] Yoshimura, S., Takagi, Y., Harada, J., Teramoto, T., Thomas, S.S., Waeber, C., Bakowska, J.C., Breakefield, X.O., Moskowitz, M.A. 2001. FGF-2 regulation of neurogenesis in adult hippocampus after brain injury. *Proc Natl Acad Sci U S A.* 98(10), 5874-9.

[116] Yoshimura, S., Teramoto, T., Whalen, M.J., Irizarry, M.C., Takagi, Y., Qiu, J., Harada, J., Waeber, C., Breakefield, X.O., Moskowitz, M.A. 2003. FGF-2 regulates neurogenesis and

degeneration in the dentate gyrus after traumatic brain injury in mice. *J Clin Invest.* 112(8), 1202-10.

[117] Hagihara, H., Hara, M., Tsunekawa, K., Nakagawa, Y., Sawada, M., Nakano, K. 2005. Tonic-clonic seizures induce division of neuronal progenitor cells with concomitant changes in expression of neurotrophic factors in the brain of pilocarpine-treated mice. *Brain Res Mol Brain Res.* 139(2), 258-66.

[118] Rai, K.S., Hattiangady, B., Shetty, A.K. 2007. Enhanced production and dendritic growth of new dentate granule cells in the middle-aged hippocampus following intracerebroventricular FGF-2 infusions. *Eur J Neurosci.* 26(7), 1765-79.

[119] Wei, D., Yang, F., Wang, Y., Yang, F., Wu, C., Wu, S.X., Jiang, W. 2015. Degeneration and regeneration of GABAergic interneurons in the dentate gyrus of adult mice in experimental models of epilepsy. *CNS Neurosci Ther.* 21(1), 52-60.

[120] Radley, J.J., & Jacobs, B.L. 2002. 5-HT1A receptor antagonist administration decreases cell proliferation in the dentate gyrus. *Brain Res.* 955(1-2), 264-7.

[121] Djavadian, R.L. 2004. Serotonin and neurogenesis in the hippocampal dentate gyrus of adult mammals. *Acta Neurobiol Exp (Wars).* 64(2), 189-200.

[122] Scharfman, H., Goodman, J., Macleod, A., Phani, S., Antonelli, C., Croll, S. 2005. Increased neurogenesis and the ectopic granule cells after intrahippocampal BDNF infusion in adult rats. *Exp Neurol.* 192(2), 348-56.

[123] Pirttila, T.J., Lukasiuk, K., Hakansson, K., Grubb, A., Abrahamson, M., Pitkanen, A. 2005. Cystatin C modulates neurodegeneration and neurogenesis following status epilepticus in mouse. *Neurobiol Dis.* 20(2), 241-53.

[124] Pirttila, T.J., Manninen, A., Jutila, L., Nissinen, J., Kalviainen, R., Vapalahti, M., Immonen, A., Paljarvi, L., Karkola, K., Alafuzoff, I., Mervaala, E., Pitkanen, A. 2005. Cystatin C expression is associated with granule cell dispersion in epilepsy. *Ann Neurol.* 58(2), 211-23.

[125] Radley, J.J., & Jacobs, B.L. 2003. Pilocarpine-induced status epilepticus increases cell proliferation in the dentate gyrus of adult rats via a 5-HT1A receptor-dependent mechanism. *Brain Res.* 966(1), 1-12.

[126] Mazarati, A., Lu, X., Kilk, K., Langel, U., Wasterlain, C., Bartfai, T. 2004. Galanin type 2 receptors regulate neuronal survival, susceptibility to seizures and seizure-induced neurogenesis in the dentate gyrus. *Eur J Neurosci.* 19(12), 3235-44.

[127] Young, S.Z., Taylor, M.M., Bordey, A. 2011. Neurotransmitters couple brain activity to subventricular zone neurogenesis. *Eur J Neurosci.* 33(6), 1123-32.

[128] Crespel, A., Coubes, P., Rousset, M.C., Alonso, G., Bockaert, J., Baldy-Moulinier, M., Lerner-Natoli, M. 2002. Immature-like astrocytes are associated with dentate granule cell migration in human temporal lobe epilepsy. *Neurosci Lett.* 330(1), 114-8.

[129] Ekdahl, C.T., Claasen, J.H., Bonde, S., Kokaia, Z., Lindvall, O. 2003. Inflammation is detrimental for neurogenesis in adult brain. *Proc Natl Acad Sci U S A.* 100(23), 13632-7.

[130] Monje, M.L., & Palmer, T. 2003. Radiation injury and neurogenesis. *Curr Opin Neurol.* 16(2), 129-34.

[131] Bonde, S., Ekdahl, C.T., Lindvall, O. 2006. Long-term neuronal replacement in adult rat hippocampus after status epilepticus despite chronic inflammation. *Eur J Neurosci.* 23(4), 965-74.

[132] Shetty, A.K., Zaman, V., Shetty, G.A. 2003. Hippocampal neurotrophin levels in a kainate model of temporal lobe epilepsy: a lack of correlation between brain-derived neurotrophic factor content and progression of aberrant dentate mossy fiber sprouting. *J Neurochem.* 87(1), 147-59.

[133] Chen, Y., Ai, Y., Slevin, J.R., Maley, B.E., Gash, D.M. 2005. Progenitor proliferation in the adult hippocampus and substantia nigra induced by glial cell line-derived neurotrophic factor. *Exp Neurol.* 196(1), 87-95.

[134] Kobayashi, T., Ahlenius, H., Thored, P., Kobayashi, R., Kokaia, Z., Lindvall, O. 2006. Intracerebral infusion of glial cell line-

derived neurotrophic factor promotes striatal neurogenesis after stroke in adult rats. *Stroke.* 37(9), 2361-7.

[135] Kanter-Schlifke, I., Georgievska, B., Kirik, D., Kokaia, M. 2007. Seizure suppression by GDNF gene therapy in animal models of epilepsy. *Mol Ther.* 15(6), 1106-13.

[136] Busceti, C.L., Biagioni, F., Aronica, E., Riozzi, B., Storto, M., Battaglia, G., Giorgi, F.S., Gradini, R., Fornai, F., Caricasole, A., Nicoletti, F., Bruno, V. 2007. Induction of the Wnt inhibitor, Dickkopf-1, is associated with neurodegeneration related to temporal lobe epilepsy. *Epilepsia.* 48(4), 694-705.

[137] Yin, J., Ma, Y., Yin, Q., Xu, H., An, N., Liu, S., Fan, X., Yang, H. 2007. Involvement of over-expressed BMP4 in pentylenetetrazol kindling-induced cell proliferation in the dentate gyrus of adult rats. *Biochem Biophys Res Commun.* 355(1), 54-60.

[138] Shu, Y., Xiao, B., Wu, Q., Liu, T., Du, Y., Tang, H., Chen, S., Feng, L., Long, L., Li, Y. 2016. The Ephrin-A5/EphA4 Interaction Modulates Neurogenesis and Angiogenesis by the p-Akt and p-ERK Pathways in a Mouse Model of TLE. *Mol Neurobiol.* 53(1), 561-576.

[139] Ma, D.K., Jang, M.H., Guo, J.U., Kitabatake, Y., Chang, M.L., Pow-Anpongkul, N., Flavell, R.A., Lu, B., Ming, G.L., Song, H. 2009. Neuronal activity-induced Gadd45b promotes epigenetic DNA demethylation and adult neurogenesis. *Science.* 323(5917), 1074-7.

[140] Jun, H., Mohammed Qasim Hussaini, S., Cho, C.H., Welby, J., Jang, M.H. 2015. Gadd45b Mediates Electroconvulsive Shock Induced Proliferation of Hippocampal Neural Stem Cells. *Brain Stimul.* 8(6), 1021-1024.

[141] Xiao, X.L., Wu, X.L., Yang, P.B., Hu, H.B., Chen, Y., Min, L., Si, K.W., Wu, F., Liu, J.X. 2020. Status epilepticus induced Gadd45b is required for augmented dentate neurogenesis. *Stem Cell Res.* 49, 102102.

[142] Lazarov, O., Demars, M.P., Zhao Kda, T., Ali, H.M., Grauzas, V., Kney, A., Larson, J. 2012. Impaired survival of neural progenitor

cells in dentate gyrus of adult mice lacking fMRP. *Hippocampus.* 22(6), 1220-4.

[143] Luo, Y., Shan, G., Guo, W., Smrt, R.D., Johnson, E.B., Li, X., Pfeiffer, R.L., Szulwach, K.E., Duan, R., Barkho, B.Z., Li, W., Liu, C., Jin, P., Zhao, X. 2010. Fragile x mental retardation protein regulates proliferation and differentiation of adult neural stem/progenitor cells. *PLoS Genet.* 6(4), e1000898.

[144] Li, Y., Stockton, M.E., Eisinger, B.E., Zhao, Y., Miller, J.L., Bhuiyan, I., Gao, Y., Wu, Z., Peng, J., Zhao, X. 2018. Reducing histone acetylation rescues cognitive deficits in a mouse model of Fragile X syndrome. *Nat Commun.* 9(1), 2494.

[145] Guo, W., Allan, A.M., Zong, R., Zhang, L., Johnson, E.B., Schaller, E.G., Murthy, A.C., Goggin, S.L., Eisch, A.J., Oostra, B.A., Nelson, D.L., Jin, P., Zhao, X. 2011. Ablation of Fmrp in adult neural stem cells disrupts hippocampus-dependent learning. *Nat Med.* 17(5), 559-65.

[146] Patzlaff, N.E., Nemec, K.M., Malone, S.G., Li, Y., Zhao, X. 2017. Fragile X related protein 1 (FXR1P) regulates proliferation of adult neural stem cells. *Hum Mol Genet.* 26(7), 1340-1352.

[147] Liu, B., Li, Y., Stackpole, E.E., Novak, A., Gao, Y., Zhao, Y., Zhao, X., Richter, J.D. 2018. Regulatory discrimination of mRNAs by FMRP controls mouse adult neural stem cell differentiation. *Proc Natl Acad Sci U S A.* 115(48), E11397-E11405.

[148] Arvola, R.M., Chang, C.T., Buytendorp, J.P., Levdansky, Y., Valkov, E., Freddolino, P.L., Goldstrohm, A.C. 2020. Unique repression domains of Pumilio utilize deadenylation and decapping factors to accelerate destruction of target mRNAs. *Nucleic Acids Res.* 48(4), 1843-1871.

[149] Zhang, M., Chen, D., Xia, J., Han, W., Cui, X., Neuenkirchen, N., Hermes, G., Sestan, N., Lin, H. 2017. Post-transcriptional regulation of mouse neurogenesis by Pumilio proteins. *Genes Dev.* 31(13), 1354-1369.

[150] Wu, X.L., Huang, H., Huang, Y.Y., Yuan, J.X., Zhou, X., Chen, Y.M. 2015. Reduced Pumilio-2 expression in patients with

temporal lobe epilepsy and in the lithium-pilocarpine induced epilepsy rat model. *Epilepsy Behav.* 50, 31-9.

[151] Follwaczny, P., Schieweck, R., Riedemann, T., Demleitner, A., Straub, T., Klemm, A.H., Bilban, M., Sutor, B., Popper, B., Kiebler, M.A. 2017. Pumilio2-deficient mice show a predisposition for epilepsy. *Dis Model Mech.* 10(11), 1333-1342.

[152] Lin, W.H., Giachello, C.N., Baines, R.A. 2017. Seizure control through genetic and pharmacological manipulation of Pumilio in Drosophila: a key component of neuronal homeostasis. *Dis Model Mech.* 10(2), 141-150.

[153] D'Mello, S.R. 2020. Histone deacetylases 1, 2 and 3 in nervous system development. *Curr Opin Pharmacol.* 50, 74-81.

[154] Jessberger, S., Nakashima, K., Clemenson, G.D., Jr., Mejia, E., Mathews, E., Ure, K., Ogawa, S., Sinton, C.M., Gage, F.H., Hsieh, J. 2007. Epigenetic modulation of seizure-induced neurogenesis and cognitive decline. *J Neurosci.* 27(22), 5967-75.

[155] Zhao, C., Sun, G., Li, S., Shi, Y. 2009. A feedback regulatory loop involving microRNA-9 and nuclear receptor TLX in neural stem cell fate determination. *Nat Struct Mol Biol.* 16(4), 365-71.

[156] Stappert, L., Klaus, F., Brustle, O. 2018. MicroRNAs Engage in Complex Circuits Regulating Adult Neurogenesis. *Front Neurosci.* 12, 707.

[157] Katz, S., Cussigh, D., Urban, N., Blomfield, I., Guillemot, F., Bally-Cuif, L., Coolen, M. 2016. A Nuclear Role for miR-9 and Argonaute Proteins in Balancing Quiescent and Activated Neural Stem Cell States. *Cell Rep.* 17(5), 1383-1398.

[158] Bielefeld, P., Mooney, C., Henshall, D.C., Fitzsimons, C.P. 2017. miRNA-Mediated Regulation of Adult Hippocampal Neurogenesis; Implications for Epilepsy. *Brain Plast.* 3(1), 43-59.

[159] Kim, D.Y., Hwang, I., Muller, F.L., Paik, J.H. 2015. Functional regulation of FoxO1 in neural stem cell differentiation. *Cell Death Differ.* 22(12), 2034-45.

[160] Zhao, C., Sun, G., Li, S., Lang, M.F., Yang, S., Li, W., Shi, Y. 2010. MicroRNA let-7b regulates neural stem cell proliferation

and differentiation by targeting nuclear receptor TLX signaling. *Proc Natl Acad Sci U S A.* 107(5), 1876-81.

[161] Risbud, R.M., & Porter, B.E. 2013. Changes in microRNA expression in the whole hippocampus and hippocampal synaptoneurosome fraction following pilocarpine induced status epilepticus. *PLoS One.* 8(1), e53464.

[162] McKiernan, R.C., Jimenez-Mateos, E.M., Bray, I., Engel, T., Brennan, G.P., Sano, T., Michalak, Z., Moran, C., Delanty, N., Farrell, M., O'Brien, D., Meller, R., Simon, R.P., Stallings, R.L., Henshall, D.C. 2012. Reduced mature microRNA levels in association with dicer loss in human temporal lobe epilepsy with hippocampal sclerosis. *PLoS One.* 7(5), e35921.

[163] Han, C.L., Liu, Y.P., Guo, C.J., Du, T.T., Jiang, Y., Wang, K.L., Shao, X.Q., Meng, F.G., Zhang, J.G. 2020. The lncRNA H19 binding to let-7b promotes hippocampal glial cell activation and epileptic seizures by targeting Stat3 in a rat model of temporal lobe epilepsy. *Cell Prolif.* 53(8), e12856.

[164] Han, C.L., Ge, M., Liu, Y.P., Zhao, X.M., Wang, K.L., Chen, N., Hu, W., Zhang, J.G., Li, L., Meng, F.G. 2018. Long non-coding RNA H19 contributes to apoptosis of hippocampal neurons by inhibiting let-7b in a rat model of temporal lobe epilepsy. *Cell Death Dis.* 9(6), 617.

[165] Esteves, M., Serra-Almeida, C., Saraiva, C., Bernardino, L. 2020. New insights into the regulatory roles of microRNAs in adult neurogenesis. *Curr Opin Pharmacol.* 50, 38-45.

[166] Jin, J., Kim, S.N., Liu, X., Zhang, H., Zhang, C., Seo, J.S., Kim, Y., Sun, T. 2016. miR-17-92 Cluster Regulates Adult Hippocampal Neurogenesis, Anxiety, and Depression. *Cell Rep.* 16(6), 1653-1663.

[167] Pan, W.L., Chopp, M., Fan, B., Zhang, R., Wang, X., Hu, J., Zhang, X.M., Zhang, Z.G., Liu, X.S. 2019. Ablation of the microRNA-17-92 cluster in neural stem cells diminishes adult hippocampal neurogenesis and cognitive function. *FASEB J.* 33(4), 5257-5267.

[168] Feng, Y., Duan, C., Luo, Z., Xiao, W., Tian, F. 2020. Silencing miR-20a-5p inhibits axonal growth and neuronal branching and prevents epileptogenesis through RGMa-RhoA-mediated synaptic plasticity. *J Cell Mol Med.* 24(18), 10573-10588.

[169] Hata, K., Fujitani, M., Yasuda, Y., Doya, H., Saito, T., Yamagishi, S., Mueller, B.K., Yamashita, T. 2006. RGMa inhibition promotes axonal growth and recovery after spinal cord injury. *J Cell Biol.* 173(1), 47-58.

[170] Letellier, M., Elramah, S., Mondin, M., Soula, A., Penn, A., Choquet, D., Landry, M., Thoumine, O., Favereaux, A. 2014. miR-92a regulates expression of synaptic GluA1-containing AMPA receptors during homeostatic scaling. *Nat Neurosci.* 17(8), 1040-2.

[171] Sakai, A., Saitow, F., Maruyama, M., Miyake, N., Miyake, K., Shimada, T., Okada, T., Suzuki, H. 2017. MicroRNA cluster miR-17-92 regulates multiple functionally related voltage-gated potassium channels in chronic neuropathic pain. *Nat Commun.* 8, 16079.

[172] Brett, J.O., Renault, V.M., Rafalski, V.A., Webb, A.E., Brunet, A. 2011. The microRNA cluster miR-106b~25 regulates adult neural stem/progenitor cell proliferation and neuronal differentiation. *Aging* (Albany NY). 3(2), 108-24.

[173] Li, R., Wen, Y., Wu, B., He, M., Zhang, P., Zhang, Q., Chen, Y. 2020. MicroRNA-25-3p suppresses epileptiform discharges through inhibiting oxidative stress and apoptosis via targeting OXSR1 in neurons. *Biochem Biophys Res Commun.* 523(4), 859-866.

[174] Liu, C., Teng, Z.Q., Santistevan, N.J., Szulwach, K.E., Guo, W., Jin, P., Zhao, X. 2010. Epigenetic regulation of miR-184 by MBD1 governs neural stem cell proliferation and differentiation. *Cell Stem Cell.* 6(5), 433-44.

[175] McKiernan, R.C., Jimenez-Mateos, E.M., Sano, T., Bray, I., Stallings, R.L., Simon, R.P., Henshall, D.C. 2012. Expression profiling the microRNA response to epileptic preconditioning

identifies miR-184 as a modulator of seizure-induced neuronal death. *Exp Neurol.* 237(2), 346-54.

[176] Cheng, L.C., Pastrana, E., Tavazoie, M., Doetsch, F. 2009. miR-124 regulates adult neurogenesis in the subventricular zone stem cell niche. *Nat Neurosci.* 12(4), 399-408.

[177] Stolt, C.C., Lommes, P., Sock, E., Chaboissier, M.C., Schedl, A., Wegner, M. 2003. The Sox9 transcription factor determines glial fate choice in the developing spinal cord. *Genes Dev.* 17(13), 1677-89.

[178] Akerblom, M., Sachdeva, R., Barde, I., Verp, S., Gentner, B., Trono, D., Jakobsson, J. 2012. MicroRNA-124 is a subventricular zone neuronal fate determinant. *J Neurosci.* 32(26), 8879-89.

[179] Krichevsky, A.M., Sonntag, K.C., Isacson, O., Kosik, K.S. 2006. Specific microRNAs modulate embryonic stem cell-derived neurogenesis. *Stem Cells.* 24(4), 857-64.

[180] Bielefeld, P., Schouten, M., Meijer, G.M., Breuk, M.J., Geijtenbeek, K., Karayel, S., Tiaglik, A., Vuuregge, A.H., Willems, R.A.L., Witkamp, D., Lucassen, P.J., Encinas, J.M., Fitzsimons, C.P. 2019. Co-administration of Anti microRNA-124 and -137 Oligonucleotides Prevents Hippocampal Neural Stem Cell Loss Upon Non-convulsive Seizures. *Front Mol Neurosci.* 12, 31.

[181] Wang, W., Wang, X., Chen, L., Zhang, Y., Xu, Z., Liu, J., Jiang, G., Li, J., Zhang, X., Wang, K., Wang, J., Chen, G., Luo, J. 2016. The microRNA miR-124 suppresses seizure activity and regulates CREB1 activity. *Expert Rev Mol Med.* 18, e4.

[182] Brennan, G.P., Dey, D., Chen, Y., Patterson, K.P., Magnetta, E.J., Hall, A.M., Dube, C.M., Mei, Y.T., Baram, T.Z. 2016. Dual and Opposing Roles of MicroRNA-124 in Epilepsy Are Mediated through Inflammatory and NRSF-Dependent Gene Networks. *Cell Rep.* 14(10), 2402-12.

[183] McClelland, S., Flynn, C., Dube, C., Richichi, C., Zha, Q., Ghestem, A., Esclapez, M., Bernard, C., Baram, T.Z. 2011. Neuron-restrictive silencer factor-mediated hyperpolarization-

activated cyclic nucleotide gated channelopathy in experimental temporal lobe epilepsy. *Ann Neurol.* 70(3), 454-64.

[184] Qiao, J., Zhao, J., Chang, S., Sun, Q., Liu, N., Dong, J., Chen, Y., Yang, D., Ye, D., Liu, X., Yu, Y., Chen, W., Zhu, S., Wang, G., Jia, W., Xi, J., Kang, J. 2020. MicroRNA-153 improves the neurogenesis of neural stem cells and enhances the cognitive ability of aged mice through the notch signaling pathway. *Cell Death Differ.* 27(2), 808-825.

[185] Gong, G.H., An, F.M., Wang, Y., Bian, M., Wang, D., Wei, C.X. 2018. MiR-153 regulates expression of hypoxia-inducible factor-1alpha in refractory epilepsy. *Oncotarget.* 9(9), 8542-8547.

[186] Li, Y., Huang, C., Feng, P., Jiang, Y., Wang, W., Zhou, D., Chen, L. 2016. Aberrant expression of miR-153 is associated with overexpression of hypoxia-inducible factor-1alpha in refractory epilepsy. *Sci Rep.* 6, 32091.

[187] Wang, G., Xie, G., Han, L., Wang, D., Du, F., Kong, X., Su, G. 2019. Involvement of hypoxia-inducible factor-1 alpha in the upregulation of P-glycoprotein in refractory epilepsy. *Neuroreport.* 30(17), 1191-1196.

[188] Li, Y., Chen, J., Zeng, T., Lei, D., Chen, L., Zhou, D. 2014. Expression of HIF-1alpha and MDR1/P-glycoprotein in refractory mesial temporal lobe epilepsy patients and pharmacoresistant temporal lobe epilepsy rat model kindled by coriaria lactone. *Neurol Sci.* 35(8), 1203-8.

[189] Li, Y., Fan, C., Gao, R., Lan, T., Wang, W., Yu, S.Y. 2021. Hippocampal miR-211-5p regulates neurogenesis and depression-like behaviors in the rat. *Neuropharmacology.* 194, 108618.

[190] Fan, C., Wu, Q., Ye, X., Luo, H., Yan, D., Xiong, Y., Zhu, H., Diao, Y., Zhang, W., Wan, J. 2016. Role of miR-211 in Neuronal Differentiation and Viability: Implications to Pathogenesis of Alzheimer's Disease. *Front Aging Neurosci.* 8, 166.

[191] Luo, Z.H., Walid, A.A., Xie, Y., Long, H., Xiao, W., Xu, L., Fu, Y., Feng, L., Xiao, B. 2019. Construction and analysis of a

dysregulated lncRNA-associated ceRNA network in a rat model of temporal lobe epilepsy. *Seizure.* 69, 105-114.

[192] Bekenstein, U., Mishra, N., Milikovsky, D.Z., Hanin, G., Zelig, D., Sheintuch, L., Berson, A., Greenberg, D.S., Friedman, A., Soreq, H. 2017. Dynamic changes in murine forebrain miR-211 expression associate with cholinergic imbalances and epileptiform activity. *Proc Natl Acad Sci U S A.* 114(25), E4996-E5005.

[193] Aranha, M.M., Santos, D.M., Sola, S., Steer, C.J., Rodrigues, C.M. 2011. miR-34a regulates mouse neural stem cell differentiation. *PLoS One.* 6(8), e21396.

[194] Fineberg, S.K., Datta, P., Stein, C.S., Davidson, B.L. 2012. MiR-34a represses Numbl in murine neural progenitor cells and antagonizes neuronal differentiation. *PLoS One.* 7(6), e38562.

[195] Agostini, M., Tucci, P., Killick, R., Candi, E., Sayan, B.S., Rivetti di Val Cervo, P., Nicotera, P., McKeon, F., Knight, R.A., Mak, T.W., Melino, G. 2011. Neuronal differentiation by TAp73 is mediated by microRNA-34a regulation of synaptic protein targets. *Proc Natl Acad Sci U S A.* 108(52), 21093-8.

[196] Morgado, A.L., Xavier, J.M., Dionisio, P.A., Ribeiro, M.F., Dias, R.B., Sebastiao, A.M., Sola, S., Rodrigues, C.M. 2015. MicroRNA-34a Modulates Neural Stem Cell Differentiation by Regulating Expression of Synaptic and Autophagic Proteins. *Mol Neurobiol.* 51(3), 1168-83.

[197] Mollinari, C., Racaniello, M., Berry, A., Pieri, M., de Stefano, M.C., Cardinale, A., Zona, C., Cirulli, F., Garaci, E., Merlo, D. 2015. miR-34a regulates cell proliferation, morphology and function of newborn neurons resulting in improved behavioural outcomes. *Cell Death Dis.* 6, e1622.

[198] Modi, P.K., Jaiswal, S., Sharma, P. 2016. Regulation of Neuronal Cell Cycle and Apoptosis by MicroRNA 34a. *Mol Cell Biol.* 36(1), 84-94.

[199] Hu, K., Xie, Y.Y., Zhang, C., Ouyang, D.S., Long, H.Y., Sun, D.N., Long, L.L., Feng, L., Li, Y., Xiao, B. 2012. MicroRNA expression profile of the hippocampus in a rat model of temporal

lobe epilepsy and miR-34a-targeted neuroprotection against hippocampal neurone cell apoptosis post-status epilepticus. *BMC Neurosci.* 13, 115.

[200] Kretschmann, A., Danis, B., Andonovic, L., Abnaof, K., van Rikxoort, M., Siegel, F., Mazzuferi, M., Godard, P., Hanon, E., Frohlich, H., Kaminski, R.M., Foerch, P., Pfeifer, A. 2015. Different microRNA profiles in chronic epilepsy versus acute seizure mouse models. *J Mol Neurosci.* 55(2), 466-79.

[201] Bencurova, P., Baloun, J., Musilova, K., Radova, L., Tichy, B., Pail, M., Zeman, M., Brichtova, E., Hermanova, M., Pospisilova, S., Mraz, M., Brazdil, M. 2017. MicroRNA and mesial temporal lobe epilepsy with hippocampal sclerosis: Whole miRNome profiling of human hippocampus. *Epilepsia.* 58(10), 1782-1793.

[202] Organista-Juarez, D., Jimenez, A., Rocha, L., Alonso-Vanegas, M., Guevara-Guzman, R. 2019. Differential expression of miR-34a, 451, 1260, 1275 and 1298 in the neocortex of patients with mesial temporal lobe epilepsy. *Epilepsy Res.* 157, 106188.

[203] Sano, T., Reynolds, J.P., Jimenez-Mateos, E.M., Matsushima, S., Taki, W., Henshall, D.C. 2012. MicroRNA-34a upregulation during seizure-induced neuronal death. *Cell Death Dis.* 3, e287.

[204] Wang, J., Zheng, Y., Cheng, X., Xu, F., Zhang, P., Zhou, X., Zhao, H. 2019. Inhibition of microRNA-34a Suppresses Epileptiform Discharges Through Regulating Notch Signaling and Apoptosis in Cultured Hippocampal Neurons. *Neurochem Res.* 44(5), 1252-1261.

[205] Vo, N., Klein, M.E., Varlamova, O., Keller, D.M., Yamamoto, T., Goodman, R.H., Impey, S. 2005. A cAMP-response element binding protein-induced microRNA regulates neuronal morphogenesis. *Proc Natl Acad Sci U S A.* 102(45), 16426-31.

[206] Nudelman, A.S., DiRocco, D.P., Lambert, T.J., Garelick, M.G., Le, J., Nathanson, N.M., Storm, D.R. 2010. Neuronal activity rapidly induces transcription of the CREB-regulated microRNA-132, in vivo. *Hippocampus.* 20(4), 492-8.

[207] Magill, S.T., Cambronne, X.A., Luikart, B.W., Lioy, D.T., Leighton, B.H., Westbrook, G.L., Mandel, G., Goodman, R.H. 2010. microRNA-132 regulates dendritic growth and arborization of newborn neurons in the adult hippocampus. *Proc Natl Acad Sci U S A.* 107(47), 20382-7.

[208] Impey, S., Davare, M., Lesiak, A., Fortin, D., Ando, H., Varlamova, O., Obrietan, K., Soderling, T.R., Goodman, R.H., Wayman, G.A. 2010. An activity-induced microRNA controls dendritic spine formation by regulating Rac1-PAK signaling. *Mol Cell Neurosci.* 43(1), 146-56.

[209] Wayman, G.A., Davare, M., Ando, H., Fortin, D., Varlamova, O., Cheng, H.Y., Marks, D., Obrietan, K., Soderling, T.R., Goodman, R.H., Impey, S. 2008. An activity-regulated microRNA controls dendritic plasticity by down-regulating p250GAP. *Proc Natl Acad Sci U S A.* 105(26), 9093-8.

[210] Luikart, B.W., Bensen, A.L., Washburn, E.K., Perederiy, J.V., Su, K.G., Li, Y., Kernie, S.G., Parada, L.F., Westbrook, G.L. 2011. miR-132 mediates the integration of newborn neurons into the adult dentate gyrus. *PLoS One.* 6(5), e19077.

[211] Yuan, J., Huang, H., Zhou, X., Liu, X., Ou, S., Xu, T., Li, R., Ma, L., Chen, Y. 2016. MicroRNA-132 Interact with p250GAP/Cdc42 Pathway in the Hippocampal Neuronal Culture Model of Acquired Epilepsy and Associated with Epileptogenesis Process. *Neural Plast.* 2016, 5108489.

[212] Huang, Y., Guo, J., Wang, Q., Chen, Y. 2014. MicroRNA-132 silencing decreases the spontaneous recurrent seizures. *Int J Clin Exp Med.* 7(7), 1639-49.

[213] Jimenez-Mateos, E.M., Bray, I., Sanz-Rodriguez, A., Engel, T., McKiernan, R.C., Mouri, G., Tanaka, K., Sano, T., Saugstad, J.A., Simon, R.P., Stallings, R.L., Henshall, D.C. 2011. miRNA Expression profile after status epilepticus and hippocampal neuroprotection by targeting miR-132. *Am J Pathol.* 179(5), 2519-32.

[214] Jia, M., Wang, X., Zhang, H., Ye, C., Ma, H., Yang, M., Li, Y., Cui, C. 2019. MicroRNA-132 in the Adult Dentate Gyrus is Involved in Opioid Addiction Via Modifying the Differentiation of Neural Stem Cells. *Neurosci Bull.* 35(3), 486-496.

[215] Chen, D., Hu, S., Wu, Z., Liu, J., Li, S. 2018. The Role of MiR-132 in Regulating Neural Stem Cell Proliferation, Differentiation and Neuronal Maturation. *Cell Physiol Biochem.* 47(6), 2319-2330.

[216] Chen, D., Liu, J., Wu, Z., Li, S.H. 2021. Role of miR-132/methyl-CpG-binding protein 2 in the regulation of neural stem cell differentiation. *Neural Regen Res.* 16(2), 345-349.

[217] Korotkov, A., Broekaart, D.W.M., Banchaewa, L., Pustjens, B., van Scheppingen, J., Anink, J.J., Baayen, J.C., Idema, S., Gorter, J.A., van Vliet, E.A., Aronica, E. 2020. microRNA-132 is overexpressed in glia in temporal lobe epilepsy and reduces the expression of pro-epileptogenic factors in human cultured astrocytes. *Glia.* 68(1), 60-75.

[218] Campbell, A., Morris, G., Heller, J.P., Langa, E., Brindley, E., Worm, J., Jensen, M.A., Miller, M.T., Henshall, D.C., Reschke, C.R. 2021. Antagomir-mediated suppression of microRNA-134 reduces kainic acid-induced seizures in immature mice. *Sci Rep.* 11(1), 340.

[219] Jimenez-Mateos, E.M., Engel, T., Merino-Serrais, P., McKiernan, R.C., Tanaka, K., Mouri, G., Sano, T., O'Tuathaigh, C., Waddington, J.L., Prenter, S., Delanty, N., Farrell, M.A., O'Brien, D.F., Conroy, R.M., Stallings, R.L., DeFelipe, J., Henshall, D.C. 2012. Silencing microRNA-134 produces neuroprotective and prolonged seizure-suppressive effects. *Nat Med.* 18(7), 1087-94.

[220] Peng, J., Omran, A., Ashhab, M.U., Kong, H., Gan, N., He, F., Yin, F. 2013. Expression patterns of miR-124, miR-134, miR-132, and miR-21 in an immature rat model and children with mesial temporal lobe epilepsy. *J Mol Neurosci.* 50(2), 291-7.

[221] Sun, J., Gao, X., Meng, D., Xu, Y., Wang, X., Gu, X., Guo, M., Shao, X., Yan, H., Jiang, C., Zheng, Y. 2017. Antagomirs

Targeting MicroRNA-134 Increase Limk1 Levels After Experimental Seizures in Vitro and in Vivo. *Cell Physiol Biochem.* 43(2), 636-643.

[222] Jimenez-Mateos, E.M., Engel, T., Merino-Serrais, P., Fernaud-Espinosa, I., Rodriguez-Alvarez, N., Reynolds, J., Reschke, C.R., Conroy, R.M., McKiernan, R.C., deFelipe, J., Henshall, D.C. 2015. Antagomirs targeting microRNA-134 increase hippocampal pyramidal neuron spine volume in vivo and protect against pilocarpine-induced status epilepticus. *Brain Struct Funct.* 220(4), 2387-99.

[223] Reschke, C.R., Silva, L.F.A., Norwood, B.A., Senthilkumar, K., Morris, G., Sanz-Rodriguez, A., Conroy, R.M., Costard, L., Neubert, V., Bauer, S., Farrell, M.A., O'Brien, D.F., Delanty, N., Schorge, S., Pasterkamp, R.J., Rosenow, F., Henshall, D.C. 2017. Potent Anti-seizure Effects of Locked Nucleic Acid Antagomirs Targeting miR-134 in Multiple Mouse and Rat Models of Epilepsy. *Mol Ther Nucleic Acids.* 6, 45-56.

[224] DeFelipe, J. 2015. The dendritic spine story: an intriguing process of discovery. *Front Neuroanat.* 9, 14.

[225] Fiore, R., Rajman, M., Schwale, C., Bicker, S., Antoniou, A., Bruehl, C., Draguhn, A., Schratt, G. 2014. MiR-134-dependent regulation of Pumilio-2 is necessary for homeostatic synaptic depression. *EMBO J.* 33(19), 2231-46.

[226] Gao, J., Wang, W.Y., Mao, Y.W., Graff, J., Guan, J.S., Pan, L., Mak, G., Kim, D., Su, S.C., Tsai, L.H. 2010. A novel pathway regulates memory and plasticity via SIRT1 and miR-134. *Nature.* 466(7310), 1105-9.

[227] Fiore, R., Khudayberdiev, S., Christensen, M., Siegel, G., Flavell, S.W., Kim, T.K., Greenberg, M.E., Schratt, G. 2009. Mef2-mediated transcription of the miR379-410 cluster regulates activity-dependent dendritogenesis by fine-tuning Pumilio2 protein levels. *EMBO J.* 28(6), 697-710.

[228] Schratt, G.M., Tuebing, F., Nigh, E.A., Kane, C.G., Sabatini, M.E., Kiebler, M., Greenberg, M.E. 2006. A brain-specific microRNA regulates dendritic spine development. *Nature.* 439(7074), 283-9.

[229] Reschke, C.R., Silva, L.F.A., Vangoor, V.R., Rosso, M., David, B., Cavanagh, B.L., Connolly, N.M.C., Brennan, G.P., Sanz-Rodriguez, A., Mooney, C., Batool, A., Greene, C., Brennan, M., Conroy, R.M., Ruber, T., Prehn, J.H.M., Campbell, M., Pasterkamp, R.J., Henshall, D.C. 2021. Systemic delivery of antagomirs during blood-brain barrier disruption is disease-modifying in experimental epilepsy. *Mol Ther.* 29(6), 2041-2052.

[230] Wang, X.M., Jia, R.H., Wei, D., Cui, W.Y., Jiang, W. 2014. MiR-134 blockade prevents status epilepticus like-activity and is neuroprotective in cultured hippocampal neurons. *Neurosci Lett.* 572, 20-5.

[231] Sun, J., Gao, X., Meng, D., Xu, Y., Wang, X., Gu, X., Guo, M., Shao, X., Yan, H., Jiang, C., Zheng, Y. 2017. Antagomirs targeting miroRNA-134 attenuates epilepsy in rats through regulation of oxidative stress, mitochondrial functions and autophagy. *Front Pharmacol.* 8, 524.

[232] Gao, X., Guo, M., Meng, D., Sun, F., Guan, L., Cui, Y., Zhao, Y., Wang, X., Gu, X., Sun, J., Qi, S. 2019. Silencing microRNA-134 alleviates hippocampal damage and occurrence of spontaneous seizures after intraventricular kainic acid-induced status epilepticus in rats. *Front Cell Neurosci.* 13, 145.

[233] Rodriguez, A.S., Engel, T., Palfi, A., Farrar, G.J., Henshall, D.C., Jimenez-Mateos, E.M. 2017. Tubby-like protein 1 (Tulp1) is a target of microRNA-134 and is down-regulated in experimental epilepsy. *Int J Physiol Pathophysiol Pharmacol.* 9(6), 178-187.

[234] Wang, W., Guo, Y., He, L., Chen, C., Luo, J., Ma, Y., Li, J., Yang, Y., Yang, Q., Du, C., Zhang, Y., Li, Z., Xu, X., Tian, X., Wang, X. 2018. Overexpression of miRNA-137 in the brain suppresses seizure activity and neuronal excitability: A new potential therapeutic strategy for epilepsy. *Neuropharmacology.* 138, 170-181.

[235] Smrt, R.D., Szulwach, K.E., Pfeiffer, R.L., Li, X., Guo, W., Pathania, M., Teng, Z.Q., Luo, Y., Peng, J., Bordey, A., Jin, P., Zhao, X. 2010. MicroRNA miR-137 regulates neuronal maturation by targeting ubiquitin ligase mind bomb-1. *Stem Cells.* 28(6), 1060-70.

[236] Schouten, M., Fratantoni, S.A., Hubens, C.J., Piersma, S.R., Pham, T.V., Bielefeld, P., Voskuyl, R.A., Lucassen, P.J., Jimenez, C.R., Fitzsimons, C.P. 2015. MicroRNA-124 and -137 cooperativity controls caspase-3 activity through BCL2L13 in hippocampal neural stem cells. *Sci Rep.* 5, 12448.

[237] Schouten, M., Bielefeld, P., Fratantoni, S.A., Hubens, C.J., Piersma, S.R., Pham, T.V., Voskuyl, R.A., Lucassen, P.J., Jimenez, C.R., Fitzsimons, C.P. 2016. Multi-omics profile of the mouse dentate gyrus after kainic acid-induced status epilepticus. *Sci Data.* 3, 160068.

[238] Gorter, J.A., Iyer, A., White, I., Colzi, A., van Vliet, E.A., Sisodiya, S., Aronica, E. 2014. Hippocampal subregion-specific microRNA expression during epileptogenesis in experimental temporal lobe epilepsy. *Neurobiol Dis.* 62, 508-20.

[239] Song, Y.J., Tian, X.B., Zhang, S., Zhang, Y.X., Li, X., Li, D., Cheng, Y., Zhang, J.N., Kang, C.S., Zhao, W. 2011. Temporal lobe epilepsy induces differential expression of hippocampal miRNAs including let-7e and miR-23a/b. *Brain Res.* 1387, 134-40.

[240] Berenguer, J., Herrera, A., Vuolo, L., Torroba, B., Llorens, F., Sumoy, L., Pons, S. 2013. MicroRNA 22 regulates cell cycle length in cerebellar granular neuron precursors. *Mol Cell Biol.* 33(14), 2706-17.

[241] Volvert, M.L., Prevot, P.P., Close, P., Laguesse, S., Pirotte, S., Hemphill, J., Rogister, F., Kruzy, N., Sacheli, R., Moonen, G., Deiters, A., Merkenschlager, M., Chariot, A., Malgrange, B., Godin, J.D., Nguyen, L. 2014. MicroRNA targeting of CoREST controls polarization of migrating cortical neurons. *Cell Rep.* 7(4), 1168-83.

[242] Beamer, E.H., Jurado-Arjona, J., Jimenez-Mateos, E.M., Morgan, J., Reschke, C.R., Kenny, A., de Leo, G., Olivos-Ore, L.A., Arribas-Blazquez, M., Madden, S.F., Merchan-Rubira, J., Delanty, N., Farrell, M.A., O'Brien, D.F., Avila, J., Diaz-Hernandez, M., Miras-Portugal, M.T., Artalejo, A.R., Hernandez, F., Henshall, D.C., Engel, T. 2018. MicroRNA-22 controls aberrant neurogenesis and changes in neuronal morphology after status epilepticus. *Front Mol Neurosci.* 11, 442.

[243] Jimenez-Mateos, E.M., Arribas-Blazquez, M., Sanz-Rodriguez, A., Concannon, C., Olivos-Ore, L.A., Reschke, C.R., Mooney, C.M., Mooney, C., Lugara, E., Morgan, J., Langa, E., Jimenez-Pacheco, A., Silva, L.F., Mesuret, G., Boison, D., Miras-Portugal, M.T., Letavic, M., Artalejo, A.R., Bhattacharya, A., Diaz-Hernandez, M., Henshall, D.C., Engel, T. 2015. microRNA targeting of the P2X7 purinoceptor opposes a contralateral epileptogenic focus in the hippocampus. *Sci Rep.* 5, 17486.

[244] Almeida Silva, L.F., Reschke, C.R., Nguyen, N.T., Langa, E., Sanz-Rodriguez, A., Gerbatin, R.R., Temp, F.R., de Freitas, M.L., Conroy, R.M., Brennan, G.P., Engel, T., Henshall, D.C. 2020. Genetic deletion of microRNA-22 blunts the inflammatory transcriptional response to status epilepticus and exacerbates epilepsy in mice. *Mol Brain.* 13(1), 114.

[245] Tauck, D.L., & Nadler, J.V. 1985. Evidence of functional mossy fiber sprouting in hippocampal formation of kainic acid-treated rats. *J Neurosci.* 5(4), 1016-22.

[246] Wenzel, H.J., Woolley, C.S., Robbins, C.A., Schwartzkroin, P.A. 2000. Kainic acid-induced mossy fiber sprouting and synapse formation in the dentate gyrus of rats. *Hippocampus.* 10(3), 244-60.

[247] Hunt, R.F., Scheff, S.W., Smith, B.N. 2010. Regionally localized recurrent excitation in the dentate gyrus of a cortical contusion model of posttraumatic epilepsy. *J Neurophysiol.* 103(3), 1490-500.

[248] Danzer, S.C. 2018. Contributions of Adult-Generated Granule Cells to Hippocampal Pathology in Temporal Lobe Epilepsy: A Neuronal Bestiary. *Brain Plast.* 3(2), 169-181.

[249] Sutula, T.P., & Dudek, F.E. 2007. Unmasking recurrent excitation generated by mossy fiber sprouting in the epileptic dentate gyrus: an emergent property of a complex system. *Prog Brain Res.* 163, 541-63.

[250] Zhan, R.Z., Timofeeva, O., Nadler, J.V. 2010. High ratio of synaptic excitation to synaptic inhibition in hilar ectopic granule cells of pilocarpine-treated rats. *J Neurophysiol.* 104(6), 3293-304.

[251] Althaus, A.L., Sagher, O., Parent, J.M., Murphy, G.G. 2015. Intrinsic neurophysiological properties of hilar ectopic and normotopic dentate granule cells in human temporal lobe epilepsy and a rat model. *J Neurophysiol.* 113(4), 1184-94.

[252] Pun, R.Y., Rolle, I.J., Lasarge, C.L., Hosford, B.E., Rosen, J.M., Uhl, J.D., Schmeltzer, S.N., Faulkner, C., Bronson, S.L., Murphy, B.L., Richards, D.A., Holland, K.D., Danzer, S.C. 2012. Excessive activation of mTOR in postnatally generated granule cells is sufficient to cause epilepsy. *Neuron.* 75(6), 1022-34.

[253] Roth, B.L. 2016. DREADDs for Neuroscientists. *Neuron.* 89(4), 683-94.

[254] Kahn, J.B., Port, R.G., Yue, C., Takano, H., Coulter, D.A. 2019. Circuit-based interventions in the dentate gyrus rescue epilepsy-associated cognitive dysfunction. *Brain.* 142(9), 2705-2721.

[255] Jung, K.H., Chu, K., Kim, M., Jeong, S.W., Song, Y.M., Lee, S.T., Kim, J.Y., Lee, S.K., Roh, J.K. 2004. Continuous cytosine-b-D-arabinofuranoside infusion reduces ectopic granule cells in adult rat hippocampus with attenuation of spontaneous recurrent seizures following pilocarpine-induced status epilepticus. *Eur J Neurosci.* 19(12), 3219-26.

[256] Jung, K.H., Chu, K., Lee, S.T., Kim, J., Sinn, D.I., Kim, J.M., Park, D.K., Lee, J.J., Kim, S.U., Kim, M., Lee, S.K., Roh, J.K. 2006. Cyclooxygenase-2 inhibitor, celecoxib, inhibits the altered hippocampal neurogenesis with attenuation of spontaneous

recurrent seizures following pilocarpine-induced status epilepticus. *Neurobiol Dis.* 23(2), 237-46.

[257] Pekcec, A., Fuest, C., Muhlenhoff, M., Gerardy-Schahn, R., Potschka, H. 2008. Targeting epileptogenesis-associated induction of neurogenesis by enzymatic depolysialylation of NCAM counteracts spatial learning dysfunction but fails to impact epilepsy development. *J Neurochem.* 105(2), 389-400.

[258] Zhu, K., Yuan, B., Hu, M., Feng, G.F., Liu, Y., Liu, J.X. 2017. Reduced abnormal integration of adult-generated granule cells does not attenuate spontaneous recurrent seizures in mice. *Epilepsy Res.* 133, 58-66.

[259] Raedt, R., Boon, P., Persson, A., Alborn, A.M., Boterberg, T., Van Dycke, A., Linder, B., De Smedt, T., Wadman, W.J., Ben-Menachem, E., Eriksson, P.S. 2007. Radiation of the rat brain suppresses seizure-induced neurogenesis and transiently enhances excitability during kindling acquisition. *Epilepsia.* 48(10), 1952-63.

[260] Pekcec, A., Lupke, M., Baumann, R., Seifert, H., Potschka, H. 2011. Modulation of neurogenesis by targeted hippocampal irradiation fails to affect kindling progression. *Hippocampus.* 21(8), 866-76.

[261] Cho, K.O., Lybrand, Z.R., Ito, N., Brulet, R., Tafacory, F., Zhang, L., Good, L., Ure, K., Kernie, S.G., Birnbaum, S.G., Scharfman, H.E., Eisch, A.J., Hsieh, J. 2015. Aberrant hippocampal neurogenesis contributes to epilepsy and associated cognitive decline. *Nat Commun.* 6, 6606.

[262] Hosford, B.E., Liska, J.P., Danzer, S.C. 2016. Ablation of Newly Generated Hippocampal Granule Cells Has Disease-Modifying Effects in Epilepsy. *J Neurosci.* 36(43), 11013-11023.

[263] Varma, P., Brulet, R., Zhang, L., Hsieh, J. 2019. Targeting Seizure-Induced Neurogenesis in a Clinically Relevant Time Period Leads to Transient But Not Persistent Seizure Reduction. *J Neurosci.* 39(35), 7019-7028.

[264] Brulet, R., Zhu, J., Aktar, M., Hsieh, J., Cho, K.O. 2017. Mice with conditional NeuroD1 knockout display reduced aberrant hippocampal neurogenesis but no change in epileptic seizures. *Exp Neurol.* 293, 190-198.

[265] Raol, Y.H., Lund, I.V., Bandyopadhyay, S., Zhang, G., Roberts, D.S., Wolfe, J.H., Russek, S.J., Brooks-Kayal, A.R. 2006. Enhancing GABA(A) receptor alpha 1 subunit levels in hippocampal dentate gyrus inhibits epilepsy development in an animal model of temporal lobe epilepsy. *J Neurosci.* 26(44), 11342-6.

[266] Goffin, K., Nissinen, J., Van Laere, K., Pitkanen, A. 2007. Cyclicity of spontaneous recurrent seizures in pilocarpine model of temporal lobe epilepsy in rat. *Exp Neurol.* 205(2), 501-5.

[267] Jung, S., Jones, T.D., Lugo, J.N., Jr., Sheerin, A.H., Miller, J.W., D'Ambrosio, R., Anderson, A.E., Poolos, N.P. 2007. Progressive dendritic HCN channelopathy during epileptogenesis in the rat pilocarpine model of epilepsy. *J Neurosci.* 27(47), 13012-21.

[268] Bumanglag, A.V., & Sloviter, R.S. 2008. Minimal latency to hippocampal epileptogenesis and clinical epilepsy after perforant pathway stimulation-induced status epilepticus in awake rats. *J Comp Neurol.* 510(6), 561-80.

[269] Liwnicz, B.H., Leach, J.L., Yeh, H.S., Privitera, M. 1990. Pericyte degeneration and thickening of basement membranes of cerebral microvessels in complex partial seizures: electron microscopic study of surgically removed tissue. *Neurosurgery.* 26(3), 409-20.

[270] Jiang, F.L., Tang, Y.C., Chia, S.C., Jay, T.M., Tang, F.R. 2007. Anticonvulsive effect of a selective mGluR8 agonist (S)-3,4-dicarboxyphenylglycine (S-3,4-DCPG) in the mouse pilocarpine model of status epilepticus. *Epilepsia.* 48(4), 783-92.

[271] Sloviter, R.S. 1987. Decreased hippocampal inhibition and a selective loss of interneurons in experimental epilepsy. *Science.* 235(4784), 73-6.

[272] Liu, S., Wang, J., Zhu, D., Fu, Y., Lukowiak, K., Lu, Y.M. 2003. Generation of functional inhibitory neurons in the adult rat hippocampus. *J Neurosci.* 23(3), 732-6.
[273] Freund, T.F., & Buzsaki, G. 1996. Interneurons of the hippocampus. *Hippocampus.* 6(4), 347-470.
[274] Kobayashi, M., & Buckmaster, P.S. 2003. Reduced inhibition of dentate granule cells in a model of temporal lobe epilepsy. *J Neurosci.* 23(6), 2440-52.
[275] Morimoto, K., Fahnestock, M., Racine, R.J. 2004. Kindling and status epilepticus models of epilepsy: rewiring the brain. *Prog Neurobiol.* 73(1), 1-60.
[276] Shetty, A.K., & Turner, D.A. 2001. Glutamic acid decarboxylase-67-positive hippocampal interneurons undergo a permanent reduction in number following kainic acid-induced degeneration of ca3 pyramidal neurons. *Exp Neurol.* 169(2), 276-97.
[277] Kempermann, G., Wiskott, L., Gage, F.H. 2004. Functional significance of adult neurogenesis. *Curr Opin Neurobiol.* 14(2), 186-91.
[278] Markakis, E.A., & Gage, F.H. 1999. Adult-generated neurons in the dentate gyrus send axonal projections to field CA3 and are surrounded by synaptic vesicles. *J Comp Neurol.* 406(4), 449-60.
[279] Stanfield, B.B., & Trice, J.E. 1988. Evidence that granule cells generated in the dentate gyrus of adult rats extend axonal projections. *Exp Brain Res.* 72(2), 399-406.
[280] Carlen, M., Cassidy, R.M., Brismar, H., Smith, G.A., Enquist, L.W., Frisen, J. 2002. Functional integration of adult-born neurons. *Curr Biol.* 12(7), 606-8.
[281] van Praag, H., Schinder, A.F., Christie, B.R., Toni, N., Palmer, T.D., Gage, F.H. 2002. Functional neurogenesis in the adult hippocampus. *Nature.* 415(6875), 1030-4.
[282] Jessberger, S., & Kempermann, G. 2003. Adult-born hippocampal neurons mature into activity-dependent responsiveness. *Eur J Neurosci.* 18(10), 2707-12.

[283] Dayer, A.G., Ford, A.A., Cleaver, K.M., Yassaee, M., Cameron, H.A. 2003. Short-term and long-term survival of new neurons in the rat dentate gyrus. *J Comp Neurol.* 460(4), 563-72.

[284] Shors, T.J., Miesegaes, G., Beylin, A., Zhao, M., Rydel, T., Gould, E. 2001. Neurogenesis in the adult is involved in the formation of trace memories. *Nature.* 410(6826), 372-6.

[285] Dodrill, C.B., & Wilensky, A.J. 1990. Intellectual impairment as an outcome of status epilepticus. *Neurology.* 40(5 Suppl 2), 23-7.

[286] Breier, J.I., Fletcher, J.M., Wheless, J.W., Clark, A., Cass, J., Constantinou, J.E. 2000. Profiles of cognitive performance associated with reading disability in temporal lobe epilepsy. *J Clin Exp Neuropsychol.* 22(6), 804-16.

[287] Lassonde, M., Sauerwein, H.C., Jambaque, I., Smith, M.L., Helmstaedter, C. 2000. Neuropsychology of childhood epilepsy: pre- and postsurgical assessment. *Epileptic Disord.* 2(1), 3-13.

[288] Dupont, S., Samson, Y., Van de Moortele, P.F., Samson, S., Poline, J.B., Adam, C., Lehericy, S., Le Bihan, D., Baulac, M. 2001. Delayed verbal memory retrieval: a functional MRI study in epileptic patients with structural lesions of the left medial temporal lobe. *Neuroimage.* 14(5), 995-1003.

[289] Giovagnoli, A.R. 2001. Relation of sorting impairment to hippocampal damage in temporal lobe epilepsy. *Neuropsychologia.* 39(2), 140-50.

[290] Gleissner, U., Helmstaedter, C., Elger, C.E. 2002. Memory reorganization in adult brain: observations in three patients with temporal lobe epilepsy. *Epilepsy Res.* 48(3), 229-34.

[291] Helmstaedter, C., Reuber, M., Elger, C.C. 2002. Interaction of cognitive aging and memory deficits related to epilepsy surgery. *Ann Neurol.* 52(1), 89-94.

[292] Hermann, B.P., Seidenberg, M., Bell, B. 2002. The neurodevelopmental impact of childhood onset temporal lobe epilepsy on brain structure and function and the risk of progressive cognitive effects. *Prog Brain Res.* 135, 429-38.

[293] Martin, P., Maestu, F., Sola, R.G. 2002. Effects of surgical treatment on intellectual performance and memory in a Spanish sample of drug-resistant partial onset-temporal lobe epilepsy patients. *Seizure.* 11(3), 151-6.

[294] Genkova-Papazova, M.G., & Lazarova-Bakarova, M.B. 1995. Pentylenetetrazole kindling impairs long-term memory in rats. *Eur Neuropsychopharmacol.* 5(1), 53-6.

[295] Rice, A.C., Floyd, C.L., Lyeth, B.G., Hamm, R.J., DeLorenzo, R.J. 1998. Status epilepticus causes long-term NMDA receptor-dependent behavioral changes and cognitive deficits. *Epilepsia.* 39(11), 1148-57.

[296] Sutula, T.P., & Hermann, B. 1999. Progression in mesial temporal lobe epilepsy. *Ann Neurol.* 45(5), 553-6.

[297] Hort, J., Brozek, G., Komarek, V., Langmeier, M., Mares, P. 2000. Interstrain differences in cognitive functions in rats in relation to status epilepticus. *Behav Brain Res.* 112(1-2), 77-83.

[298] Hannesson, D.K., Mohapel, P., Corcoran, M.E. 2001. Dorsal hippocampal kindling selectively impairs spatial learning/short-term memory. *Hippocampus.* 11(3), 275-86.

[299] Wu, C.L., Huang, L.T., Liou, C.W., Wang, T.J., Tung, Y.R., Hsu, H.Y., Lai, M.C. 2001. Lithium-pilocarpine-induced status epilepticus in immature rats result in long-term deficits in spatial learning and hippocampal cell loss. *Neurosci Lett.* 312(2), 113-7.

[300] Sogawa, Y., Monokoshi, M., Silveira, D.C., Cha, B.H., Cilio, M.R., McCabe, B.K., Liu, X., Hu, Y., Holmes, G.L. 2001. Timing of cognitive deficits following neonatal seizures: relationship to histological changes in the hippocampus. *Brain Res Dev Brain Res.* 131(1-2), 73-83.

[301] Rutten, A., van Albada, M., Silveira, D.C., Cha, B.H., Liu, X., Hu, Y.N., Cilio, M.R., Holmes, G.L. 2002. Memory impairment following status epilepticus in immature rats: time-course and environmental effects. *Eur J Neurosci.* 16(3), 501-13.

[302] Kubova, H., Mares, P., Suchomelova, L., Brozek, G., Druga, R., Pitkanen, A. 2004. Status epilepticus in immature rats leads to

behavioural and cognitive impairment and epileptogenesis. *Eur J Neurosci.* 19(12), 3255-65.

[303] Kinoshameg, S.E., & Persinger, M.A. 2002. Working memory and reference memory in adult rats following limbic seizures induced at 21 or 90 days of age. *Psychol Rep.* 91(3 Pt 1), 729-30.

[304] Brooks-Kayal, A.R., Bath, K.G., Berg, A.T., Galanopoulou, A.S., Holmes, G.L., Jensen, F.E., Kanner, A.M., O'Brien, T.J., Whittemore, V.H., Winawer, M.R., Patel, M., Scharfman, H.E. 2013. Issues related to symptomatic and disease-modifying treatments affecting cognitive and neuropsychiatric comorbidities of epilepsy. *Epilepsia.* 54 Suppl 4, 44-60.

[305] Alessio, A., Damasceno, B.P., Camargo, C.H., Kobayashi, E., Guerreiro, C.A., Cendes, F. 2004. Differences in memory performance and other clinical characteristics in patients with mesial temporal lobe epilepsy with and without hippocampal atrophy. *Epilepsy Behav.* 5(1), 22-7.

[306] Brown-Croyts, L.M., Caton, P.W., Radecki, D.T., McPherson, S.L. 2000. Phenobarbital pre-treatment prevents kainic acid-induced impairments in acquisition learning. *Life Sci.* 67(6), 643-50.

[307] Santarelli, L., Saxe, M., Gross, C., Surget, A., Battaglia, F., Dulawa, S., Weisstaub, N., Lee, J., Duman, R., Arancio, O., Belzung, C., Hen, R. 2003. Requirement of hippocampal neurogenesis for the behavioral effects of antidepressants. *Science.* 301(5634), 805-9.

[308] Engel, J., Jr., Thompson, P.M., Stern, J.M., Staba, R.J., Bragin, A., Mody, I. 2013. Connectomics and epilepsy. *Curr Opin Neurol.* 26(2), 186-94.

[309] Song, H., Stevens, C.F., Gage, F.H. 2002. Astroglia induce neurogenesis from adult neural stem cells. *Nature.* 417(6884), 39-44.

[310] Gonzalez-Perez, O., & Quinones-Hinojosa, A. 2012. Astrocytes as neural stem cells in the adult brain. *J Stem Cells.* 7(3), 181-8.

[311] Staley, K. 2004. Neuroscience. Epileptic neurons go wireless. *Science.* 305(5683), 482-3.

[312] Bernard, C., Anderson, A., Becker, A., Poolos, N.P., Beck, H., Johnston, D. 2004. Acquired dendritic channelopathy in temporal lobe epilepsy. *Science*. 305(5683), 532-5.

[313] Wang, N., Mi, X., Gao, B., Gu, J., Wang, W., Zhang, Y., Wang, X. 2015. Minocycline inhibits brain inflammation and attenuates spontaneous recurrent seizures following pilocarpine-induced status epilepticus. *Neuroscience*. 287, 144-56.

In: The Dentate Gyrus
Editor: Feng-Ru Tang
ISBN: 978-1-68507-212-4

Chapter 7

THE DENTATE GYRUS AND ITS INVOLVEMENT IN ALZHEIMER'S DISEASE

Lee Rui Xue*

Radiation Physiology Lab,
Singapore Nuclear Research and Safety Initiative,
National University of Singapore, Singapore

ABSTRACT

As one of the most common forms of dementia globally with ever-growing number of diagnosed individuals, Alzheimer's disease (AD) is becoming a public health crisis. AD patients often suffer from memory loss and other cognitive impairments that severely lower their quality of life as the disease progresses. Current therapeutic methods have largely been ineffective and the search for viable treatment options remains urgent. Located in the temporal lobe, the dentate gyrus has been demonstrated to be implicated in AD. Loss of volume and altered adult neurogenesis in the dentate gyrus have been reported in AD animal models and human samples. Impaired pattern separation, altered synaptic signaling and astrocytic changes in the dentate gyrus may also

* Corresponding Author's Email: leerx4@gmail.com.

be associated with the cognitive impairments observed in AD patients. Understanding the involvement of the dentate gyrus in AD could aid us in elucidating the aetiology and pathophysiology of AD, thereby providing avenues for more drug targets to be discovered. Thus, in this chapter, we will outline the alterations observed in the dentate gyrus, with a focus on the associations of AD-related changes to altered adult neurogenesis.

Keywords: dentate gyrus, Alzheimer's disease, adult neurogenesis

1. Introduction

As the most common form of dementia worldwide, Alzheimer's disease (AD) is a progressive and multifactorial neurodegenerative disease, characterized by cognitive and memory impairments, that eventually come to severely impact a patient's quality of life [1]. Despite being the most widely studied form of dementia and affecting almost 50 million people globally [2], current therapeutic methods against AD have largely been ineffective. The inability to deliver drugs across the impassable blood-brain barrier, coupled with contradicting hypotheses proposed about AD aetiology and the complex physiology of the neurological system, pose great challenges in the identification and development of successful therapies [3]. Thus, there is a pressing need to resolve the underlying pathophysiology of AD, identify potential biomarkers and develop diagnostic tools and effective therapies for AD.

AD usually presents itself in patients with two particular histopathological hallmarks: the abnormal extracellular accumulation of amyloid plaques and the presence of intracellular neurofibrillary tangles (NFTs) due to hyperphosphorylated tau proteins [4-7]. Other common findings of AD include neuronal degeneration [8, 9] particularly in the hippocampus [10, 11], synaptic loss [12, 13] and altered synaptic signalling [14, 15]. Early studies show that NFTs initially form in medial temporal lobe structures such as the hippocampus and spread to the temporal, parietal and frontal lobes. On the other hand, amyloid plaque deposition starts in the parietal, temporal and frontal regions [16, 17]. As the core region responsible for human episodic memory, alterations to the structures and functions of the medial temporal lobe have been demonstrated to be associated with AD progression [18-20].

Residing in the temporal lobe, the dentate gyrus is a crucial member of the hippocampal trisynaptic circuit [21]. The dentate gyrus is widely believed to play a key role in hippocampus-related functions such as learning, mnemonic processing and episodic memory [22-24]. The subgranular zone (SGZ) of the dentate gyrus is one of the two regions of adult neurogenesis [25, 26]. Neural stem cells (NSCs) within the SGZ continuously proliferates throughout adulthood, with some of its daughter cells differentiating into dentate granule cells (DGCs). These neurons are highly abundant within the dentate gyrus and they integrate into pre-existing neural networks of the brain [27]. Within the trisynaptic circuit, DGCs receive sensory inputs from the entorhinal cortex and process them into spatial and non-spatial information [28]. The information is subsequently conveyed to Cornu Ammonis (CA) 3 of the hippocampus [29] via mossy fibre projections of DGCs [30]. The ability of these neurons to convert similar cortical neural inputs into non-overlapping output patterns [31], coupled with their low firing rates [32] and sparse encoding system contribute to the differentiation of similar memories and help to keep memories distinct [31-34]. As such, the dentate gyrus carries out pattern separation [22, 35] and acts as a pre-processing region to facilitate information storage in the CA3 [36].

Several studies have proposed that adult neurogenesis may be involved in mediating pattern separation. A reduction of adult neurogenesis in the dentate gyrus has also been shown to be associated with pattern separation deficits [37, 38], while elevating levels of adult neurogenesis in a mouse model conferred an improved ability to differentiate overlapping contextual representations and sufficiently enhanced pattern separation [39]. Incidentally, impairments in pattern separation have been found to be implicated in AD [34]. Compromised or diminished adult neurogenesis in the dentate gyrus compared to age-matched controls is also a common finding in AD animal models [40-42]. Likewise, similar findings have recently been observed in human samples [43]. Furthermore, gross abnormalities in the dentate gyrus was observed in AD sufferers. Simultaneous [^{18}F] fluorodeoxyglucose-positron emission tomography (FGD-PET) magnetic resonance imaging (MRI) scans showed that dentate gyrus volume negatively associated with AD and changes in metabolic activity in the diseased dentate gyrus was also observed [44, 45]. Functional MRI studies on individuals genetically predisposed to AD; i.e., carriers of the apolipoprotein E ε4 (APOEε4) allele, revealed that these individuals exhibited decreased dentate gyrus activity [46]. Altogether, these findings suggest that the dentate gyrus is implicated in the pathophysiology of AD.

In this chapter, the pathophysiological hallmarks of AD observed in the dentate gyrus will be discussed, with an emphasis on how these AD-associated changes may be related to altered adult neurogenesis in the dentate gyrus. Other modifications to the dentate gyrus in AD and their contributions to AD-related cognitive impairments will also be considered.

2. AD-Related Alterations in the Dentate Gyrus and Their Association with the Dysregulation of Adult Neurogenesis in AD

Over decades of AD research, multiple hypotheses pertaining to the aetiology of AD have been proposed and served as a foundation of AD therapies [47]. However, the exact mechanisms underlying the manifestation of this disease have yet to be fully elucidated. Nonetheless, it is clear that AD is multifactorial. There are two distinct types of AD, the rare ‘early-onset’ familial AD (FAD) and the pervasive ‘late-onset’ sporadic AD (SAD). The former is commonly associated with mutations in amyloid precursor protein (APP), presenilin 1 (PS1) and presenilin 2

(PS2), while the latter is frequently linked to APOEε4, as well as other genetic and environmental factors [48, 49]. Both forms of AD share common clinical presentations as well as the abnormal accumulation of extracellular amyloid plaques and intraneuronal NFTs [50, 51].

Furthermore, reduced neurogenesis appears to be a frequent observation in AD animal models and human samples [40-43]. Reduction in doublecortin (DCX) positive cells also correlated with the severity of disease progression in AD patients [52]. On the other hand, there were several reports of increased hippocampal neurogenesis [53-55] in AD mouse models, this discrepancy may be due to off-target effects from genetic alterations or the combination of mutations in the mouse models [56, 57]. Nonetheless, studies have indicated an age-related decline in normal adult hippocampal neurogenesis [58, 59]. Thus, it is necessary to differentiate between healthy physiological and pathological reductions in neurogenesis [60, 61]. Evaluation of the dentate gyrus in human AD patients revealed drastic declines in immature neuron numbers and maturation compared to age-matched healthy human controls, thereby supporting the notion that adult neurogenesis is implicated in AD [43]. Here, we will focus on the AD-related alterations to the dentate gyrus, including the classical hallmarks, and their relationship with impaired adult neurogenesis.

2.1. Accumulation of Amyloid Plaques

The abnormal build-up of amyloid plaques in the brain is a classic indicator of AD. These plaques are composed of β-amyloid peptides (Aβ) accumulates. Generally, Aβ peptides are thought to be formed by the sequential cleavage of APP by β- and γ-secretase via the amyloidogenic pathway [62, 63]. In the hippocampus, it seems that Aβ peptides released by neurons in the entorhinal cortex of transgenic AD mice with double mutations in PS-1 and APP were transported to the dentate gyrus via the perforant pathway, where they formed amyloid plaques [64]. Many studies have ascribed the AD-related impairments in neurogenesis to the extracellular accumulation of Aβ. At 12-14 months of age, transgenic mice overexpressing the Swedish APP (APP^{Swe}) mutant experienced reduced neurogenesis where proliferation and survival of neural progenitor cells (NPCs) were diminished only in the presence of abundant amyloid deposits. Prior to any discernible deposits, these 3-month-old transgenic mice did not show signs of impaired neurogenesis [65]. Another study using double transgenic mutant mice ($APP^{Swe}/PS1^{L166P}$) revealed that amyloid deposits possibly disrupted neurogenesis by altering the biology of NSCs as morphologically abnormal quiescent nestin-positive astrocyte-like stem cells and transient amplifying progenitor cells were observed in these mice [66].

Amyloid plaques were also observed in the granule cell layer (GCL) of the dentate gyrus in aged APP-PS1 mice, with a concomitant loss of GCL volume, likely attributed to neuronal loss [67]. Double "knock-in" mice with mutations in APP and PS1 also suffered from long term impairment of adult neurogenesis [68]. Further, *in vitro* treatment of human and murine neurospheres with $A\beta_{42}$ disrupted NPC proliferation and differentiation [65], perhaps due to the induction of senescent phenotype via the activation of formylpeptide receptor 2, a target of $A\beta_{42}$ [69]. Similarly, bilateral intrahippocampal injection of human $A\beta_{1-42}$ to adult mouse brain also reduced neurogenesis, as demonstrated by a significant reduction in bromodeoxyuridine (BrdU)/DCX double positive cells in the SGZ of the dentate gyrus, with concomitant decreases in interferon-γ (IFNγ) and nuclear factor-kappa B (NF-κB) levels [70]. In addition, PDAPP mice (APP^{V717F}) exhibited abnormal maturation of newborn DGCs and reduced SGZ proliferation [40]. Altogether, accumulation of amyloid plaques seems to alter the neurogenesis process in the dentate gyrus through multiple mechanisms, that ultimately lead to reduced neurogenesis.

However, it was also reported that neurogenesis impairment in the dentate gyrus may have occurred prior to the accumulation of amyloid plaques. APPswe/PS1ΔE9 transgenic mice, age as young as two months, suffered significantly diminished neurogenesis with impaired NPC proliferation and neuronal differentiation, in the absence of any observable amyloid deposits [71]. Moreover, while investigations involving APPswe/PS1ΔE9 and Tg2576 mouse models revealed hyperproliferation of neuroblasts in the SGZ of young individuals (3 months old) without amyloid plaques, these cells exhibited an immature morphology with significantly lowered survival and maturation capabilities compared to age-matched wild type mice [67]. Similarly, impairments in neurogenesis and reduced numbers of new neurons in the hippocampus of young Tg2576 mice were also observed [72]. Furthermore, triple transgenic (3xTg) AD mouse models had diminished numbers of proliferating cells, NPCs and neuroblasts at pre-plaque stages as well [73]. While these data suggest that impaired neurogenesis may precede the formation of amyloid plaques, the extent of plaque accumulation is inextricably linked to the severity of neurogenesis impairment, as demonstrated in a time course study of 3xTg mice [41]. Overall, it is undeniable that the presence and accumulation of amyloid plaques negatively impacts neurogenesis in the dentate gyrus.

2.2. Hyperphosphorylated Tau and NFTs

Another classic neuropathological hallmark of AD is the progressive formation of NFTs. These tangles are composed of microtubule-associated protein tau (MAPT). In neurons, tau proteins are known to associate with microtubules for their stabilization and for axonal growth and integrity [74-76]. Under physiological conditions, tau proteins may also be involved in the migration of newborn neurons from the SGZ to the granular layer [77] as well as adult neurogenesis in the dentate gyrus [78], as demonstrated by the deficiencies of these processes observed in Tau knockout mice [77, 78]. In a group of neurodegenerative diseases including AD, known as tauopathy, tau proteins are aberrantly hyperphosphorylated. Hyperphosphorylated tau dissociates from microtubules and form insoluble aggregates, leading to the formation of NFTs [79]. Despite being highly associated with the progression of AD, surprisingly little has been done to elucidate the relationship between hyperphosphorylated tau and NFTs to adult neurogenesis. Early studies showed that AD-associated neurofibrillary changes first begin in the hippocampus and its associated regions. Furthermore, several AD patients and tauopathy mouse models displayed NFT depositions in the dentate gyrus [80-83]. Tauopathy mice expressing human tau (hTau) proteins suffered reduced neurogenesis in the dentate gyrus starting at 2 months of age, with a 31% decrease in proliferating DCX/BrdU double positive cells in the dentate gyrus, indicating deficiencies in neural progenitor proliferation [84].

Mice expressing tau^{P301L} displayed NFTs that worsened with age, along with neuronal loss and memory deficits similar to those observed in AD [85]. Transplantation of NSCs into the hippocampus of tau^{P301L} mice resulted in increased levels of proteins related to neurogenesis, along with improvements of cognitive abilities [86]. Additionally, tau knockout in the Tg30 tauopathy murine model rescued the reductions in numbers of Ki-67-positive and DCX-positive cells in the SGZ of the dentate gyrus. Moreover, these tau knockout-Tg30 mice had a lower density of phopshotau positive cells in the dentate gyrus, compared to Tg30 mice [87]. Furthermore, $mapt^{-/-}$ mice exhibited increased neurogenesis in the dentate gyrus, demonstrated by elevated numbers of BrdU+ cells and increased expression levels of proteins related to neuronal growth and proliferation, as well as neurite development and branching [88]. Altogether, the data indicates that presence of tau pathology in the dentate gyrus likely causes a reduction of hippocampal neurogenesis by disrupting the proliferation of neural progenitor cells.

Although murine models of tauopathy revealed impaired adult neurogenesis along with cognitive decline similar to that of AD, these data may not necessarily imply that reduced neurogenesis in AD was due to similar causes. In fact, many common AD animal models with impaired neurogenesis do not exhibit NFT formations [89, 90], thereby suggesting that the impairments may be tau-independent. Nonetheless, phosphorylated tau proteins were observed in γ-aminobutyric acid

(GABA)-ergic interneurons of the SGZ and hilus of the dentate gyrus of AD patients and 3xTg AD mice. In addition, overexpression of hTau in dentate gyrus GABAergic interneurons repressed GABAergic transmission, leading to impaired neurogenesis [91]. Furthermore, an AD mouse model expressing the Osaka mutation (E693Δ) in APP, in addition to tau264 with low levels of 3- and 4-repeat human tau, experienced tau hyperphosphorylation and NFT accumulation at 6 and 18 months of age respectively, along with Aβ oligomer accumulation. Neuronal loss was also observed at 18 months [92]. Thus, it is possible that amyloid plaques and NFTs are involved in exacerbating the pathogenesis of AD. Administration of exogenous amyloid peptides into tau transgenic mice with NFTs further worsened the tau pathology [93, 94]. Overall, how hyperphosphorylated tau and NFT formation affects adult neurogenesis in AD remains unclear. Further investigations using transgenic AD models expressing hTau may elucidate the contributions and mechanisms of tauopathy to altered neurogenesis. As tau ablation was demonstrated to increase adult neurogenesis, anti-tau therapy may be a promising option for AD treatment.

2.3. Neuroinflammation

Apart from amyloid plaques and NFTs, neuroinflammation, mediated mostly by astrocytes and microglia, is also a common finding in AD [95]. Microglia and astrocytes become reactive in the presence of Aβ and NFT and secrete a variety of proinflammatory cytokines such as tumour necrosis factor α (TNFα), interleukin 1β (IL-1β) [96, 97] and IL-6 [96, 98]. Similar pro-inflammatory cytokines were also detected at elevated levels in AD patients [99, 100]. A recent longitudinal PET imaging study of AD patients with mild cognitive impairments revealed that neuroinflammation in AD is biphasic. Initially, microglial activation increased as Aβ load increased. Once Aβ load approached AD levels, microglial activation reduces and subsequently increases again as NFT load rose [101]. Unfortunately, secretion of proinflammatory cytokines by reactive microglia and astrocytes, particularly TNFα, seemed to further worsen amyloid deposition and tau pathology [102-104]. NLR family pyrin domain containing 3 (NLRP3) inflammasome activation in microglia also contributes to this vicious cycle in the APP/PS1 double transgenic AD mice [104]. Thus, with persistent neuroinflammation and its ability to modify the neurogenic microenvironment [105], coupled with the sensitivity of NSCs and NPCs to cytokines and immune molecules [106], it is highly likely that neuroinflammation is a factor that contributes to altered neurogenesis in AD.

Previously, neuroinflammation was commonly associated with a reduction in neurogenesis. Now, with increasing evidence showing that microglial support is required for neurogenesis [107, 108], it is possible that the effects of inflammation on neurogenesis depends the balance between the actions of secreted pro- and anti-inflammatory molecules [106]. Nonetheless, the pro-inflammatory cytokines secreted by activated microglia and astrocytes in AD are known to have a negative impact on neurogenesis. Intracerebroventricular streptozotocin injections in rats, used to mimic SAD, resulted in microgliosis and astrogliosis, supported by the increased immunoreactivity to ionized calcium binding adaptor molecule 1 (Iba1) and glial fibrillary acidic protein (GFAP) respectively [109, 110]. The same rodent model also suffered from acute and sustained neuroinflammation and concomitant reductions in cellular proliferation of NSCs and immature neuron numbers in the dentate gyrus as well as diminished survival, differentiation and survival of newly generated neurons [110]. In addition, microglia-derived TNFα promoted the death of hippocampal-specific progenitor cells *in vitro* [111]. Chronic expression of TNFα in the hippocampus of 3xTg AD mice using stereotactically introduced recombinant adeno-associated virus (AAV) vector expressing TNFα promoted localised neuroinflammation with Aβ and hyperphosphorylated tau, and resulted in neuronal death in the dentate gyrus [112].

Incidentally, not only did impaired neurogenesis occur early before any discernible amyloid deposits in APP/PS1 double transgenic mice, it seemed to be altered prior to microglial activation and neuroinflammation as well [113]. This further supports the notion that altered hippocampal neurogenesis could be an early pathology of AD. Nonetheless, AAV serotype 2/1-mediated gene delivery of IL-10, an anti-inflammatory cytokine into the hippocampus of APP/PS1 AD mice reduced gliosis and enhanced neurogenesis by promoting NSC proliferation [114]. Administration of metformin, a drug commonly prescribed for type II diabetes, to APPswe/PS1ΔE9 mice reduced amyloid plaque load, attenuated chronic inflammation and hippocampal neuron loss and improved neurogenesis via the adenosine monophosphate-activate protein kinase/mammalian target of rapamycin/S6 kinase/β-secretase 1 (AMPK/mTOR/S6K/Bace1) and AMPK/P65 NF-κB hippocampal signalling pathways [115]. Altogether, the relationship between neurogenesis and neuroinflammation is highly complex. Further investigations are required to elucidate the exact causal mechanism between these events. Nevertheless, anti-inflammatory agents may provide another potential avenue for AD therapy.

2.4. Overactivity of GSK3β

Glycogen synthase kinase 3 (GSK3) is a serine/threonine kinase with two mammalian isoforms, GSK3α and GSK3β [116]. Expression levels of the latter was observed to be elevated in brains of AD patients [117]. Overactivity of GSK3β is believed to be associated with various pathological hallmarks of AD including hyperphosphorylation of tau, increased production of Aβ and activation of inflammatory responses, thus giving rise to the "GSK3 hypothesis of AD" [118]. GSK3β is also commonly regarded to be the molecular bridge between the amyloid and tau hypotheses [119, 120], where GSK3β mediates Aβ production and Aβ-related neuronal death while Aβ activates GSK3β to phosphorylate tau [121, 122]. Inhibition of GSK3β overactivity in $PDAPP^{+/-}$ mice has been demonstrated to reverse several AD-related modifications such as reducing levels of hyperphosphorylated tau and amyloid plaques [123].

Normal physiological activity of GSK3 is highly important for processes in neural development, such as neurogenesis and neuronal survival [124]. However, overexpression of GSK3β was found to be correlated with increased levels of hyperphosphorylated tau proteins in dentate gyrus neurons [125], neurodegeneration [126], altered neuronal maturation and depletion of neurogenic niches in the dentate gyrus [127]. Interestingly, overexpression of GSK3β in BG6 mice during adulthood seemed to increase the number of DCX+ cells in the dentate gyrus, indicating increased adult neurogenesis. However, this observation may be a compensatory mechanism to replace dying neurons observed in this model [125].

Furthermore, overexpression of GSK3β resulted in alterations to the dendritic tree and post-synaptic densities of newborn neurons in the dentate gyrus, similar to that observed in AD patients [128, 129]. Reversal of GSK3β overexpression resulted in regression of the altered morphologies in DGCs [128] and led to the amelioration of AD-related pathologies with normal GSK3β activity and reduced neuronal death [130]. Moreover, chemical inhibition of GSK3β increased neurosphere proliferation and induced NSC differentiation *in vitro* and tideglusib-inhibition of GSK3β enhanced neurogenesis in the dentate gyrus of adult rats [131]. Competitive inhibition of GSK3β in APPswe/PS1ΔE9 double transgenic AD mice using andrographolide increased DGC numbers through the activation of Wnt signalling [132]. Interestingly, enhancing GSK3β activity by intermittent fasting of 3xTg AD mice promoted neurogenesis in the dentate gyrus via the activation of adenosine monophosphate-activated protein kinase and brain-derived neurotrophic factor pathways, an effect that was abolished when GSK3β was knocked down [133]. Overall, GSK3β is a promising target for AD treatment based on its pleiotropic roles in AD pathophysiology. More work has to be done to elucidate the effects of GSK3β overactivity on adult neurogenesis in the context of AD through the use of AD transgenic models.

2.5. Other Factors

The brain is highly complex with intricate interactions and cross-talks between different neural cell types. Hence, it is highly possible that there are other factors and modifications in AD, besides the aforementioned factors, that alter adult neurogenesis in the dentate gyrus.

Elevated GABAergic signalling influenced by Aβ or an imbalance between GABAergic and glutamatergic transmission in the dentate gyrus of human APP-J20 AD mice was observed to be associated with impaired neurogenesis, where adult-born DGCs had compromised morphologies and functions during maturation [134]. Further, AD patients were found to experience dysregulated leptin signalling within the hippocampus as leptin receptors were localized to NFTs [135]. Leptin is an adipose-derived hormone that has neuroprotective effects [136] and may participate in adult neurogenesis [137]. Treatment with leptin increased NSC proliferation and differentiation in the dentate gyrus of APP/PS1 AD mice and attenuated the pathological features of AD [138]. Hence, it is possible that a resistance to leptin signalling contributes to altered neurogenesis in AD. However, this association remains to be established.

Post-mortem analysis of human AD brains also revealed reduced levels of fibroblast growth factor (FGF) 2 [139]. Declines in FGF signalling in aged mice correlated with aging-related reductions in hippocampal neurogenesis [140]. Delivery of FGF2 gene to the hippocampus of APP/PS1 mice using AAV serotype 2/1 improved neurogenesis and reinstituted hippocampal functions [141]. This suggests that FGF signalling may be altered in AD brains, thereby contributing to altered neurogenesis.

Furthermore, decreased microRNA (miR)-132 levels were observed in AD mouse models and patients, and may play a role in AD pathology [142, 143]. miR-132 is necessary for normal NPC proliferation and adult neurogenesis in the dentate gyrus [144, 145]. Overexpression of miR-132 in knock-in humanized $App^{NL\text{-}G\text{-}F}$ and APP/PS1 transgenic AD mice rescued adult neurogenesis in the dentate gyrus and restored associated memory deficits in these animals [146]. Similarly, upregulation of miR-

132 in rats with AD also improved cognitive performance by inhibiting the expression of mitogen-activated protein kinase (MAPK) 1 [147]. Thus, not only can miR-132 expression levels be a potential biomarker for AD diagnosis, it is also a promising therapeutic target for AD therapy.

Altogether, the factors contributing to altered neurogenesis in AD that have been discussed in this section is non-exhaustive. However, as these factors often interact and influence each other, it will be challenging to isolate a causal mechanism for targeted AD therapy. Further investigations will be warranted to understand the true mechanism underlying AD-related altered neurogenesis. Nonetheless, combinatorial therapies targeting different factors influencing adult neurogenesis may be a promising avenue for AD treatment.

3. Contributions of Altered Adult Neurogenesis to AD Pathology

As mentioned in the introduction, the dentate gyrus and adult neurogenesis play important roles in learning and memory [148]. With cognitive impairments being one of the most common presentations of AD, it is only natural to wonder if altered adult neurogenesis in the dentate gyrus contributes to the pathogenesis of AD. Many studies have observed that decreased adult hippocampal neurogenesis preceded the accumulation of amyloid plaques and NFTs in various AD models [67, 71-73]. Impairments in neurogenesis also occurred prior to neuroinflammation and altered dentate gyrus function in APP/PS1 [113] and Tg2576 AD mice [72] respectively. Furthermore, cognitive impairments of APP/PS1 AD mice were observed to develop after reductions of NSCs and intermediate progenitor cell numbers [149]. Thus, impairment of adult neurogenesis seems to be an early occurrence in AD pathology and may underlie the cognitive deficits associated with AD. This was demonstrated in APPswe/PS1ΔE9 and 5xFAD mouse models where ablation of neurogenesis in the dentate gyrus exacerbated cognitive deficits [150, 151]. Decreased neurogenesis in APPswe/ PS1ΔE9 AD mice was also suggested to induce cognitive deficits in AD by promoting overactivations of neurons in the dentate gyrus and hippocampal CA1 and CA3 regions [150].

Furthermore, improvement in neurogenesis through AAV serotype 2/1 gene delivery of IL-10 into the hippocampus also enhanced spatial learning in APP/PS1 mice [114]. Transplantation of adipose-derived mesenchymal stem cells also increased the number of DCX+/BrdU+ neuroblasts in the SGZ and improved cognitive function in the same model [152]. On the contrary, while adult hippocampal neurogenesis was indeed compromised in hAPP-20 and APP/PS1 AD mice, drug-induced and genetic ablation of adult NSCs improved cognitive function in these models via the restoration of synaptic transmission among DGCs, without reducing Aβ load [153]. Regardless, with evidence that impaired neurogenesis could occur before the emergence of AD hallmarks and the importance of adult hippocampal neurogenesis in learning and memory, it is possible that impaired neurogenesis may in fact, be causative of the cognitive decline seen in AD patients and mouse models. Early changes in neurogenesis may have sensitized the dentate gyrus and hippocampus to further damage in late stage AD. However, more studies are required to determine whether impaired hippocampal neurogenesis is one of the causal factors in AD pathology, or if it is a repercussion of other AD-related hallmarks.

4. Other Alterations to the Dentate Gyrus in AD

Aside from altered neurogenesis in the dentate gyrus, several other changes to the dentate gyrus have been observed in AD models and patients. Here, these modifications and their contributions to AD pathology will be briefly discussed. A graphical summary of these alterations as well as the factors influencing adult neurogenesis in the dentate gyrus is included in Figure 1.

Synaptic changes in the dentate gyrus have been reported in AD [154]. Electron microscopy of the outer molecular layer in the dentate gyrus of APP/PS1 mice showed reduced synaptic density compared to wild type mice [155]. Post-mortem electron microscopy analysis of AD patients also revealed a signification decrease in synaptic density and reduction in width of the entire molecular layer compared to non-demented age match controls [156,157]. Interestingly, an earlier study reported that the levels of synaptophysin, a marker for synaptic terminals, were higher in 19 months old Tg2576 AD mice compared to age-matched controls. The elevated synaptophysin level was associated with impaired synaptic function which contributed to cognitive dysfunction [158]. Nonetheless, synaptic loss and dysfunction in other parts of the brain have been closely associated with the cognitive impairments observed in AD [159-161]. Hence, such changes in the dentate gyrus would likely contribute to this phenomenon as well.

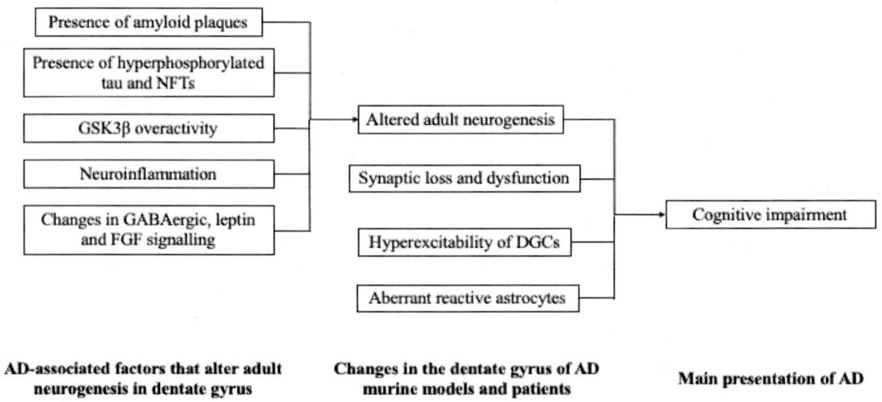

Figure 1. Graphical summary of the factors influencing adult neurogenesis within the dentate gyrus and contributions of alterations in the dentate gyrus to cognitive impairment in AD. NFTs: neurofibrillary tangles; GSK3β: glycogen synthase kinase 3; GABA: γ-aminobutyric acid; FGF: fibroblast growth factor; DGCs: dentate granule cells.

Another frequent observation in the dentate gyrus of AD brains is the hyperexcitability of DGCs. In fact, hyperexcitability of the hippocampal network has been considered as an early sign of memory impairment in AD [162-164]. As mentioned in the introduction, sparse firing in the dentate gyrus is crucial for pattern separation and keeping memories distinct [31-34]. Hyperexcitability of DGCs in Tg2576 AD mice was associated with impaired pattern separation, likely due to decreased expression of Kv4.1 ion channels in the DGCs [165, 166]. This suggests that DGC hyperactivity could be one of the causal mechanisms underlying cognitive deficits observed in AD [165]. A separate study using the same model showed that Tg2576 DGCs had a higher frequency of excitatory postsynaptic currents, which was indicative that the hyperactivity could be due to disrupted communication between the entorhinal cortex and dentate gyrus. Treatment with a peroxisome proliferator-activated receptor γ (PPARγ) agonist restored DGC presynaptic function and improved cognitive functions in treated mice [167]. In support of a pre-synaptic mechanism for DGC hyperexcitability, several presynaptic proteins related to neurotransmitter release were found to be at reduced levels in the outer molecular layer of the dentate gyrus [168, 169], a main region of input into the hippocampus [170].

Furthermore, another study revealed that DGC hyperexcitability in Tg2576 AD mice is an early phenomenon. The hyperactivity of these DGCs was reduced upon administration of atropine, a non-selective muscarinic receptor antagonist, showing that these hyperactive neurons also exhibited muscarinic cholinergic dysregulation [171]. Intriguingly, reduced adult hippocampal neurogenesis seem to have preceded the alterations in the excitatory and inhibitory neuronal circuits in the dentate gyrus of Tg2576 AD mice [72], thereby suggesting that altered neurogenesis may have a role in AD hippocampal dysfunction. Altogether, these data suggest that the hyperactivity of neurons in the dentate gyrus very likely contributes to hippocampal hyperexcitability in AD. Understanding the underlying mechanism of this abnormality could aid in the development of treatment options that can alleviate the cognitive impairments suffered by AD patients.

Apart from changes in the neural properties of the dentate gyrus in AD, research focusing on the changes of astrocytes in AD has become increasingly popular. Atrophy of astrocytes were observed in the dentate gyrus of 3xTg AD mice, with lowered GFAP-positive volume and surface area [172]. Astrocyte-neuron interactions were also significantly decreased in the dentate gyrus of 5xFAD mice, which was ameliorated by Stattic, a STAT3 phosphorylation inhibitor. Reduced colocalization of astrocytes and neurons in the dentate gyrus may have impaired memory formation in these mice [173]. Reactive astrocytes around amyloid plaques found in the dentate gyrus of APP/PS1 AD mice abnormally released the inhibitory gliotransmitter GABA that decreased the spike probability of DGCs. This contributed to impaired learning and memory in the mice [174]. A similar finding was reported in 5xFAD mice where a high level of astrocytic GABA imposed tonic inhibition of DGCs and impaired long-term potentiation and memory [175]. In human AD patients, accumulation of tau proteins was discovered in astrocytes of the dentate gyrus hilus. Similar tau accumulation in mice resulted in alterations to mitochondrial physiology in these cells which resulted in decreased adult neurogenesis and impaired spatial memory [176]. Together, these data suggest that astrocytes could have an important role in AD pathogenesis by influencing neuronal networks in the dentate gyrus. Furthermore, astrocytes in the dentate gyrus influence adult neurogenesis and their compromised functions in AD likely also contribute to the impairment of adult neurogenesis [177].

Conclusion and Future Directions

In this chapter, we have outlined how the dentate gyrus is altered in AD. It is evident that the dentate gyrus is implicated in the pathogenesis of AD. Hallmarks of AD such as the presence of hyperphosphorylated tau, NFTs and amyloid plaques negatively impact adult neurogenesis in the dentate gyrus, possibly leading to impaired memory and cognitive functions, a phenomenon characteristic of AD. Other alterations in the dentate gyrus such as neuroinflammation, overactivity of GSK3β and altered GABAergic or leptin signalling were also described to alter adult hippocampal neurogenesis. As further research is conducted on AD models and post-mortem human AD brains, more factors associated with impaired neurogenesis are revealed.

Many studies have considered altered neurogenesis as an early sign in AD and this process may also be possibly implicated in the development of cognitive dysfunctions as well. In addition, modifications apart from impaired neurogenesis, such as synaptic alterations, hyperactivity of DGCs and astrocytic changes in the dentate gyrus could also contribute to the dysfunctions. Given the complexity and intricacies of the factors involved in AD pathogenesis, pinpointing the exact cause of AD will be challenging. However, by understanding the various factors involved and the interactions between them, we will gain a clearer picture on the pathogenesis of AD. Eventually, novel drugs and combinatorial therapies targeting the pathological and molecular changes in the AD dentate gyrus can be developed.

References

[1] Querfurth, H. W., LaFerla, F. M. 2010. Alzheimer's disease. *N. Engl. J. Med.* 362, 329-44.

[2] Guzman-Martinez, L., Calfio, C., Farias, G. A., Vilches, C., Prieto, R., Maccioni, R. B. 2021. New frontiers in the prevention, diagnosis, and treatment of Alzheimer's disease. *J. Alzheimers.* Dis. 82, S51-S63.

[3] Se Thoe, E., Fauzi, A., Tang, Y. Q., Chamyuang, S., Chia, A. Y. Y. 2021. A review on advances of treatment modalities for Alzheimer's disease. *Life. Sci.* 276, 119129.

[4] Minter, M. R., Taylor, J. M., Crack, P. J. 2016. The contribution of neuroinflammation to amyloid toxicity in Alzheimer's disease. *J. Neurochem*. 136, 457-74.

[5] Blennow, K., de Leon, M. J., Zetterberg, H. 2006. Alzheimer's disease. *Lancet*. 368, 387-403.

[6] Gouras, G. K., Olsson, T. T., Hansson, O. 2015. Beta-amyloid peptides and amyloid plaques in Alzheimer's disease. *Neurotherapeutics*. 12, 3-11.

[7] Gao, Y., Tan, L., Yu, J. T., Tan, L. 2018. Tau in Alzheimer's disease: Mechanisms and therapeutic strategies. *Curr. Alzheimer. Res*. 15, 283-300.

[8] Bondareff, W., Mountjoy, C. Q., Roth, M., Hauser, D. L. 1989. Neurofibrillary degeneration and neuronal loss in Alzheimer's disease. *Neurobiol. Aging*. 10, 709-15.

[9] Pei, J. J., Sjogren, M., Winblad, B. 2008. Neurofibrillary degeneration in Alzheimer's disease: From molecular mechanisms to identification of drug targets. *Curr. Opin. Psychiatry*. 21, 555-61.

[10] Doebler, J. A., Markesbery, W. R., Anthony, A., Rhoads, R. E. 1987. Neuronal rna in relation to neuronal loss and neurofibrillary pathology in the hippocampus in Alzheimer's disease. *J.* Neuropathol. *Exp. Neurol*. 46, 28-39.

[11] Fukutani, Y., Cairns, N. J., Shiozawa, M., Sasaki, K., Sudo, S., Isaki, K., Lantos, P. L. 2000. Neuronal loss and neurofibrillary degeneration in the hippocampal cortex in late-onset sporadic Alzheimer's disease. *Psychiatry. Clin. Neurosci*. 54, 523-9.

[12] Arendt, T. 2009. Synaptic degeneration in Alzheimer's disease. *Acta. Neuropathol*. 118, 167-79.

[13] Terry, R. D., Masliah, E., Salmon, D. P., Butters, N., DeTeresa, R., Hill, R., Hansen, L. A., Katzman, R. 1991. Physical basis of cognitive alterations in Alzheimer's disease: Synapse loss is the major correlate of cognitive impairment. *Ann. Neurol*. 30, 572-80.

[14] Pozueta, J., Lefort, R., Shelanski, M. L. 2013. Synaptic changes in Alzheimer's disease and its models. *Neuroscience*. 251, 51-65.

[15] Li, K., Wei, Q., Liu, F. F., Hu, F., Xie, A. J., Zhu, L. Q., Liu, D. 2018. Synaptic dysfunction in Alzheimer's disease: Abeta, tau, and epigenetic alterations. *Mol. Neurobiol*. 55, 3021-3032.

[16] Braak, H., Braak, E. 1998. Evolution of neuronal changes in the course of Alzheimer's disease. *J. Neural. Transm. Suppl*. 53, 127-40.

[17] Braak, E., Griffing, K., Arai, K., Bohl, J., Bratzke, H., Braak, H. 1999. Neuropathology of Alzheimer's disease: What is new since a. Alzheimer? *Eur. Arch. Psychiatry. Clin. Neurosci*. 249 Suppl 3, 14-22.

[18] Cavedo, E., Pievani, M., Boccardi, M., Galluzzi, S., Bocchetta, M., Bonetti, M., Thompson, P. M., Frisoni, G. B. 2014. Medial temporal atrophy in early and late-onset Alzheimer's disease. *Neurobiol. Aging*. 35, 2004-12.

[19] Grajski, K. A., Bressler, S. L., Alzheimer's Disease Neuroimaging, I. 2019. Differential medial temporal lobe and default-mode network functional connectivity and morphometric changes in Alzheimer's disease. *Neuroimage. Clin*. 23, 101860.

[20] Berron, D., van Westen, D., Ossenkoppele, R., Strandberg, O., Hansson, O. 2020. Medial temporal lobe connectivity and its associations with cognition in early Alzheimer's disease. *Brain*. 143, 1233-1248.

[21] Amaral, D. G., Scharfman, H. E., Lavenex, P. 2007. The dentate gyrus: Fundamental neuroanatomical organization (dentate gyrus for dummies). *Prog. Brain. Res*. 163, 3-22.

[22] Lee, J. W., Jung, M. W. 2017. Separation or binding? Role of the dentate gyrus in hippocampal mnemonic processing. *Neurosci. Biobehav. Rev*. 75, 183-194.

[23] Kesner, R. P. 2007. A behavioral analysis of dentate gyrus function. *Prog. Brain. Res*. 163, 567-76.

[24] Kesner, R. P. 2018. An analysis of dentate gyrus function (an update). *Behav. Brain. Res*. 354, 84-91.

[25] Altman, J., Das, G. D. 1965. Autoradiographic and histological evidence of postnatal hippocampal neurogenesis in rats. *J. Comp. Neurol.* 124, 319-35.

[26] Urban, N., Guillemot, F. 2014. Neurogenesis in the embryonic and adult brain: Same regulators, different roles. *Front. Cell. Neurosci.* 8, 396.

[27] Abbott, L. C., Nigussie, F. 2020. Adult neurogenesis in the mammalian dentate gyrus. *Anat. Histol. Embryol.* 49, 3-16.

[28] Zhang, X., Jonas, P. 2020. Integration of spatial and non-spatial information by heterogeneous dentate gyrus granule cells. *J. Life. Sci.* (Westlake Village). 2, 19-24.

[29] Prince, L. Y., Bacon, T. J., Tigaret, C. M., Mellor, J. R. 2016. Neuromodulation of the feedforward dentate gyrus-ca3 microcircuit. *Front. Synaptic. Neurosci.* 8, 32.

[30] Rolls, E. T. 2013. The mechanisms for pattern completion and pattern separation in the hippocampus. *Front. Syst. Neurosci.* 7, 74.

[31] Madar, A. D., Ewell, L. A., Jones, M. V. 2019. Temporal pattern separation in hippocampal neurons through multiplexed neural codes. *PLoS. Comput. Biol.* 15, e1006932.

[32] Piatti, V. C., Ewell, L. A., Leutgeb, J. K. 2013. Neurogenesis in the dentate gyrus: Carrying the message or dictating the tone. *Front. Neurosci.* 7, 50.

[33] Leutgeb, J. K., Leutgeb, S., Moser, M. B., Moser, E. I. 2007. Pattern separation in the dentate gyrus and ca3 of the hippocampus. *Science.* 315, 961-6.

[34] Chavlis, S., Petrantonakis, P. C., Poirazi, P. 2017. Dendrites of dentate gyrus granule cells contribute to pattern separation by controlling sparsity. *Hippocampus.* 27, 89-110.

[35] Berron, D., Schutze, H., Maass, A., Cardenas-Blanco, A., Kuijf, H. J., Kumaran, D., Duzel, E. 2016. Strong evidence for pattern separation in human dentate gyrus. *J. Neurosci.* 36, 7569-79.

[36] Neunuebel, J. P., Knierim, J. J. 2014. Ca3 retrieves coherent representations from degraded input: Direct evidence for ca3 pattern completion and dentate gyrus pattern separation. *Neuron*. 81, 416-27.

[37] Faghihi, F., Moustafa, A. A. 2016. Impaired neurogenesis of the dentate gyrus is associated with pattern separation deficits: A computational study. *J. Integr. Neurosci*. 15, 277-293.

[38] Castillon, C., Lunion, S., Desvignes, N., Hanauer, A., Laroche, S., Poirier, R. 2018. Selective alteration of adult hippocampal neurogenesis and impaired spatial pattern separation performance in the rsk2-deficient mouse model of coffin-lowry syndrome. *Neurobiol. Dis*. 115, 69-81.

[39] Sahay, A., Scobie, K. N., Hill, A. S., O'Carroll, C. M., Kheirbek, M. A., Burghardt, N. S., Fenton, A. A., Dranovsky, A., Hen, R. 2011. Increasing adult hippocampal neurogenesis is sufficient to improve pattern separation. *Nature*. 472, 466-70.

[40] Donovan, M. H., Yazdani, U., Norris, R. D., Games, D., German, D. C., Eisch, A. J. 2006. Decreased adult hippocampal neurogenesis in the pdapp mouse model of Alzheimer's disease. *J. Comp. Neurol*. 495, 70-83.

[41] Rodriguez, J. J., Jones, V. C., Tabuchi, M., Allan, S. M., Knight, E. M., LaFerla, F. M., Oddo, S., Verkhratsky, A. 2008. Impaired adult neurogenesis in the dentate gyrus of a triple transgenic mouse model of Alzheimer's disease. *PLoS. One*. 3, e2935.

[42] Poirier, R., Veltman, I., Pflimlin, M. C., Knoflach, F., Metzger, F. 2010. Enhanced dentate gyrus synaptic plasticity but reduced neurogenesis in a mouse model of amyloidosis. *Neurobiol. Dis*. 40, 386-93.

[43] Moreno-Jimenez, E. P., Flor-Garcia, M., Terreros-Roncal, J., Rabano, A., Cafini, F., Pallas-Bazarra, N., Avila, J., Llorens-Martin, M. 2019. Adult hippocampal neurogenesis is abundant in neurologically healthy subjects and drops sharply in patients with Alzheimer's disease. *Nat. Med*. 25, 554-560.

[44] Carlson, M. L., DiGiacomo, P. S., Fan, A. P., Goubran, M., Khalighi, M. M., Chao, S. Z., Vasanawala, M., Wintermark, M., Mormino, E., Zaharchuk, G., James, M. L., Zeineh, M. M. 2020. Simultaneous fdg-pet/mri detects hippocampal subfield metabolic differences in ad/mci. *Sci. Rep*. 10, 12064.

[45] Yan, S., Zheng, C., Cui, B., Qi, Z., Zhao, Z., An, Y., Qiao, L., Han, Y., Zhou, Y., Lu, J. 2020. Multiparametric imaging hippocampal neurodegeneration and functional connectivity with simultaneous pet/mri in Alzheimer's disease. *Eur. J. Nucl. Med. Mol. Imaging*. 47, 2440-2452.

[46] Suthana, N. A., Krupa, A., Donix, M., Burggren, A., Ekstrom, A. D., Jones, M., Ercoli, L. M., Miller, K. J., Siddarth, P., Small, G. W., Bookheimer, S. Y. 2010. Reduced hippocampal ca2, ca3, and dentate gyrus activity in asymptomatic people at genetic risk for Alzheimer's disease. *Neuroimage*. 53, 1077-84.

[47] Du, X., Wang, X., Geng, M. 2018. Alzheimer's disease hypothesis and related therapies. *Transl. Neurodegener*. 7, 2.

[48] Bekris, L. M., Yu, C. E., Bird, T. D., Tsuang, D. W. 2010. Genetics of alzheimer disease. *J. Geriatr. Psychiatry. Neurol*. 23, 213-27.

[49] Piaceri, I., Nacmias, B., Sorbi, S. 2013. Genetics of familial and sporadic Alzheimer's disease. *Front. Biosci*. (Elite Ed). 5, 167-77.

[50] Armstrong, R. A. 2009. The molecular biology of senile plaques and neurofibrillary tangles in Alzheimer's disease. *Folia. Neuropathol*. 47, 289-99.

[51] Iqbal, K., Liu, F., Gong, C. X. 2014. Alzheimer disease therapeutics: Focus on the disease and not just plaques and tangles. *Biochem. Pharmacol*. 88, 631-9.

[52] Tobin, M. K., Musaraca, K., Disouky, A., Shetti, A., Bheri, A., Honer, W. G., Kim, N., Dawe, R. J., Bennett, D. A., Arfanakis, K., Lazarov, O. 2019. Human hippocampal neurogenesis persists in aged adults and Alzheimer's disease patients. *Cell. Stem. Cell*. 24, 974-982 e3.

[53] Jin, K., Peel, A. L., Mao, X. O., Xie, L., Cottrell, B. A., Henshall, D. C., Greenberg, D. A. 2004. Increased hippocampal neurogenesis in Alzheimer's disease. *Proc. Natl. Acad. Sci. USA.* 101, 343-7.

[54] Yu, Y., He, J., Zhang, Y., Luo, H., Zhu, S., Yang, Y., Zhao, T., Wu, J., Huang, Y., Kong, J., Tan, Q., Li, X. M. 2009. Increased hippocampal neurogenesis in the progressive stage of Alzheimer's disease phenotype in an app/ps1 double transgenic mouse model. *Hippocampus*. 19, 1247-53.

[55] Gan, L., Qiao, S., Lan, X., Chi, L., Luo, C., Lien, L., Yan Liu, Q., Liu, R. 2008. Neurogenic responses to amyloid-beta plaques in the brain of Alzheimer's disease-like transgenic (ppdgf-appsw,ind) mice. *Neurobiol. Dis*. 29, 71-80.

[56] Disouky, A., Lazarov, O. 2021. Adult hippocampal neurogenesis in Alzheimer's disease. *Prog. Mol. Biol. Transl. Sci.* 177, 137-156.

[57] Li Puma, D. D., Piacentini, R., Grassi, C. 2020. Does impairment of adult neurogenesis contribute to pathophysiology of Alzheimer's disease? A still open question. *Front. Mol. Neurosci.* 13, 578211.

[58] Galvan, V., Jin, K. 2007. Neurogenesis in the aging brain. *Clin. Interv. Aging*. 2, 605-10.

[59] Katsimpardi, L., Lledo, P. M. 2018. Regulation of neurogenesis in the adult and aging brain. *Curr. Opin. Neurobiol*. 53, 131-138.

[60] Baptista, P., Andrade, J. P. 2018. Adult hippocampal neurogenesis: Regulation and possible functional and clinical correlates. *Front. Neuroanat*. 12, 44.

[61] Babcock, K. R., Page, J. S., Fallon, J. R., Webb, A. E. 2021. Adult hippocampal neurogenesis in aging and Alzheimer's disease. *Stem. Cell. Reports*. 16, 681-693.

[62] Octave, J. N. 2005. [alzheimer disease: Cellular and molecular aspects]. *Bull. Mem. Acad. R. Med. Belg*. 160, 445-9; discussion 450-1.

[63] Takahashi, R. H., Nagao, T., Gouras, G. K. 2017. Plaque formation and the intraneuronal accumulation of beta-amyloid in Alzheimer's disease. *Pathol. Int.* 67, 185-193.

[64] Lazarov, O., Lee, M., Peterson, D. A., Sisodia, S. S. 2002. Evidence that synaptically released beta-amyloid accumulates as extracellular deposits in the hippocampus of transgenic mice. *J. Neurosci.* 22, 9785-93.

[65] Haughey, N. J., Nath, A., Chan, S. L., Borchard, A. C., Rao, M. S., Mattson, M. P. 2002. Disruption of neurogenesis by amyloid beta-peptide, and perturbed neural progenitor cell homeostasis, in models of Alzheimer's disease. *J. Neurochem.* 83, 1509-24.

[66] Ermini, F. V., Grathwohl, S., Radde, R., Yamaguchi, M., Staufenbiel, M., Palmer, T. D., Jucker, M. 2008. Neurogenesis and alterations of neural stem cells in mouse models of cerebral amyloidosis. *Am. J. Pathol.* 172, 1520-8.

[67] Unger, M. S., Marschallinger, J., Kaindl, J., Hofling, C., Rossner, S., Heneka, M. T., Van der Linden, A., Aigner, L. 2016. Early changes in hippocampal neurogenesis in transgenic mouse models for Alzheimer's disease. *Mol. Neurobiol.* 53, 5796-806.

[68] Zhang, C., McNeil, E., Dressler, L., Siman, R. 2007. Long-lasting impairment in hippocampal neurogenesis associated with amyloid deposition in a knock-in mouse model of familial Alzheimer's disease. *Exp. Neurol.* 204, 77-87.

[69] He, N., Jin, W. L., Lok, K. H., Wang, Y., Yin, M., Wang, Z. J. 2013. Amyloid-beta(1-42) oligomer accelerates senescence in adult hippocampal neural stem/progenitor cells via formylpeptide receptor 2. *Cell. Death. Dis.* 4, e924.

[70] Zheng, M., Liu, J., Ruan, Z., Tian, S., Ma, Y., Zhu, J., Li, G. 2013. Intrahippocampal injection of abeta1-42 inhibits neurogenesis and down-regulates ifn-gamma and nf-kappab expression in hippocampus of adult mouse brain. *Amyloid.* 20, 13-20.

[71] Demars, M., Hu, Y. S., Gadadhar, A., Lazarov, O. 2010. Impaired neurogenesis is an early event in the etiology of familial

Alzheimer's disease in transgenic mice. *J. Neurosci. Res*. 88, 2103-17.

[72] Krezymon, A., Richetin, K., Halley, H., Roybon, L., Lassalle, J. M., Frances, B., Verret, L., Rampon, C. 2013. Modifications of hippocampal circuits and early disruption of adult neurogenesis in the tg2576 mouse model of Alzheimer's disease. *PLoS. One*. 8, e76497.

[73] Hamilton, L. K., Aumont, A., Julien, C., Vadnais, A., Calon, F., Fernandes, K. J. 2010. Widespread deficits in adult neurogenesis precede plaque and tangle formation in the 3xtg mouse model of Alzheimer's disease. *Eur. J. Neurosci*. 32, 905-20.

[74] Binder, L. I., Frankfurter, A., Rebhun, L. I. 1985. The distribution of tau in the mammalian central nervous system. *J. Cell. Biol*. 101, 1371-8.

[75] Black, M. M., Slaughter, T., Moshiach, S., Obrocka, M., Fischer, I. 1996. Tau is enriched on dynamic microtubules in the distal region of growing axons. *J. Neurosci*. 16, 3601-19.

[76] Barbier, P., Zejneli, O., Martinho, M., Lasorsa, A., Belle, V., Smet-Nocca, C., Tsvetkov, P. O., Devred, F., Landrieu, I. 2019. Role of tau as a microtubule-associated protein: Structural and functional aspects. *Front. Aging. Neurosci*. 11, 204.

[77] Fuster-Matanzo, A., de Barreda, E. G., Dawson, H. N., Vitek, M. P., Avila, J., Hernandez, F. 2009. Function of tau protein in adult newborn neurons. *FEBS. Lett*. 583, 3063-8.

[78] Hong, X. P., Peng, C. X., Wei, W., Tian, Q., Liu, Y. H., Yao, X. Q., Zhang, Y., Cao, F. Y., Wang, Q., Wang, J. Z. 2010. Essential role of tau phosphorylation in adult hippocampal neurogenesis. *Hippocampus*. 20, 1339-49.

[79] Zempel, H., Mandelkow, E. 2014. Lost after translation: Missorting of tau protein and consequences for alzheimer disease. Trends. *Neurosci*. 37, 721-32.

[80] Kowall, N. W., Beal, M. F. 1991. Glutamate-, glutaminase-, and taurine-immunoreactive neurons develop neurofibrillary tangles in Alzheimer's disease. *Ann. Neurol*. 29, 162-7.

[81] Hof, P. R., Bouras, C., Perl, D. P., Morrison, J. H. 1994. Quantitative neuropathologic analysis of pick's disease cases: Cortical distribution of pick bodies and coexistence with Alzheimer's disease. *Acta. Neuropathol.* 87, 115-24.

[82] Dickson, D. W., Yen, S. H., Horoupian, D. S. 1986. Pick body-like inclusions in the dentate fascia of the hippocampus in Alzheimer's disease. *Acta. Neuropathol.* 71, 38-45.

[83] Wakabayashi, K., Hansen, L. A., Vincent, I., Mallory, M., Masliah, E. 1997. Neurofibrillary tangles in the dentate granule cells of patients with Alzheimer's disease, lewy body disease and progressive supranuclear palsy. *Acta. Neuropathol.* 93, 7-12.

[84] Komuro, Y., Xu, G., Bhaskar, K., Lamb, B. T. 2015. Human tau expression reduces adult neurogenesis in a mouse model of tauopathy. *Neurobiol. Aging*. 36, 2034-42.

[85] Ramsden, M., Kotilinek, L., Forster, C., Paulson, J., McGowan, E., SantaCruz, K., Guimaraes, A., Yue, M., Lewis, J., Carlson, G., Hutton, M., Ashe, K. H. 2005. Age-dependent neurofibrillary tangle formation, neuron loss, and memory impairment in a mouse model of human tauopathy (p301l). *J. Neurosci.* 25, 10637-47.

[86] Zhang, H. A., Yuan, C. X., Liu, K. F., Yang, Q. F., Zhao, J., Li, H., Yang, Q. H., Song, D., Quan, Z. Z., Qing, H. 2022. Neural stem cell transplantation alleviates functional cognitive deficits in a mouse model of tauopathy. *Neural. Regen. Res.* 17, 152-162.

[87] Houben, S., Leroy, K., Ando, K., Yilmaz, Z., Widomski, C., Buee, L., Brion, J. P. 2019. Genetic ablation of tau in postnatal neurons rescues decreased adult hippocampal neurogenesis in a tauopathy model. *Neurobiol. Dis.* 127, 131-141.

[88] Criado-Marrero, M., Sabbagh, J. J., Jones, M. R., Chaput, D., Dickey, C. A., Blair, L. J. 2020. Hippocampal neurogenesis is enhanced in adult tau deficient mice. *Cells*. 9.

[89] Drummond, E., Wisniewski, T. 2017. Alzheimer's disease: Experimental models and reality. *Acta. Neuropathol.* 133, 155-175.

[90] Jankowsky, J. L., Zheng, H. 2017. Practical considerations for choosing a mouse model of Alzheimer's disease. *Mol. Neurodegener.* 12, 89.

[91] Zheng, J., Li, H. L., Tian, N., Liu, F., Wang, L., Yin, Y., Yue, L., Ma, L., Wan, Y., Wang, J. Z. 2020. Interneuron accumulation of phosphorylated tau impairs adult hippocampal neurogenesis by suppressing gabaergic transmission. *Cell. Stem. Cell*. 26, 331-345 e6.

[92] Umeda, T., Maekawa, S., Kimura, T., Takashima, A., Tomiyama, T., Mori, H. 2014. Neurofibrillary tangle formation by introducing wild-type human tau into app transgenic mice. *Acta. Neuropathol.* 127, 685-98.

[93] Gotz, J., Chen, F., van Dorpe, J., Nitsch, R. M. 2001. Formation of neurofibrillary tangles in p3011 tau transgenic mice induced by abeta 42 fibrils. *Science*. 293, 1491-5.

[94] Bolmont, T., Clavaguera, F., Meyer-Luehmann, M., Herzig, M. C., Radde, R., Staufenbiel, M., Lewis, J., Hutton, M., Tolnay, M., Jucker, M. 2007. Induction of tau pathology by intracerebral infusion of amyloid-beta -containing brain extract and by amyloid-beta deposition in app x tau transgenic mice. *Am. J. Pathol.* 171, 2012-20.

[95] Hensley, K. 2010. Neuroinflammation in Alzheimer's disease: Mechanisms, pathologic consequences, and potential for therapeutic manipulation. *J. Alzheimers*. Dis. 21, 1-14.

[96] Benzing, W. C., Wujek, J. R., Ward, E. K., Shaffer, D., Ashe, K. H., Younkin, S. G., Brunden, K. R. 1999. Evidence for glial-mediated inflammation in aged app(sw) transgenic mice. *Neurobiol. Aging*. 20, 581-9.

[97] Apelt, J., Schliebs, R. 2001. Beta-amyloid-induced glial expression of both pro- and anti-inflammatory cytokines in cerebral cortex of aged transgenic tg2576 mice with alzheimer plaque pathology. *Brain. Res*. 894, 21-30.

[98] Quintanilla, R. A., Orellana, D. I., Gonzalez-Billault, C., Maccioni, R. B. 2004. Interleukin-6 induces alzheimer-type phosphorylation

of tau protein by deregulating the cdk5/p35 pathway. *Exp. Cell. Res.* 295, 245-57.

[99] Smith, J. A., Das, A., Ray, S. K., Banik, N. L. 2012. Role of pro-inflammatory cytokines released from microglia in neurodegenerative diseases. *Brain. Res. Bull.* 87, 10-20.

[100] Zheng, C., Zhou, X. W., Wang, J. Z. 2016. The dual roles of cytokines in Alzheimer's disease: Update on interleukins, tnf-alpha, tgf-beta and ifn-gamma. *Transl. Neurodegener.* 5, 7.

[101] Ismail, R., Parbo, P., Madsen, L. S., Hansen, A. K., Hansen, K. V., Schaldemose, J. L., Kjeldsen, P. L., Stokholm, M. G., Gottrup, H., Eskildsen, S. F., Brooks, D. J. 2020. The relationships between neuroinflammation, beta-amyloid and tau deposition in Alzheimer's disease: A longitudinal pet study. *J. Neuroinflammation.* 17, 151.

[102] Liao, Y. F., Wang, B. J., Cheng, H. T., Kuo, L. H., Wolfe, M. S. 2004. Tumor necrosis factor-alpha, interleukin-1beta, and interferon-gamma stimulate gamma-secretase-mediated cleavage of amyloid precursor protein through a jnk-dependent mapk pathway. *J. Biol. Chem.* 279, 49523-32.

[103] Decourt, B., Lahiri, D. K., Sabbagh, M. N. 2017. Targeting tumor necrosis factor alpha for Alzheimer's disease. *Curr. Alzheimer. Res.* 14, 412-425.

[104] Heneka, M. T., Kummer, M. P., Stutz, A., Delekate, A., Schwartz, S., Vieira-Saecker, A., Griep, A., Axt, D., Remus, A., Tzeng, T. C., Gelpi, E., Halle, A., Korte, M., Latz, E., Golenbock, D. T. 2013. Nlrp3 is activated in Alzheimer's disease and contributes to pathology in app/ps1 mice. *Nature.* 493, 674-8.

[105] Chintamen, S., Imessadouene, F., Kernie, S. G. 2020. Immune regulation of adult neurogenic niches in health and disease. *Front. Cell. Neurosci.* 14, 571071.

[106] Ekdahl, C. T., Kokaia, Z., Lindvall, O. 2009. Brain inflammation and adult neurogenesis: The dual role of microglia. *Neuroscience.* 158, 1021-9.

[107] Diaz-Aparicio, I., Paris, I., Sierra-Torre, V., Plaza-Zabala, A., Rodriguez-Iglesias, N., Marquez-Ropero, M., Beccari, S., Huguet, P., Abiega, O., Alberdi, E., Matute, C., Bernales, I., Schulz, A., Otrokocsi, L., Sperlagh, B., Happonen, K. E., Lemke, G., Maletic-Savatic, M., Valero, J., Sierra, A. 2020. Microglia actively remodel adult hippocampal neurogenesis through the phagocytosis secretome. *J. Neurosci.* 40, 1453-1482.

[108] Araki, T., Ikegaya, Y., Koyama, R. 2020. The effects of microglia- and astrocyte-derived factors on neurogenesis in health and disease. *Eur. J. Neurosci.*

[109] Bassani, T. B., Turnes, J. M., Moura, E. L. R., Bonato, J. M., Coppola-Segovia, V., Zanata, S. M., Oliveira, R., Vital, M. 2017. Effects of curcumin on short-term spatial and recognition memory, adult neurogenesis and neuroinflammation in a streptozotocin-induced rat model of dementia of Alzheimer's type. *Behav. Brain. Res.* 335, 41-54.

[110] Bassani, T. B., Bonato, J. M., Machado, M. M. F., Coppola-Segovia, V., Moura, E. L. R., Zanata, S. M., Oliveira, R., Vital, M. 2018. Decrease in adult neurogenesis and neuroinflammation are involved in spatial memory impairment in the streptozotocin-induced model of sporadic Alzheimer's disease in rats. *Mol. Neurobiol.* 55, 4280-4296.

[111] Cacci, E., Claasen, J. H., Kokaia, Z. 2005. Microglia-derived tumor necrosis factor-alpha exaggerates death of newborn hippocampal progenitor cells in vitro. *J. Neurosci. Res.* 80, 789-97.

[112] Janelsins, M. C., Mastrangelo, M. A., Park, K. M., Sudol, K. L., Narrow, W. C., Oddo, S., LaFerla, F. M., Callahan, L. M., Federoff, H. J., Bowers, W. J. 2008. Chronic neuron-specific tumor necrosis factor-alpha expression enhances the local inflammatory environment ultimately leading to neuronal death in 3xtg-ad mice. *Am. J. Pathol.* 173, 1768-82.

[113] Liu, L., Liu, Y., Li, N., Huang, R., Zheng, X., Huang, L., Hou, S., Yuan, Q. 2020. Multiple inflammatory profiles of microglia and

altered neuroimages in app/ps1 transgenic ad mice. *Brain. Res. Bull.* 156, 86-104.

[114] Kiyota, T., Ingraham, K. L., Swan, R. J., Jacobsen, M. T., Andrews, S. J., Ikezu, T. 2012. Aav serotype 2/1-mediated gene delivery of anti-inflammatory interleukin-10 enhances neurogenesis and cognitive function in app+ps1 mice. *Gene. Ther.* 19, 724-33.

[115] Ou, Z., Kong, X., Sun, X., He, X., Zhang, L., Gong, Z., Huang, J., Xu, B., Long, D., Li, J., Li, Q., Xu, L., Xuan, A. 2018. Metformin treatment prevents amyloid plaque deposition and memory impairment in app/ps1 mice. *Brain. Behav. Immun.* 69, 351-363.

[116] Sayas, C. L., Avila, J. 2021. Gsk-3 and tau: A key duet in Alzheimer's disease. *Cells.* 10.

[117] Leroy, K., Yilmaz, Z., Brion, J. P. 2007. Increased level of active gsk-3beta in Alzheimer's disease and accumulation in argyrophilic grains and in neurones at different stages of neurofibrillary degeneration. Neuropathol. *Appl. Neurobiol.* 33, 43-55.

[118] Hooper, C., Killick, R., Lovestone, S. 2008. The gsk3 hypothesis of Alzheimer's disease. *J. Neurochem.* 104, 1433-9.

[119] Hernandez, F., Gomez de Barreda, E., Fuster-Matanzo, A., Lucas, J. J., Avila, J. 2010. Gsk3: A possible link between beta amyloid peptide and tau protein. *Exp. Neurol.* 223, 322-5.

[120] Proctor, C. J., Gray, D. A. 2012. A unifying hypothesis for familial and sporadic Alzheimer's disease. *Int. J. Alzheimers. Dis.* 2012, 978742.

[121] Mines, M. A., Beurel, E., Jope, R. S. 2011. Regulation of cell survival mechanisms in Alzheimer's disease by glycogen synthase kinase-3. *Int. J. Alzheimers. Dis.* 2011, 861072.

[122] Cai, Z., Zhao, Y., Zhao, B. 2012. Roles of glycogen synthase kinase 3 in Alzheimer's disease. *Curr. Alzheimer. Res.* 9, 864-79.

[123] Hurtado, D. E., Molina-Porcel, L., Carroll, J. C., Macdonald, C., Aboagye, A. K., Trojanowski, J. Q., Lee, V. M. 2012. Selectively

silencing gsk-3 isoforms reduces plaques and tangles in mouse models of Alzheimer's disease. *J. Neurosci.* 32, 7392-402.

[124] Hur, E. M., Zhou, F. Q. 2010. Gsk3 signalling in neural development. *Nat. Rev. Neurosci.* 11, 539-51.

[125] Rodriguez-Matellan, A., Avila, J., Hernandez, F. 2020. Overexpression of gsk-3beta in adult tet-off gsk-3beta transgenic mice, and not during embryonic or postnatal development, induces tau phosphorylation, neurodegeneration and learning deficits. *Front. Mol. Neurosci.* 13, 561470.

[126] Lucas, J. J., Hernandez, F., Gomez-Ramos, P., Moran, M. A., Hen, R., Avila, J. 2001. Decreased nuclear beta-catenin, tau hyperphosphorylation and neurodegeneration in gsk-3beta conditional transgenic mice. *EMBO. J. 20*, 27-39.

[127] Sirerol-Piquer, M., Gomez-Ramos, P., Hernandez, F., Perez, M., Moran, M. A., Fuster-Matanzo, A., Lucas, J. J., Avila, J., Garcia-Verdugo, J. M. 2011. Gsk3beta overexpression induces neuronal death and a depletion of the neurogenic niches in the dentate gyrus. *Hippocampus.* 21, 910-22.

[128] Llorens-Martin, M., Fuster-Matanzo, A., Teixeira, C. M., Jurado-Arjona, J., Ulloa, F., Defelipe, J., Rabano, A., Hernandez, F., Soriano, E., Avila, J. 2013. Gsk-3beta overexpression causes reversible alterations on postsynaptic densities and dendritic morphology of hippocampal granule neurons in vivo. *Mol. Psychiatry.* 18, 451-60.

[129] de Ruiter, J. P., Uylings, H. B. 1987. Morphometric and dendritic analysis of fascia dentata granule cells in human aging and senile dementia. *Brain. Res.* 402, 217-29.

[130] Engel, T., Hernandez, F., Avila, J., Lucas, J. J. 2006. Full reversal of Alzheimer's disease-like phenotype in a mouse model with conditional overexpression of glycogen synthase kinase-3. *J. Neurosci.* 26, 5083-90.

[131] Morales-Garcia, J. A., Luna-Medina, R., Alonso-Gil, S., Sanz-Sancristobal, M., Palomo, V., Gil, C., Santos, A., Martinez, A., Perez-Castillo, A. 2012. Glycogen synthase kinase 3 inhibition

promotes adult hippocampal neurogenesis in vitro and in vivo. ACS. *Chem. Neurosci.* 3, 963-71.

[132] Varela-Nallar, L., Arredondo, S. B., Tapia-Rojas, C., Hancke, J., Inestrosa, N. C. 2015. Andrographolide stimulates neurogenesis in the adult hippocampus. *Neural. Plast.* 2015, 935403.

[133] Li, W., Wu, M., Zhang, Y., Wei, X., Zang, J., Liu, Y., Wang, Y., Gong, C. X., Wei, W. 2020. Intermittent fasting promotes adult hippocampal neuronal differentiation by activating gsk-3beta in 3xtg-ad mice. *J. Neurochem.* 155, 697-713.

[134] Sun, B., Halabisky, B., Zhou, Y., Palop, J. J., Yu, G., Mucke, L., Gan, L. 2009. Imbalance between gabaergic and glutamatergic transmission impairs adult neurogenesis in an animal model of Alzheimer's disease. *Cell. Stem. Cell.* 5, 624-33.

[135] Bonda, D. J., Stone, J. G., Torres, S. L., Siedlak, S. L., Perry, G., Kryscio, R., Jicha, G., Casadesus, G., Smith, M. A., Zhu, X., Lee, H. G. 2014. Dysregulation of leptin signaling in alzheimer disease: Evidence for neuronal leptin resistance. *J. Neurochem.* 128, 162-72.

[136] Fujita, Y., Yamashita, T. 2019. The effects of leptin on glial cells in neurological diseases. *Front. Neurosci.* 13, 828.

[137] Whitfield, J. F., Chiarini, A., Dal Pra, I., Armato, U., Chakravarthy, B. 2015. The possible roles of the dentate granule cell's leptin and other ciliary receptors in Alzheimer's neuropathology. *Cells.* 4, 253-74.

[138] Calio, M. L., Mosini, A. C., Marinho, D. S., Salles, G. N., Massinhani, F. H., Ko, G. M., Porcionatto, M. A. 2021. Leptin enhances adult neurogenesis and reduces pathological features in a transgenic mouse model of Alzheimer's disease. *Neurobiol. Dis.* 148, 105219.

[139] Katsouri, L., Ashraf, A., Birch, A. M., Lee, K. K., Mirzaei, N., Sastre, M. 2015. Systemic administration of fibroblast growth factor-2 (fgf2) reduces bace1 expression and amyloid pathology in app23 mice. *Neurobiol. Aging.* 36, 821-31.

[140] Kang, W., Hebert, J. M. 2015. Fgf signaling is necessary for neurogenesis in young mice and sufficient to reverse its decline in old mice. *J. Neurosci*. 35, 10217-23.

[141] Kiyota, T., Ingraham, K. L., Jacobsen, M. T., Xiong, H., Ikezu, T. 2011. Fgf2 gene transfer restores hippocampal functions in mouse models of Alzheimer's disease and has therapeutic implications for neurocognitive disorders. *Proc. Natl. Acad. Sci. USA*. 108, E1339-48.

[142] Zhang, M., Bian, Z. 2021. Alzheimer's disease and microrna-132: A widespread pathological factor and potential therapeutic target. *Front. Neurosci*. 15, 687973.

[143] Cha, D. J., Mengel, D., Mustapic, M., Liu, W., Selkoe, D. J., Kapogiannis, D., Galasko, D., Rissman, R. A., Bennett, D. A., Walsh, D. M. 2019. Mir-212 and mir-132 are downregulated in neurally derived plasma exosomes of Alzheimer's patients. *Front. Neurosci*. 13, 1208.

[144] Luikart, B. W., Bensen, A. L., Washburn, E. K., Perederiy, J. V., Su, K. G., Li, Y., Kernie, S. G., Parada, L. F., Westbrook, G. L. 2011. Mir-132 mediates the integration of newborn neurons into the adult dentate gyrus. *PLoS. One*. 6, e19077.

[145] Magill, S. T., Cambronne, X. A., Luikart, B.W ., Lioy, D. T., Leighton, B. H., Westbrook, G. L., Mandel, G., Goodman, R. H. 2010. Microrna-132 regulates dendritic growth and arborization of newborn neurons in the adult hippocampus. *Proc. Natl. Acad. Sci. USA*. 107, 20382-7.

[146] Walgrave, H., Balusu, S., Snoeck, S., Vanden Eynden, E., Craessaerts, K., Thrupp, N., Wolfs, L., Horre, K., Fourne, Y., Ronisz, A., Silajdzic, E., Penning, A., Tosoni, G., Callaerts-Vegh, Z., D'Hooge, R., Thal, D. R., Zetterberg, H., Thuret, S., Fiers, M., Frigerio, C. S., De Strooper, B., Salta, E. 2021. Restoring mir-132 expression rescues adult hippocampal neurogenesis and memory deficits in Alzheimer's disease. *Cell. Stem. Cell*.

[147] Deng, Y., Zhang, J., Sun, X., Ma, G., Luo, G., Miao, Z., Song, L. 2020. Mir-132 improves the cognitive function of rats with

Alzheimer's disease by inhibiting the mapk1 signal pathway. *Exp. Ther. Med.* 20, 159.

[148] Yau, S. Y., Li, A., So, K. F. 2015. Involvement of adult hippocampal neurogenesis in learning and forgetting. *Neural. Plast*. 2015, 717958.

[149] Baglietto-Vargas, D., Sanchez-Mejias, E., Navarro, V., Jimenez, S., Trujillo-Estrada, L., Gomez-Arboledas, A., Sanchez-Mico, M., Sanchez-Varo, R., Vizuete, M., Davila, J. C., Garcia-Verdugo, J. M., Vitorica, J., Gutierrez, A. 2017. Dual roles of abeta in proliferative processes in an amyloidogenic model of Alzheimer's disease. *Sci. Rep*. 7, 10085.

[150] Hollands, C., Tobin, M. K., Hsu, M., Musaraca, K., Yu, T. S., Mishra, R., Kernie, S. G., Lazarov, O. 2017. Depletion of adult neurogenesis exacerbates cognitive deficits in Alzheimer's disease by compromising hippocampal inhibition. *Mol. Neurodegener*. 12, 64.

[151] Choi, S. H., Bylykbashi, E., Chatila, Z. K., Lee, S. W., Pulli, B., Clemenson, G. D., Kim, E., Rompala, A., Oram, M. K., Asselin, C., Aronson, J., Zhang, C., Miller, S. J., Lesinski, A., Chen, J. W., Kim, D. Y., van Praag, H., Spiegelman, B. M., Gage, F. H., Tanzi, R. E. 2018. Combined adult neurogenesis and bdnf mimic exercise effects on cognition in an Alzheimer's mouse model. *Science*. 361.

[152] Yan, Y., Ma, T., Gong, K., Ao, Q., Zhang, X., Gong, Y. 2014. Adipose-derived mesenchymal stem cell transplantation promotes adult neurogenesis in the brains of Alzheimer's disease mice. *Neural. Regen. Res*. 9, 798-805.

[153] Zhang, X., Mei, Y., He, Y., Wang, D., Wang, J., Wei, X., Yang, E., Zhou, D., Shen, H., Peng, G., Shu, Q., Li, X., Luo, B., Zhou, Y., Sun, B. 2021. Ablating adult neural stem cells improves synaptic and cognitive functions in alzheimer models. *Stem. Cell. Reports.* 16, 89-105.

[154] Scheff, S. W., Price, D. A. 2006. Alzheimer's disease-related alterations in synaptic density: Neocortex and hippocampus. *J. Alzheimers. Dis*. 9, 101-15.

[155] Alonso-Nanclares, L., Merino-Serrais, P., Gonzalez, S., DeFelipe, J. 2013. Synaptic changes in the dentate gyrus of app/ps1 transgenic mice revealed by electron microscopy. *J. Neuropathol. Exp. Neurol*. 72, 386-95.

[156] Scheff, S. W., Price, D. A. 1998. Synaptic density in the inner molecular layer of the hippocampal dentate gyrus in alzheimer disease. *J. Neuropathol. Exp. Neurol*. 57, 1146-53.

[157] Scheff, S. W., Sparks, D. L., Price, D. A. 1996. Quantitative assessment of synaptic density in the outer molecular layer of the hippocampal dentate gyrus in Alzheimer's disease. *Dementia*. 7, 226-32.

[158] King, D. L., Arendash, G. W. 2002. Maintained synaptophysin immunoreactivity in tg2576 transgenic mice during aging: Correlations with cognitive impairment. *Brain. Res*. 926, 58-68.

[159] Colom-Cadena, M., Spires-Jones, T., Zetterberg, H., Blennow, K., Caggiano, A., DeKosky, S. T., Fillit, H., Harrison, J. E., Schneider, L. S., Scheltens, P., de Haan, W., Grundman, M., van Dyck, C. H., Izzo, N. J., Catalano, S. M., Synaptic Health Endpoints Working, G. 2020. The clinical promise of biomarkers of synapse damage or loss in Alzheimer's disease. *Alzheimers. Res*. Ther. 12, 21.

[160] DeKosky, S. T., Scheff, S. W. 1990. Synapse loss in frontal cortex biopsies in Alzheimer's disease: Correlation with cognitive severity. *Ann. Neurol*. 27, 457-64.

[161] Blennow, K., Bogdanovic, N., Alafuzoff, I., Ekman, R., Davidsson, P. 1996. Synaptic pathology in Alzheimer's disease: Relation to severity of dementia, but not to senile plaques, neurofibrillary tangles, or the apoe4 allele. *J. Neural. Transm* (Vienna). 103, 603-18.

[162] Palop, J. J., Chin, J., Roberson, E. D., Wang, J., Thwin, M. T., Bien-Ly, N., Yoo, J., Ho, K. O., Yu, G. Q., Kreitzer, A., Finkbeiner, S., Noebels, J. L., Mucke, L. 2007. Aberrant excitatory

neuronal activity and compensatory remodeling of inhibitory hippocampal circuits in mouse models of Alzheimer's disease. *Neuron*. 55, 697-711.

[163] Putcha, D., Brickhouse, M., O'Keefe, K., Sullivan, C., Rentz, D., Marshall, G., Dickerson, B., Sperling, R. 2011. Hippocampal hyperactivation associated with cortical thinning in Alzheimer's disease signature regions in non-demented elderly adults. *J. Neurosci*. 31, 17680-8.

[164] Kazim, S. F., Chuang, S. C., Zhao, W., Wong, R. K., Bianchi, R., Iqbal, K. 2017. Early-onset network hyperexcitability in presymptomatic Alzheimer's disease transgenic mice is suppressed by passive immunization with anti-human app/abeta antibody and by mglur5 blockade. *Front. Aging. Neurosci*. 9, 71.

[165] Kim, K. R., Kim, Y., Jeong, H. J., Kang, J. S., Lee, S. H., Kim, Y., Lee, S. H., Ho, W. K. 2021. Impaired pattern separation in tg2576 mice is associated with hyperexcitable dentate gyrus caused by kv4.1 downregulation. *Mol. Brain*. 14, 62.

[166] Kim, K. R., Lee, S. Y., Yoon, S. H., Kim, Y., Jeong, H. J., Lee, S., Suh, Y. H., Kang, J. S., Cho, H., Lee, S. H., Kim, M. H., Ho, W. K. 2020. Kv4.1, a key ion channel for low frequency firing of dentate granule cells, is crucial for pattern separation. *J. Neurosci*. 40, 2200-2214.

[167] Nenov, M. N., Laezza, F., Haidacher, S. J., Zhao, Y., Sadygov, R. G., Starkey, J. M., Spratt, H., Luxon, B. A., Dineley, K. T., Denner, L. 2014. Cognitive enhancing treatment with a ppargamma agonist normalizes dentate granule cell presynaptic function in tg2576 app mice. *J. Neurosci*. 34, 1028-36.

[168] Haytural, H., Jorda-Siquier, T., Winblad, B., Mulle, C., Tjernberg, L. O., Granholm, A. C., Frykman, S., Barthet, G. 2021. Distinctive alteration of presynaptic proteins in the outer molecular layer of the dentate gyrus in Alzheimer's disease. *Brain. Commun*. 3, fcab079.

[169] Haytural, H., Mermelekas, G., Emre, C., Nigam, S. M., Carroll, S. L., Winblad, B., Bogdanovic, N., Barthet, G., Granholm, A. C., Orre, L. M., Tjernberg, L. O., Frykman, S. 2020. The proteome of the dentate terminal zone of the perforant path indicates presynaptic impairment in alzheimer disease. *Mol. Cell. Proteomics*. 19, 128-141.

[170] Hirano-Sakamaki, W., Sugiyama, E., Hayasaka, T., Ravid, R., Setou, M., Taki, T. 2015. Alzheimer's disease is associated with disordered localization of ganglioside gm1 molecular species in the human dentate gyrus. *FEBS. Lett*. 589, 3611-6.

[171] Alcantara-Gonzalez, D., Chartampila, E., Criscuolo, C., Scharfman, H. E. 2021. Early changes in synaptic and intrinsic properties of dentate gyrus granule cells in a mouse model of Alzheimer's disease neuropathology and atypical effects of the cholinergic antagonist atropine. *Neurobiol. Dis*. 152, 105274.

[172] Olabarria, M., Noristani, H. N., Verkhratsky, A., Rodriguez, J. J. 2010. Concomitant astroglial atrophy and astrogliosis in a triple transgenic animal model of Alzheimer's disease. *Glia*. 58, 831-8.

[173] Choi, M., Lee, S. M., Kim, D., Im, H. I., Kim, H. S., Jeong, Y. H. 2021. Disruption of the astrocyte-neuron interaction is responsible for the impairments in learning and memory in 5xfad mice: An Alzheimer's disease animal model. *Mol. Brain*. 14, 111.

[174] Jo, S., Yarishkin, O., Hwang, Y. J., Chun, Y. E., Park, M., Woo, D. H., Bae, J. Y., Kim, T., Lee, J., Chun, H., Park, H. J., Lee, D. Y., Hong, J., Kim, H. Y., Oh, S. J., Park, S. J., Lee, H., Yoon, B. E., Kim, Y., Jeong, Y., Shim, I., Bae, Y. C., Cho, J., Kowall, N. W., Ryu, H., Hwang, E., Kim, D., Lee, C. J. 2014. Gaba from reactive astrocytes impairs memory in mouse models of Alzheimer's disease. *Nat. Med*. 20, 886-96.

[175] Wu, Z., Guo, Z., Gearing, M., Chen, G. 2014. Tonic inhibition in dentate gyrus impairs long-term potentiation and memory in an Alzheimer's [corrected] disease model. *Nat. Commun*. 5, 4159.

[176] Richetin, K., Steullet, P., Pachoud, M., Perbet, R., Parietti, E., Maheswaran, M., Eddarkaoui, S., Begard, S., Pythoud, C., Rey,

M., Caillierez, R., K, Q. D., Halliez, S., Bezzi, P., Buee, L., Leuba, G., Colin, M., Toni, N., Deglon, N. 2020. Tau accumulation in astrocytes of the dentate gyrus induces neuronal dysfunction and memory deficits in Alzheimer's disease. *Nat. Neurosci*. 23, 1567-1579.

[177] Young, J. K. 2020. Neurogenesis makes a crucial contribution to the neuropathology of Alzheimer's disease. *J. Alzheimers. Dis. Rep*. 4, 365-371.

In: The Dentate Gyrus
Editor: Feng-Ru Tang
ISBN: 978-1-68507-212-4

Chapter 8

NEUROGENESIS IN THE DENTATE GYRUS AS AN EMOTIONAL REGULATOR THROUGH CIRCUITS MODIFICATION

***Alonso Martínez-Canabal*[1,*], *Grecia López-Oropeza*[1], *Jimena Arroyo-Perez*[2] *and Pilar Durán*[1]**
[1]Cell Biology Department Faculty of Sciences,
[2]Faculty of Psychology, National Autonomous University of Mexico, Mexico City, Mexico

ABSTRACT

The hippocampus's dentate gyrus is a critical structure for memory acquisition and emotional processing in the brain. This structure is unique as it is one of the areas with a higher density of excitatory neurons and contains some of the largest known axonic terminals. Those terminals form the unique synaptic structures known as thorny excrescences with the pyramidal neurons of the critical memory processing area, the third layer of the Cornu Ammonis (CA3). However, the most intriguing characteristic of the dentate gyrus is its

* Corresponding Author's Email: acanabal@ciencias.unam.mx.

continual addition of newborn neurons through the lifetime of most mammals, and there is substantial evidence that the same occurs in humans. The continuous addition of newborn cells confers the dentate gyrus with an extraordinary and unique source of plasticity. This feature facilitates cognitive flexibility, critical for the proper acquisition of new memories over old schemes. The failure of the dentate gyrus' unique plasticity features can be critical to understanding the etiology of depression and the continuous fear relapse characteristic of post-traumatic stress disorder (PTSD). There is compelling evidence that depression and PTSD onset rely on the decreased hippocampus and dentate gyrus- CA3 complex, and apparently, neurogenesis can be beneficial for the treatment of those ailments. This chapter aims to explain how the dentate gyrus circuits and their neurogenesis modulation can generate interesting insights to treat psychopathologies of emotional nature.

INTRODUCTION

In 1962 Altman et al. showed that adult brains were capable of generating new neurons and astrocytes; in 1965, Altman and Das showed that the hippocampus's dentate gyrus is one of two main structures that generate newborn cells at postnatal ages [1, 2]. These findings ended a neuroscience dogma established half a century earlier by Ramón y Cajal, which stated that the nervous system could not generate new cells after development [3]. Today there is extensive evidence that most mammals produce new brain cells, both neurons, and astroglia, in the postnatal and adult dentate gyrus [4]. However, there is a current debate on whether dentate gyrus neurogenesis in humans continues beyond early adulthood through life or ends in early life stages [5]. Nevertheless, most works, using both endogenous markers [6] and incorporation of traceable elements in DNA [7], indicate that humans can produce new brain cells during the whole life, although at reduced quantities during adulthood and senescence.

The main question that remains is, why is there neurogenesis in the dentate gyrus? Many studies have reported a possible role of newborn neurons in memory acquisition [8], storage [9], and consolidation [10]. However, the hippocampus's remaining layers, the frontal lobes, the amygdala, and other critical areas for cognition do not present newborn neurons during postnatal and adult stages. Therefore, adult neurogenesis is not an obligatory feature for memory systems to perform correctly but an active constituent of the dentate gyrus dynamics, a critical structure for cognition [11].

The dentate gyrus is a unique structure in the forebrain of humans and other mammals. It contains a remarkably high cell density where most of its neurons share the excitatory granule phenotype. Contrary to most brain areas, such cells only receive projections from the perforant pathway axons coming from the entorhinal cortex and only project, through the mossy bundle, to the CA3 layer [12]. The peculiar connectivity organization suggests that the dentate gyrus is just a bridge structure between the entorhinal cortex and the hippocampus's cornu ammonis (CA1,2,3); nevertheless, the dentate gyrus has unique properties. The granule cell layer of the dentate gyrus has a very high neural density; its cells have strong excitatory output and scarce activation, qualities that enable the dentate gyrus to work as a filter that only allows the pass of robust and repetitive patterns while filtering the most random and transient patterns [13]. The presence of newborn neurons can contribute to this proposed model of the dentate gyrus by increasing excitability and allowing more storage for new patterns in neurons not previously associated with any circuit; notably, these neurons can degrade previously established circuits with CA3 by forming new connections able to disrupt synaptic contacts in which those circuits rely on [9, 14]. The dentate gyrus can then function as a structure capable of filtering only the most robust patterns and can modify previously established circuits; these peculiar features strongly suggest an important role in memory flexibility or the capability to acquire fresh memories without interference. Such cognitive flexibility allows individuals to adapt to a continually changing environment [15].

There is a large body of evidence that shows the hippocampus as one of the structures that suffer a significant modification during chronic mental health problems. Patients that suffer from chronic depression [16, 17] or post-traumatic stress disorder (PTSD) [18] show a decreased hippocampal size. Both patients suffering major depression or PTSD are characterized by not adapting to change and forming long-lasting extinction memories capable of competing with previous fear-associated and trauma memories in context, spatial, or narrative frames [19, 20]. In both cases, the evidence of a relation between those diseases and the dentate gyrus neurogenesis is strong. It is well established that many antidepressants stimulate the generation of more newborn neurons able to integrate into memory circuits [21], the same as aerobic exercise, which also has an antidepressant effect [22]. Other results point that newborn neurons increase resilience to stress and decrease depressive-like behaviors in animals [23]. Finally, neurogenesis facilitates extinction [24], prevents the return of fear, and favors retaining the extinction memory in the long term [25]. In the present chapter, we aim to present an extensive body of evidence supporting the idea that newborn neurons in the dentate gyrus can help understand emotional disorders' etiology in animal models and human patients. They can also play a positive role in the recovery in both animal models and patients suffering emotional disorders such as chronic depression and PTSD, considering dentate gyrus' newborn neurons' strong ability to facilitate cognitive flexibility.

Roles of Postnatal and Adult Neurogenesis in Learning and Memory

More than twenty years after their discovery, the neuroscience community started to study if the newborn hippocampal neurons were just an artifact of surviving stem cells from development or if these cells performed a function within the hippocampal circuits. The first line of approach was to observe if ablation or increased adult neurogenesis would directly impact learning and memory in hippocampal-dependent tasks. Initially, it became clear that hippocampal-dependent learning tasks in laboratory animals would promote neurogenesis [26]. However, if neurogenesis changes affect the outcome of learning and memory, needed to be further investigated.

In the first cohort of published data, the approach was to modify - increase or decrease- neurogenesis and evaluate learning and memory retention. Many initial reports confirmed an initial link between adult new-born neurons and learning and memory retention [27-29]; nevertheless, other studies showed no neurogenesis impact in some hippocampal-dependent learning and memory tasks [30, 31]. After those initial publications, many groups adopted the idea to use transgenic mice to increase or reduce neurogenesis and, therefore, prevent the noise caused by invasive techniques such as toxic drugs or harmful irradiation; however, these experiments, again, did not provide a clear answer about a direct role of neurogenesis in learning and memory retention [32-34].

Posteriorly, some authors have suggested that hippocampal neurogenesis could have a role in pattern separation and completion, a process associated with the DG. In the adult DG, there is a mixture of mature and immature granule cells. Aimone et al. [35], using computational models, showed that mature granule cells could encode selected contextual information with high precision, whereas immature cells could encode much more information but with lower precision. The proposed differentiated role implies that newborn neurons are transiently more excitable during maturation and have a lower threshold for LTP formation than fully mature cells [36]. According to this model, these two cell populations would separate and complete contexts more efficiently than only mature cells could.

Some studies have tested Aimone's hypothesis using a paradigm of neurogenesis increase by running. One report showed that running enhanced hippocampal neurogenesis facilitated pattern separation in mice [37]; nevertheless, another study indicated that this effect was not related to neurogenesis [38]. Another approach showed an increase in pattern separation when neurogenesis was increased by ablating a proapoptotic factor [39]. However, using the ablation of newborn neurons, a different study showed that those neurons could be part of the circuits supporting pattern separation, but in their absence, the pattern separation task was still performed successfully [40]. Then, several research groups started to look for different approaches to evaluate newborn neurons' possible roles. Some groups considered the possibility that more than having an effect during learning and memory encoding, neurogenesis could have a role in long term internal memory processing and memory circuits reconfiguration.

In 2009, Kitamura et al. reported that high rates of neurogenesis could decrease the time in which context memories can cease to be hippocampal-dependent and rely more on cortical circuits, while lower neurogenesis rates increase the hippocampal-dependent memory storage by extending the time point in which contextual memories become entirely dependent on cortical structures [41]. This paradigm-changing experiment shows that studies on neurogenesis' role should not focus on the impact in learning and memory acquisition but rather on how the emergence of new neurons and new synaptic contacts can modify previously established memory circuits. Weisz and Argibay [9], using an in silico model, proposed that the dentate gyrus's storage sites that process patterns are the synaptic contacts formed between the mossy fibers and the basal pyramidal dendrites of CA3 [42]. Accordingly to their model, when high neurogenesis rates are present, recent memories show a slightly better performance; nevertheless, remote memories suffer from substantial interference decreasing their retrieval performance dramatically. This finding showed consistency with a previous study of Feng et al. [43]. When they studied a knockout mouse lacking presenilin with decreased neurogenesis, they observed that running impaired remote memory retention only in wild-type mice. Consequently, proposing that neurogenesis could be a mechanism to clear out hippocampal information.

These studies yielded a new developmental hypothesis in which large amounts of newborn neurons generated during early childhood led to infantile amnesia, or the failure to retrieve early childhood episodic-like memories [44]. According to this hypothesis, newborn neurons s would also facilitate the forgetting of old memories in adults, too [45]. Akers et al. successfully proved this hypothesis [46], showing that neurogenesis ablation in early life stages can prevent infantile amnesia. They also showed that increased neurogenesis in adults caused forgetting in different hippocampus-dependent memory tasks. Posteriorly, follow-up studies corroborated these findings [15, 47].

The structural and molecular mechanisms that allow newborn neurons to modify previously established circuits are not fully understood. Besides the observations in quantified proliferating cells and the somata of immature newborn neurons, no other comprehensive studies have used a causal or even correlative approach. Meltzer et al. proposed that an accumulation of newborn neurons would cause a catastrophic failure of remote memory retrieval due to compromised circuit homeostasis [48]. They further proposed that a correction for such an anomaly should occur, including interneurons' neurogenesis, conversion of excitatory neurons to interneurons, or synaptic scaling by decreasing their excitatory output. So far, no empirical data has proven any of those mechanisms. Similar in silico data has been shown by Weisz and Argibay [9] and Akers, Martinez-Canabal, Restivo, et al. [46]. At this moment, morphological evidence -provided by Toni et al.- shows that newborn neurons establish new and functional synaptic contacts with CA3 dendrites, and those new synaptic contacts compete with previously established synapses [49]. That competition means removing the previously established synaptic contact or adding a new synaptic terminal to the same post-synaptic space; both cases would disrupt the synapses' recruitment with established memory engrams [36].

The Role of Hippocampal Neurogenesis in Cognitive Flexibility

The research on adult hippocampal neurogenesis's role has focused on how newborn neurons improve the acquisition of hippocampal-dependent memories [35, 50-53]. However, recent investigations have suggested that adult neurogenesis may also contribute to cognitive flexibility [15, 46, 53-56]. In the next paragraphs, we will discuss cognitive flexibility implications through neurogenesis regulation.

The definition of cognitive flexibility is the capacity to adapt learned behavioral responses to a continually changing environment [57, 58]. Cognitive flexibility is associated with enhanced capacity for behavioral reconfiguration facilitating the more rapid shifting between different memory traces or engrams; meanwhile, some studies suggest that an absence of behavior shifting affects cognitive performance [59, 60]. Following this idea, it is crucial to understand where and how memory traces are encoded, modified, and recalled. The prefrontal cortex is the center of executive functions, an essential region for cognitive flexibility [61, 62]. As a result, recall and reconfiguration of hippocampal-dependent memories are controlled mostly by prefrontal areas once they are consolidated [61, 63, 64]. Nevertheless, Kitamura et al. have demonstrated that hippocampal-formation circuits are necessary during remote memory recall as the prefrontal cortex is during initial memory encoding [65]. This interaction between cortical and hippocampal areas is essential for memory consolidation and cognitive flexibility.

Establishing a clearer understanding of cognitive flexibility's associated apparatus and functioning rests on investigating how the hippocampus, through neurogenesis, regulates memory consolidation [46, 54-56]. As has been aforementioned, memory firstly encodes within hippocampal areas and, over-time, it migrates toward cortical areas, where it is stored permanently, and hippocampal memory trace becomes silent [41, 61, 65]. However, a significant proportion of an organism's memories seemingly need to be accessible at any moment. In contrast, non-significant memories' erasure is important to facilitate the continuous encoding of novel, relevant information as a perfect example of cognitive flexibility [58]. During the past decade, evidence emerged that hippocampal neurogenesis modifies hippocampal-dependent memory consolidation [41]. In a first study, low neurogenesis levels in mice prevented migration of hippocampal-dependent memory to cortical areas. On the contrary, mice with high neurogenesis levels with voluntary exercise showed improvement in their capacity to migrate memory to the prefrontal cortex [41]. As a result, this experiment suggests that hippocampus neurogenesis modulates memory dependency on the hippocampus and cortical circuits, suggesting a neurogenesis implication in cognitive flexibility.

Additionally, after the study of Kitamura et al. [65], a study explored how hippocampal neurogenesis affects memory persistence in mice. The associated animals underwent a hippocampal-dependent task, called contextual fear conditioning, in which animals learn to predict an aversive stimulus due to their exposure to a specific context. After the training, some adult mice had free access to a running wheel for a month, and, afterward, they were returned to their conditional chamber to test fear memory. Consequently, the running exercise was associated with an increase in hippocampal neurogenesis and reduced contextual fear memory. Importantly this finding was reproduced on a study conducted on transgenic mice with high levels of hippocampal neurogenesis. Moreover, the result disappeared in transgenic mice that lacked hippocampal neurogenesis [46]. Together these results indicate that memory persistence depends on the number of newborn neurons in the hippocampus.

In addition to the experiments mentioned above, in order to test cognitive flexibility, some authors have conducted an interesting analysis using the water maze task. In the task, animals learn to find, during several training trials, a dry platform within an opaque water tank using distal contextual clues. In such a context, eventually, it has been inferred that these animals establish a cognitive map of the maze. After several trials, mice reduce their time finding the platform and arrive at the platform's location, even when it is no longer present. After learning, the mice were allowed to voluntarily run for a month and a half and then tested in the same water maze. As expected, these mice had increased neurogenesis and forgot the original platform location. The animals then searched for the platform located in another place, those with higher neurogenesis performed better in finding the new location than controls [15].

These results are consistent with other studies that have found that hippocampal neurogenesis improves behavior flexibility when a task is reconfigured [54, 55]. Therefore, a circuit reconfiguration within the hippocampus must be necessary to accomplish this. A possible mechanism that can explain the hippocampal circuit reconfiguration is replacing old DG-CA3 connections that encode previous memories for new DG-CA3 connections. Newborn neurons generate new mossy axons, and new large mossy terminals sought new connection places with CA3 neurons [14]. The newly established connections, not previously used for memory storage, can facilitate new memory acquisition over a schema previously used, a process in which significant hippocampal-dependent memories remain accessible all the time while non-significant ones are forgotten [66].

Interestingly, in a recent study, hippocampal neurogenesis showed facilitation of prefrontal cortices recruitment in fear regulation. In this study, researchers performed contextual fear conditioning followed by an extinction protocol to test spontaneous fear recovery [67]. Spontaneous fear recovery is a phenomenon in which fear memory resurges overtime despite new learning that the conditioned stimulus is no longer a threat [68]. After a month of enrichment and running wheel treatment, an increment of hippocampal neurogenesis was improved and associated with the prevention of spontaneous fear recovery. Furthermore, a decreased in hippocampal neurogenesis due to focal x-ray irradiation promoted fear-related responses. In this situation, animals cannot shift between safe memory trace (extinction engram) and danger memory trace (fear conditioning engram), which is related to the absence of flexibility in behavior. Additionally, impairment of fear responses was associated with the prelimbic cortex activation and improving fear responses dependent on the activation of the infralimbic cortex [67]. In conclusion, this study suggested that hippocampal neurogenesis through cortical-hippocampal engram activation modulates fear and extinction memories.

NEUROGENESIS AND AFFECTIVE DISORDERS

Mood and anxiety disorders are linked to psychological flexibility deficiencies, including cognitive flexibility alterations [19, 20, 69, 70]. According to Kashdan and Rottenberg [20], psychological flexibility involves the capacity to make mental and behavioral shifts. Thus, psychological flexibility refers to an ensemble of "dynamic processes that unfold over time." When interacting with an environment, these dynamic processes involve four principal aspects of a person's mental and behavioral capabilities [20]:

- Adapting to fluctuating situational demands (e.g., modify behavioral responses in concordance to the situation and goals);
- Reconfiguring mental resources means "accepting and being open about "emotional experiences" instead of "devoting finite attentional resources and energy to regulating emotions."
- Being able to shift perspective (e.g., deciding between problem-focused or emotion-focused coping strategy when encountering a stressful situation.
- Making a balance between desires, needs, and life domains [20].

The first three aspects of psychological flexibility mentioned above go in line with the neuropsychological definition of cognitive flexibility [71]. Neuropsychological research refers to cognitive flexibility as "the ability to shift avenues of thought and action in order to perceive, process, and respond to situations in different ways" [72]. Also, cognitive flexibility encloses the production of new ideas and different ways of thinking, enables the consideration of response alternatives, and modifies plans and behaviors [71, 72]. Furthermore, some studies have related cognitive flexibility with the executive function system [73].

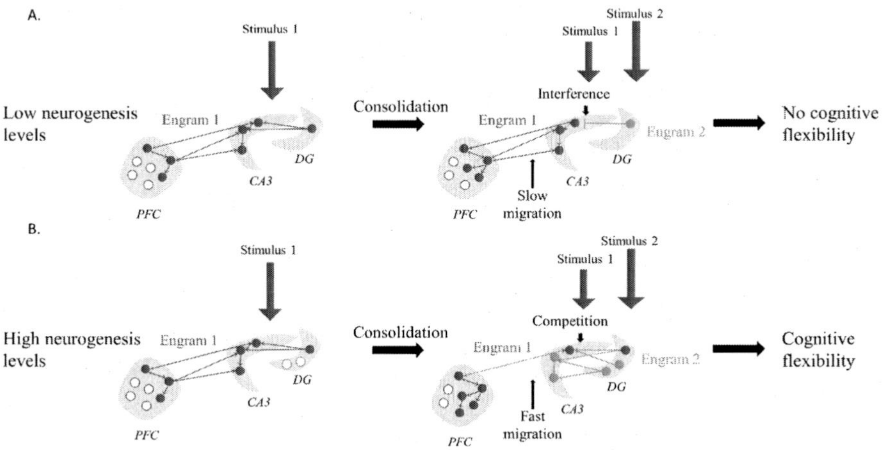

Figure 1. The cognitive flexibility of episodic-like memories depends on hippocampal neurogenesis. A) Lower neurogenesis rates increase the hippocampal-dependent episodic memories (engram 1) and thus prevent that a new contextual memory encodes in the dentate gyrus (engram 2); as a result, there is no cognitive flexibility. B) Higher neurogenesis rates decrease the hippocampal-dependent of contextual memories (engram 1) and thus promote that a new contextual memory encodes in the dentate gyrus (engram 2); as a result, there is cognitive flexibility. PFC = prefrontal cortex, DG = dentate gyrus, CA3 = Cornu amonis 3.

Executive functions are a set of control mechanisms that enable an individual to self-control and self-regulate his cognitions and actions according to short and long-term goals in his everyday life [73]. Additionally, these self-control and self-regulation capacities associate with emotion regulation strategies in clinical psychological research [74, 75]. Therefore, cognitive control processes are significant abilities when it comes to adequate emotion regulation. Such cognitive control processes include inhibition of reactive emotional responses and disengagement from processing irrelevant material no longer critical [73, 75]. Conversely, as viewed from a neuropsychological perspective, cognitive inflexibility comprises impairments in inhibition, disengagement, and shifting of cognitive sets [71]. Although cognitive flexibility commonly corresponds to prefrontal cortex executive functions [71, 76, 77], recent works showed that it is also related to hippocampal neurogenesis [78].

Anacker and Hen proposed a model in which hippocampal neurogenesis could be a potential target for facilitating cognitive flexibility in mood and anxiety disorders [78]. Fear conditioning-studies in rodents show that the inhibition or activation of a previously formed memory (e.g., memory trace or engram) of an aversive context is sufficient to suppress or activate contextual-conditioned fear expression [79]. Moreover, hippocampal neurogenesis plays a part in the inhibition of a previously formed contextual fear association [80] and the prevention of spontaneous recovery of a previous contextual fear conditioned-response in favor of a safe-context association [25]. Therefore, concerning human psychopathology, hippocampal neurogenesis could inhibit previously learned negative and traumatic memories (or associations), facilitating the ability to shift and learn new, more adaptive ones.

Previously learned associations such as negative core beliefs, intrusive, harmful, or traumatic memories, and inadequate emotion regulation strategies are all implicated in neuropsychiatric disorders like Major Depressive Disorder (MDD) and Post Traumatic Stress Disorder [81-84]. These maladaptive and pervasive learned associations might be consequences of hippocampal neurogenesis-cognitive flexibility deficits. Moreover, both disorders show impairments in cognitive flexibility tasks [85, 86]; and also, both disorders share similar structural hippocampal alterations [82, 87] that return to normal levels with therapeutic pharmacological [88, 89] and non-pharmacological treatment [90].

Major Depressive Disorder has a strong association with psychological inflexibility in general [19]. MDD patients also have impaired cognitive flexibility, lacking the ability to inhibit negative emotional irrelevant stimuli when solving a cognitive task [81, 91]. They also show impairments in shifting cognitive sets (especially with affective stimuli) when it comes to cognitive flexibility tasks that measure the capacity to change previously learned rules to a new set of rules [85, 92]. Also, rumination, which is "the process of thinking perseveratively about one's feelings and problems" [93], has been strongly associated with depressive and anxiety symptoms [93-95]. Rumination is a maladaptive emotion regulation strategy [19] related to cognitive flexibility deficits [81, 96, 97]. Furthermore, the evidence shows that MDD patients seem to be unable to disengage from negative rumination, making them unable to solve task-related problems and respond adequately to the environment (due to lack of cognitive flexibility) [98, 99].

Recent clinical research in PTSD has shown that cognitive flexibility turned out to be a significant predictor for symptom severity and positively correlates with clinical improvement [86, 100]. Cognitive flexibility impairments in PTSD have been observed and measured in patients, e.g., impairments in inhibition of processing irrelevant but threatening stimuli [101], shifting cognitive set [86, 102], and rumination [103]. If a person is exposed to a traumatic event and develops PTSD, they exhibit trauma-related intrusion symptoms, which involve "recurrent, involuntary, and intrusive distressing memories of the traumatic event" as well as "traumatic event-related flashbacks" [104]. These symptoms are associated with cognitive inflexibility because of the inability to inhibit and disengage from the trauma's rumination [105].

Table 1. Clinical data showing dentate gyrus and neurogenesis response to psychiatric disorders and treatment

Psychiatric disorder	Type of Study	Observation	Treatment	Results
MDD	Post-mortem tissue		Treatment with TCA or SSRI (before death)	SSRI treated patients had more neural progenitor cells dentate gyrus than MDD untreated patients. Treated patients had larger DG volume compared with untreated MDD or controls [124].
		Reduced number in neural progenitor cells in depressed patients against controls, regardless of medication [112].		
			Treatment with TCA or SSRI (before death)	SSRI-treated patients had more neural progenitor cells and angiogenesis in the dentate gyrus [125].
	MRI		SSRI/SNRI or and bupropion for six months or more before examination	Unmedicated patients had lower dentate gyrus volume against controls, and medicated patients; unmedicated patients had lower CA1-3 volume than controls [114].
		Reduced hippocampal grey matter in untreated patients against controls	Depressed patients underwent eight weeks with SSRI citalopram	Increase in hippocampal grey after citalopram treatment [123].
	Post-mortem tissue	Fewer granule neurons and smaller dentate gyrus in untreated patients compared to controls.	SSRI or TCA at least three months before death	Unmedicated patients had fewer granule cells in the dentate gyrus than SSRI-treated patients. SSRI treated patients showed a larger granule cell layer than patients treated with TCA and controls [109].
		Untreated patients had fewer granule neurons compared to controls in the anterior and mid dentate gyrus.	SSRI/TCA/bupropion/lithium during last three months before death	Treated patients increased progenitor and granule cells compared to untreated and controls [110].
		Post-mortem suicide patients had smaller dentate gyrus with fewer granule neurons and neural progenitor cells.		Exposure to early life adversity before death was associated with more granule neurons in the whole dentate gyrus in MDD suicide decedents and controls [125].

Table 1. (Continued)

Psychiatric disorder	Type of Study	Observation	Treatment	Results
MDD	MRI		SSRI or SNRI for six months or more	Volume increase of left CA3 and dentate gyrus granule cell layer compared to measures at baseline [89].
PTSD	MRI		Paroxetine for 9-12 months	Increase in mean hippocampal volume [88].
		Smaller CA3/dentate gyrus and total hippocampal volume in PTSD war veterans against control veterans [142].		
		Smaller hippocampal and orbitofrontal cortex volume compared to controls.	CBT	After CBT, Increased hippocampal volume [90].
		Smaller dentate gyrus subfield volume in veterans with PTSD against trauma-exposed controls [82].		

Structural alterations in MDD and PTSD patients are related, in part, to hippocampal neurogenesis changes. These neuroanatomical disturbances among MDD and PTSD patients are related to both disorders, and the effects of pharmacological and psychological treatment can reverse the neuroanatomical changes [90, 106]. Both MDD and PTSD patients have an overall reduced hippocampal volume likely related to reduced hippocampal neurogenesis. A recent meta-analysis using data from 15 magnetic resonance imaging (MRI) studies worldwide found significantly lower hippocampal volumes among MDD patients (specifically those with recurrent episodes) against healthy controls [107]. About PTSD, a meta-analysis study with pooled data from 13 MRI studies found significantly lower bilateral hippocampal volumes [108]. Although smaller hippocampal volume could be due to other plasticity changes aside from neurogenesis, as dendritic arbor reduction, some studies show a particular relation to the CA-3-dentate gyrus connecting fibers with such volume decrease. For example, hippocampal brain sections of unmedicated MDD patients contained fewer granule neurons in the anterior and mid dentate gyrus, which were smaller in volume in the anterior and mid granule cell layer against controls [109, 110]; as granule neurons are unlikely to die spontaneously or by neurodegeneration in adults, this reduction is likely due to reduced neurogenesis [111]. Furthermore, a study found a significant reduction in progenitor cell numbers within the dentate gyrus' subgranular layer in tissues from elderly depressed patients compared to same-age controls [112]. Furthermore, high-resolution MRI studies have found smaller CA3/dentate gyrus volumes in PTSD-diagnosed veterans [82, 113] and smaller volumes in the dentate gyrus and cornu ammonis (CA1-3) of unmedicated MDD patients versus medicated patients and control subjects [114].

Apart from the effects on cognitive flexibility seen in animal research, neurogenesis has also proven to be sufficient for decreasing anxiety and depressive-like behaviors [115, 116]. Interestingly, antidepressant treatments such as selective serotonin reuptake inhibitors (SSRI), tricyclic antidepressants (TCA), and electroconvulsive therapy

(ECT) have proven to increase hippocampal neurogenesis in animal models [116-119]. Specifically, sertraline, an SSRI, showed increased neurogenesis in a human hippocampal progenitor cell line HPC03A/07 [120]. Indeed, SSRIs are the first-line pharmacological treatment option for MDD [121] and PTSD [122]. Moreover, remitted and depressed patients treated with SSRI show increased hippocampal grey matter against untreated currently depressed patients [123]. MDD patients treated with antidepressants have a larger granule cell layer and DG volume than unmedicated patients [89, 114]. PTSD patients also show an increase in mean hippocampal volume after chronic treatment with SSRI [88]. As well, postmortem hippocampal sections of MDD patients treated with antidepressants, including SSRIs, have larger dentate gyrus volume [124], a larger number of neural progenitor cells in the dentate gyrus [110, 124, 125], increased granule neuron number [110], and larger anterior/mid granule cell layer volume [109] than unmedicated MDD patients.

Concerning non-pharmacological treatments, therapeutic effects of Cognitive Behavioral Therapy (CBT), physical exercise, and environmental enrichment could also be related to hippocampal neurogenesis changes. CBT is an evidence-based validated psychological treatment for MDD [126, 127] and PTSD [128]. CBT improves psychological flexibility by making the patient aware of and changing negative biased cognitive processing of information about the self, the world, and the future [83, 129]. Mental representations of these negative biased cognitive processes are called schemas [83]. Negative schemas are modified and replaced with more adaptive ones by CBT interventions such as cognitive restructuring, behavioral modification techniques, and biased attention and biased recalling of memory modification techniques [83, 130]. After CBT treatment MRI hippocampal volumetric changes appear in PTSD patients; such changes could be related to hippocampal neurogenesis [90, 131].

Furthermore, extinction and reconsolidation, the most effective behavioral techniques for treating PTSD, depend on hippocampal neurogenesis in its fear regulation, as shown by recent animal experiments [25, 132]. Physical exercise, which increases neurogenesis in animal models [133], has improved clinical outcomes when used in parallel with CBT and SSRIs [134]. Finally, environmental enrichment, which also increases neurogenesis and enhances cognitive flexibility in animal models [135], has also started to be used as a treatment for reducing rumination [136].

There are some controversies regarding the neurogenic effect of antidepressants [112, 137, 138]; also, CBT has shown to be effective despite cognitive flexibility tasks-deficits at baseline and without making any significant improvement in those tasks after treatment, although the age of the sample ranged from 61-78 years old [70]. Additionally, other non-neurogenic processes could play a part in the effects of antidepressants and CBT, such as dendritic arborization and enhanced LTD [139]; and activation of prefrontal areas in the cognitive control network [140]. However, hippocampal neurogenesis is another contributor factor that participates in the therapeutic effects of antidepressants [115] and other non-pharmacological treatments like CBT [26], physical exercise, and environmental enrichment [133]. In this sense, we posit that hippocampal neurogenesis plays an essential role in mood and anxiety disorders because of its cognitive flexibility enhancement. By making available and enhancing psychological flexibility processes, we increase the person's likelihood of achieving significant clinical improvement [141], and most importantly, we could prevent relapse [25] and promote sustained remission [116, 123]. Mental health professionals should be aware of all the potential strategies that can be combined and deployed depending on each patient's situation to guarantee therapeutic success.

Conclusion

The study of hippocampal neurogenesis shows a novel, substantial and dynamic mechanism of memory regulation. More importantly, it shows a dynamic plasticity mechanism capable of modifying previously established circuits and allows paradigm-shiftings to be critical for survival. Paradigm-shifting capabilities or cognitive flexibility are a central part of the etiology of many mental illnesses. This chapter centered on MDD and PTSD for brevity; nevertheless, misadjustment of cognitive flexibility also appears in other forms of depression, bipolar disorder, and even schizophrenia.

The recent findings on the relevance of hippocampal neurogenesis for cognitive flexibility can translate to a better understanding of mental illnesses due to an extensive body of evidence, which includes the regulation of neurogenesis by antidepressants, the consistent decrease in hippocampal size, dentate gyrus, and progenitor cells in patients suffering from mental illnesses and the observed recovery of those symptoms after pharmacological (as SSRIs antidepressants) and non-pharmacological (As CBT therapy) treatments. All these biological and medical associations strongly suggest the need for more translational studies to systematize the possible advantages that neurogenesis modulation could implicate for people with mental health conditions. The biological and medical links between neurogenesis, cognitive flexibility, and mental health suggest the need for new therapeutical approaches, including aerobic exercise, environmental enrichment, and other neurogenesis increasing drugs not considered antidepressants as memantine. Therefore, the scenery for using a naturalistic plasticity structured strategy to treat mental health problems is promising. However, it is critical to obtain more evidence of the biological mechanisms of neurogenesis circuit modification, its influence on memory consolidation, cognitive flexibility, and emotional responses; in parallel to developing structured clinical studies on the therapeutic impact of different neurogenesis modulation strategies.

REFERENCES

[1] Altman, J. & Das, G. D. (1965). Autoradiographic and histological evidence of postnatal hippocampal neurogenesis in rats. *The Journal of Comparative Neurology*, *124* (3), 319-35.

[2] Altman, J. (1962). Are new neurons formed in the brains of adult mammals? *Science*, *135* (3509), 1127-8.

[3] Ramón y Cajal, S. (1914). *Estudios sobre la degeneración y regeneración del sistema nervioso*. [*Studies on the degeneration and regeneration of the nervous system*.] Madrid,: Impr. de hijos de N. Moya.

[4] Amrein, I., Isler, K. & Lipp, H. P. (2011). Comparing adult hippocampal neurogenesis in mammalian species and orders: influence of chronological age and life history stage. *The European Journal of Neuroscience*, *34* (6), 978-87.

[5] Sorrells, S. F., Paredes, M. F., Cebrian-Silla, A., Sandoval, K., Qi, D., Kelley, K. W., James, D., Mayer, S., Chang, J., Auguste, K. I., Chang, E. F., Gutierrez, A. J., Kriegstein, A. R., Mathern, G. W., Oldham, M. C., Huang, E. J., Garcia-Verdugo, J. M., Yang, Z. & Alvarez-Buylla, A. (2018). Human hippocampal neurogenesis drops sharply in children to undetectable levels in adults. *Nature*, *555* (7696), 377-81.

[6] Moreno-Jimenez, E. P., Flor-Garcia, M., Terreros-Roncal, J., Rabano, A., Cafini, F., Pallas-Bazarra, N., Avila, J. & Llorens-Martin, M. (2019). Adult hippocampal neurogenesis is abundant in neurologically healthy subjects and drops sharply in patients with Alzheimer's disease. *Nature Medicine*, *25* (4), 554-60.

[7] Spalding, K. L., Bergmann, O., Alkass, K., Bernard, S., Salehpour, M., Huttner, H. B., Bostrom, E., Westerlund, I., Vial,

C., Buchholz, B. A., Possnert, G., Mash, D. C., Druid, H. & Frisen, J. (2013). Dynamics of hippocampal neurogenesis in adult humans. *Cell*, *153* (6), 1219-27

[8] Leuner, B., Gould, E. & Shors, T. J. (2006). Is there a link between adult neurogenesis and learning? *Hippocampus*, *16* (3), 216-24.

[9] Weisz, V. I. & Argibay, P. F. (2012). Neurogenesis interferes with the retrieval of remote memories: forgetting in neuro-computational terms. *Cognition*, *125* (1), 13-25.

[10] Kitamura, R. i., Yoshii, T. & Yamamoto, T. (2009). The expanding sphere of travel behaviour research: selected papers from the 11th *International Conference on Travel Behaviour Research*. Bingley: Emerald.

[11] Kesner, R. P. (2018). An analysis of dentate gyrus function (an update). *Behavioural Brain Research*, *354*, 84-91.

[12] Amaral, D. G. (1993). Emerging principles of intrinsic hippocampal organization. *Current Opinion in Neurobiology*, *3* (2), 225-9.

[13] Hsu, D. (2007). *The dentate gyrus as a filter or gate: a look back and a look ahead.*, *163*, 601-13.

[14] Toni, N., Teng, E. M., Bushong, E. A., Aimone, J. B., Zhao, C., Consiglio, A., van Praag, H., Martone, M. E., Ellisman, M. H. & Gage, F. H. (2007). Synapse formation on neurons born in the adult hippocampus. *Nature Neuroscience*, *10* (6), 727-34.

[15] Epp, J. R., Silva Mera, R., Kohler, S., Josselyn, S. A. & Frankland, P. W. (2016). Neurogenesis-mediated forgetting minimizes proactive interference. *Nature Communications*, *7*, 10838.

[16] Cao, B., Passos, I. C., Mwangi, B., Amaral-Silva, H., Tannous, J., Wu, M. J., Zunta-Soares, G. B. & Soares, J. C. (2017). Hippocampal subfield volumes in mood disorders. *Molecular Psychiatry*, *22* (9), 1352-8.

[17] Santos, M. A. O., Bezerra, L. S., Carvalho, A. & Brainer-Lima, A. M. (2018). Global hippocampal atrophy in major depressive disorder: a meta-analysis of magnetic resonance imaging studies. *Trends Psychiatry Psychother*, *40* (4), 369-78.

[18] Bromis, K., Calem, M., Reinders, A., Williams, S. C. R. & Kempton, M. J. (2018). Meta-Analysis of 89 Structural MRI Studies in Posttraumatic Stress Disorder and Comparison With Major Depressive Disorder. *The American Journal of Psychiatry*, *175* (10), 989-98.

[19] Stange, J. P., Alloy, L. B. & Fresco, D. M. (2017). Inflexibility as a Vulnerability to Depression: A Systematic Qualitative Review. *Clin Psychol (New York)*, *24* (3), 245-76.

[20] Kashdan, T. B. & Rottenberg, J. (2010). Psychological flexibility as a fundamental aspect of health. *Clin Psychol Rev*, *30* (7), 865-78.

[21] Santarelli, L., Saxe, M., Gross, C., Surget, A., Battaglia, F., Dulawa, S., Weisstaub, N., Lee, J., Duman, R., Arancio, O., Belzung, C. & Hen, R. (2003). Requirement of hippocampal neurogenesis for the behavioral effects of antidepressants. *Science*, *301*, (5634), 805-9.

[22] Lee, H. J. & Baek, S. S. (2017). Role of exercise on molecular mechanisms in the regulation of antidepressant effects. *J. Exerc. Rehabil.*, *13* (6), 617-20.

[23] Anacker, C., Luna, V. M., Stevens, G. S., Millette, A., Shores, R., Jimenez, J. C., Chen, B. & Hen, R. (2018). Hippocampal neurogenesis confers stress resilience by inhibiting the ventral dentate gyrus. *Nature*, *559* (7712), 98-102.

[24] Pan, Y. W., Chan, G. C., Kuo, C. T., Storm, D. R. & Xia, Z. (2012). Inhibition of adult neurogenesis by inducible and targeted deletion of ERK5 mitogen-activated protein kinase specifically in adult neurogenic regions impairs contextual fear extinction and remote fear memory. *The Journal of Neuroscience*, *32* (19), 6444-55.

[25] Martínez-Canabal, A., López-Oropeza, G., Gaona-Gamboa, A., Ballesteros-Zebadua, P., de la Cruz, O. G., Moreno-Jimenez, S. & Sotres-Bayon, F. (2019). Hippocampal neurogenesis regulates recovery of defensive responses by recruiting threat- and extinction-signalling brain networks. *Scientific Reports*, *9* (1), 2939.

[26] Gould, E., Beylin, A., Tanapat, P., Reeves, A. & Shors, T. J. (1999). Learning enhances adult neurogenesis in the hippocampal formation. *Nature Neuroscience*, *2* (3), 260-5.

[27] Snyder, J. S., Hong, N. S., McDonald, R. J. & Wojtowicz, J. M. (2005). A role for adult neurogenesis in spatial long-term memory. *Neuroscience*, *130* (4), 843-52.

[28] van Praag, H., Christie, B. R., Sejnowski, T. J. & Gage, F. H. (1999). Running enhances neurogenesis, learning, and long-term potentiation in mice. *Proceedings of the National Academy of Sciences of the United States of America*, *96* (23), 13427-31.

[29] Drapeau, E., Mayo, W., Aurousseau, C., Le Moal, M., Piazza, P. V. & Abrous, D. N. (2003). Spatial memory performances of aged rats in the water maze predict levels of hippocampal neurogenesis. *Proceedings of the National Academy of Sciences of the United States of America*, *100* (24), 14385-90.

[30] Shors, T. J., Townsend, D. A., Zhao, M., Kozorovitskiy, Y. & Gould, E. (2002). Neurogenesis may relate to some but not all types of hippocampal-dependent learning. *Hippocampus*, *12* (5), 578-84.

[31] Merrill, D. A., Karim, R., Darraq, M., Chiba, A. A. & Tuszynski, M. H. (2003). Hippocampal cell genesis does not correlate with spatial learning ability in aged rats. *The Journal of comparative neurology*, *459* (2), 201-7.

[32] Imayoshi, I., Sakamoto, M., Ohtsuka, T., Takao, K., Miyakawa, T., Yamaguchi, M., Mori, K., Ikeda, T., Itohara, S. & Kageyama, R. (2008). Roles of continuous neurogenesis in the structural and

functional integrity of the adult forebrain. *Nature neuroscience, 11* (10), 1153-61.

[33] Zhang, C. L., Zou, Y., He, W., Gage, F. H. & Evans, R. M. (2008). A role for adult TLX-positive neural stem cells in learning and behaviour. *Nature*, *451* (7181), 1004-7.

[34] Jaholkowski, P., Kiryk, A., Jedynak, P., Ben Abdallah, N. M., Knapska, E., Kowalczyk, A., Piechal, A., Blecharz-Klin, K., Figiel, I., Lioudyno, V., Widy-Tyszkiewicz, E., Wilczynski, G. M., Lipp, H. P., Kaczmarek, L. & Filipkowski, R. K. (2009). New hippocampal neurons are not obligatory for memory formation; cyclin D2 knockout mice with no adult brain neurogenesis show learning. *Learning & memory*, *16* (7), 439-51.

[35] Aimone, J. B., Deng, W. & Gage, F. H. (2011). Resolving new memories: a critical look at the dentate gyrus, adult neurogenesis, and pattern separation. *Neuron*, *70* (4), 589-96.

[36] Toni, N. & Schinder, A. F. (2015). Maturation and Functional Integration of New Granule Cells into the Adult Hippocampus. *Cold Spring Harbor perspectives in biology*, *8* (1), a018903.

[37] Creer, D. J., Romberg, C., Saksida, L. M., van Praag, H. & Bussey, T. J. (2010). Running enhances spatial pattern separation in mice. *Proceedings of the National Academy of Sciences of the United States of America*, *107* (5), 2367-72.

[38] Lazic, S. E. (2012). Using causal models to distinguish between neurogenesis-dependent and -independent effects on behaviour. *J. R. Soc. Interface*, *9* (70), 907-17.

[39] Sahay, A., Scobie, K. N., Hill, A. S., O'Carroll, C. M., Kheirbek, M. A., Burghardt, N. S., Fenton, A. A., Dranovsky, A. & Hen, R. (2011). Increasing adult hippocampal neurogenesis is sufficient to improve pattern separation. *Nature*, *472* (7344), 466-70.

[40] Arruda-Carvalho, M., Sakaguchi, M., Akers, K. G., Josselyn, S. A. & Frankland, P. W. (2011). Posttraining ablation of adult-generated neurons degrades previously acquired memories. *The Journal of neuroscience: the official journal of the Society for Neuroscience*, *31* (42), 15113-27.

[41] Kitamura, T., Saitoh, Y., Takashima, N., Murayama, A., Niibori, Y., Ageta, H., Sekiguchi, M., Sugiyama, H. & Inokuchi, K. (2009). Adult neurogenesis modulates the hippocampus-dependent period of associative fear memory. *Cell*, *139* (4), 814-27.

[42] Weisz, V. I. & Argibay, P. F. (2009). A putative role for neurogenesis in neuro-computational terms: inferences from a hippocampal model. *Cognition*, *112* (2), 229-40.

[43] Feng, R., Rampon, C., Tang, Y. P., Shrom, D., Jin, J., Kyin, M., Sopher, B., Miller, M. W., Ware, C. B., Martin, G. M., Kim, S. H., Langdon, R. B., Sisodia, S. S. & Tsien, J. Z. (2001). Deficient neurogenesis in forebrain-specific presenilin-1 knockout mice is associated with reduced clearance of hippocampal memory traces. *Neuron*, *32* (5), 911-26.

[44] Josselyn, S. A. & Frankland, P. W. (2012). Infantile amnesia: a neurogenic hypothesis. *Learning & NMemory*, *19* (9), 423-33.

[45] Frankland, P. W., Kohler, S. & Josselyn, S. A. (2013). Hippocampal neurogenesis and forgetting. *Trends in Neurosciences*, *36* (9), 497-503.

[46] Akers, K. G., Martinez-Canabal, A., Restivo, L., Yiu, A. P., De Cristofaro, A., Hsiang, H. L., Wheeler, A. L., Guskjolen, A., Niibori, Y., Shoji, H., Ohira, K., Richards, B. A., Miyakawa, T., Josselyn, S. A. & Frankland, P. W. (2014). Hippocampal neurogenesis regulates forgetting during adulthood and infancy. *Science*, *344* (6184), 598-602.

[47] Guskjolen, A., Josselyn, S. A. & Frankland, P. W. (2017). Age-dependent changes in spatial memory retention and flexibility in mice. *Neurobiology of Learning and Memory*, *143*, 59-66.

[48] Meltzer, L. A., Yabaluri, R. & Deisseroth, K. (2005). A role for circuit homeostasis in adult neurogenesis. *Trends in Neurosciences*, *28* (12), 653-60.

[49] Toni, N., Laplagne, D. A., Zhao, C., Lombardi, G., Ribak, C. E., Gage, F. H. & Schinder, A. F. (2008). Neurons born in the adult

dentate gyrus form functional synapses with target cells. *Nature Neuroscience*, *11* (8), 901-7.

[50] Kitamura, T. & Inokuchi, K. (2014). Role of adult neurogenesis in hippocampal-cortical memory consolidation. *Molecular Brain*, *7*, 13.

[51] Ko, H. G., Jang, D. J., Son, J., Kwak, C., Choi, J. H., Ji, Y. H., Lee, Y. S., Son, H. & Kaang, B. K. (2009). Effect of ablated hippocampal neurogenesis on the formation and extinction of contextual fear memory. *Molecular Brain*, *2*, 1.

[52] Koehl, M. & Abrous, D. N. (2011). A new chapter in the field of memory: adult hippocampal neurogenesis. *The European Journal of Neuroscience*, *33* (6), 1101-14.

[53] Leuner, B., Mendolia-Loffredo, S., Kozorovitskiy, Y., Samburg, D., Gould, E. & Shors, T. J. (2004). Learning enhances the survival of new neurons beyond the time when the hippocampus is required for memory. *The Journal of Neuroscience*, *24* (34), 7477-81.

[54] Garthe, A., Behr, J. & Kempermann, G. (2009). Adult-generated hippocampal neurons allow the flexible use of spatially precise learning strategies. *PloS one*, *4* (5), e5464.

[55] Garthe, A., Roeder, I. & Kempermann, G. (2016). Mice in an enriched environment learn more flexibly because of adult hippocampal neurogenesis. *Hippocampus*, *26* (2), 261-71.

[56] Burghardt, N. S., Park, E. H., Hen, R. & Fenton, A. A. (2012). Adult-born hippocampal neurons promote cognitive flexibility in mice. *Hippocampus*, *22* (9), 1795-808.

[57] Crone, E. A., Ridderinkhof, K. R., Worm, M., Somsen, R. J. & van der Molen, M. W. (2004). Switching between spatial stimulus-response mappings: a developmental study of cognitive flexibility. *Dev. Sci.*, *7* (4), 443-55.

[58] Ridderinkhof, K. R., Ullsperger, M., Crone, E. A. & Nieuwenhuis, S. (2004). The role of the medial frontal cortex in cognitive control. *Science*, *306* (5695), 443-7.

[59] Clarke, H. F., Dalley, J. W., Crofts, H. S., Robbins, T. W. & Roberts, A. C. (2004). Cognitive inflexibility after prefrontal serotonin depletion. *Science*, *304*, (5672), 878-80.

[60] Lacreuse, A., Parr, L., Chennareddi, L. & Herndon, J. G. (2018). Age-related decline in cognitive flexibility in female chimpanzees. *Neurobiology of Aging*, *72*, 83-8.

[61] Frankland, P. W. & Bontempi, B. (2005). The organization of recent and remote memories. *Nature reviews Neuroscience*, *6* (2), 119-30.

[62] Logue, S. F. & Gould, T. J. (2014). The neural and genetic basis of executive function: attention, cognitive flexibility, and response inhibition. *Pharmacol. Biochem. Behav.*, *123*, 45-54.

[63] Rudy, J. W., Biedenkapp, J. C. & O'Reilly, R. C. (2005). Prefrontal cortex and the organization of recent and remote memories: an alternative view. *Learning & memory*, *12* (5), 445-6.

[64] Wang, S. H., Teixeira, C. M., Wheeler, A. L. & Frankland, P. W. (2009). The precision of remote context memories does not require the hippocampus. *Nature Neuroscience*, *12* (3), 253-5.

[65] Kitamura, T., Ogawa, S. K., Roy, D. S., Okuyama, T., Morrissey, M. D., Smith, L. M., Redondo, R. L. & Tonegawa, S. (2017). Engrams and circuits crucial for systems consolidation of a memory. *Science*, *356* (6333), 73-8.

[66] Richards, B. A. & Frankland, P. W. (2017). The Persistence and Transience of Memory. *Neuron*, *94* (6), 1071-84.

[67] Martinez-Canabal, A., Lopez-Oropeza, G., Gaona-Gamboa, A., Ballesteros-Zebadua, P., de la Cruz, O. G., Moreno-Jimenez, S. & Sotres-Bayon, F. (2019). Hippocampal neurogenesis regulates recovery of defensive responses by recruiting threat- and extinction-signalling brain networks. *Scientific Reports*, *9* (1), 2939.

[68] Rescorla, R. A. (2004). Spontaneous recovery. *Learning & memory*, *11* (5), 501-9.

[69] Yu, Y., Yu, Y. & Lin, Y. (2020). Anxiety and depression aggravate impulsiveness: the mediating and moderating role of cognitive flexibility. *Psychol Health Med*, *25* (1), 25-36.

[70] Johnco, C., Wuthrich, V. M. & Rapee, R. M. (2014). The influence of cognitive flexibility on treatment outcome and cognitive restructuring skill acquisition during cognitive behavioural treatment for anxiety and depression in older adults: Results of a pilot study. *Behaviour research and therapy*, *57*, 55-64.

[71] Rende, B. (2000). Cognitive Flexibility: Theory, Assessment, and Treatment. *Seminars in Speech and Language*, Volume *21*, (Number 02), 0121-53.

[72] Eslinger, P. J. & Grattan, L. M. (1993). Frontal lobe and frontal-striatal substrates for different forms of human cognitive flexibility. *Neuropsychologia*, *31* (1), 17-28.

[73] Miyake, A. & Friedman, N. P. (2012). The Nature and Organization of Individual Differences in Executive Functions: Four General Conclusions. *Curr Dir Psychol Sci*, *21* (1), 8-14.

[74] Joormann, J. & Vanderlind, W. M. (2014). Emotion Regulation in Depression. *Clinical Psychological Science*, *2* (4), 402-21.

[75] Joormann, J. & Stanton, C. H. (2016). Examining emotion regulation in depression: A review and future directions. *Behaviour Research and Therapy*, *86*, 35-49.

[76] Miyake, A., Friedman, N. P., Emerson, M. J., Witzki, A. H., Howerter, A. & Wager, T. D. (2000). The Unity and Diversity of Executive Functions and Their Contributions to Complex "Frontal Lobe" Tasks: A Latent Variable Analysis. *Cognitive Psychology*, *41* (1), 49-100.

[77] Zaehringer, J., Falquez, R., Schubert, A. L., Nees, F. & Barnow, S. (2018). Neural correlates of reappraisal considering working memory capacity and cognitive flexibility. *Brain Imaging and Behavior*, *12* (6), 1529-43.

[78] Anacker, C. & Hen, R. (2017). Adult hippocampal neurogenesis and cognitive flexibility - linking memory and mood. *Nature Reviews Neuroscience*, *18* (6), 335-46.

[79] Josselyn, S. A., Köhler, S. & Frankland, P. W. (2015). Finding the engram. *Nature Reviews Neuroscience*, *16* (9), 521-34.

[80] Gao, A., Xia, F., Guskjolen, A. J., Ramsaran, A. I., Santoro, A., Josselyn, S. A. & Frankland, P. W. (2018). Elevation of Hippocampal Neurogenesis Induces a Temporally Graded Pattern of Forgetting of Contextual Fear Memories. *The Journal of Neuroscience*, *38* (13), 3190-8.

[81] Joormann, J. & Gotlib, I. H. (2010). Emotion regulation in depression: relation to cognitive inhibition. *Cogn. Emot.*, *24* (2), 281-98.

[82] Hayes, J. P., Hayes, S., Miller, D. R., Lafleche, G., Logue, M. W. & Verfaellie, M. (2017). Automated measurement of hippocampal subfields in PTSD: Evidence for smaller dentate gyrus volume. *J. Psychiatr. Res.*, *95*, 247-52.

[83] Beck, A. T. & Haigh, E. A. P. (2014). Advances in Cognitive Theory and Therapy: The Generic Cognitive Model. *Annual review of clinical psychology*, *10* (1), 1-24.

[84] Aldao, A., Nolen-Hoeksema, S. & Schweizer, S. (2010). Emotion-regulation strategies across psychopathology: A meta-analytic review. *Clinical Psychology Review*, *30* (2), 217-37.

[85] Deveney, C. M. & Deldin, P. J. (2006). A preliminary investigation of cognitive flexibility for emotional information in major depressive disorder and non-psychiatric controls. *Emotion*, *6* (3), 429-37.

[86] Ben-Zion, Z., Fine, N. B., Keynan, N. J., Admon, R., Green, N., Halevi, M., Fonzo, G. A., Achituv, M., Merin, O., Sharon, H., Halpern, P., Liberzon, I., Etkin, A., Hendler, T. & Shalev, A. Y. (2018). Cognitive Flexibility Predicts PTSD Symptoms: Observational and Interventional Studies. *Front Psychiatry*, *9*, 477.

[87] Huang, A. C., Shyu, B. C., Hsiao, S., Chen, T. C. & He, A. B. (2013). Neural substrates of fear conditioning, extinction, and spontaneous recovery in passive avoidance learning: a c-fos study in rats. *Behavioural Brain Research*, *237*, 23-31.

[88] Vermetten, E., Vythilingam, M., Southwick, S. M., Charney, D. S. & Bremner, J. D. (2003). Long-term treatment with paroxetine increases verbal declarative memory and hippocampal volume in posttraumatic stress disorder. *Biological psychiatry*, *54* (7), 693-702.

[89] Katsuki, A., Watanabe, K., Nguyen, L., Otsuka, Y., Igata, R., Ikenouchi, A., Kakeda, S., Korogi, Y. & Yoshimura, R. (2020). Structural changes in hippocampal subfields in patients with continuous remission of drug-naive major depressive disorder. *International Journal of Molecular Sciences*, *21* (9), 3032.

[90] Levy-Gigi, E., Szabó, C., Kelemen, O. & Kéri, S. (2013). Association Among Clinical Response, Hippocampal Volume, and FKBP5 Gene Expression in Individuals with Posttraumatic Stress Disorder Receiving Cognitive Behavioral Therapy. *Biological psychiatry*, *74* (11), 793-800.

[91] Kaiser, R. H., Andrews-Hanna, J. R., Spielberg, J. M., Warren, S. L., Sutton, B. P., Miller, G. A., Heller, W. & Banich, M. T. (2015). Distracted and down: neural mechanisms of affective interference in subclinical depression. *Soc Cogn Affect Neurosci*, *10* (5), 654-63.

[92] Murphy, F. C., Michael, A. & Sahakian, B. J. (2011). Emotion modulates cognitive flexibility in patients with major depression. *Psychological Medicine*, *42* (7), 1373-82.

[93] Nolen-Hoeksema, S., Wisco, B. E. & Lyubomirsky, S. (2008). Rethinking Rumination. *Perspectives on Psychological Science*, *3* (5), 400-24.

[94] Michl, L. C., McLaughlin, K. A., Shepherd, K. & Nolen-Hoeksema, S. (2013). Rumination as a mechanism linking stressful life events to symptoms of depression and anxiety:

longitudinal evidence in early adolescents and adults. *J. Abnorm. Psychol.*, *122* (2), 339-52.

[95] McLaughlin, K. A. & Nolen-Hoeksema, S. (2011). Rumination as a transdiagnostic factor in depression and anxiety. *Behaviour research and therapy*, *49* (3), 186-93.

[96] Davis, R. N. & Nolen-Hoeksema, S. (2000). *Cognitive Therapy and Research*, *24* (6), 699-711.

[97] Owens, M. & Derakshan, N. (2013). The effects of dysphoria and rumination on cognitive flexibility and task selection. *Acta Psychologica*, *142* (3), 323-31.

[98] Demeyer, I., De Lissnyder, E., Koster, E. H. W. & De Raedt, R. (2012). Rumination mediates the relationship between impaired cognitive control for emotional information and depressive symptoms: A prospective study in remitted depressed adults. *Behaviour Research and Therapy*, *50* (5), 292-7.

[99] Koster, E. H. W., De Lissnyder, E., Derakshan, N. & De Raedt, R. (2011). Understanding depressive rumination from a cognitive science perspective: The impaired disengagement hypothesis. *Clinical Psychology Review*, *31* (1), 138-45.

[100] Walter, K. H., Palmieri, P. A. & Gunstad, J. (2010). More than symptom reduction: Changes in executive function over the course of PTSD treatment. *Journal of Traumatic Stress n/a-n/a.*

[101] Cisler, J. M., Wolitzky-Taylor, K. B., Adams, T. G., Jr., Babson, K. A., Badour, C. L. & Willems, J. L. (2011). The emotional Stroop task and posttraumatic stress disorder: a meta-analysis. *Clinical Psychology Review*, *31* (5), 817-28.

[102] Hausman, C., Meffert, B. N., Mosich, M. K. & Heinz, A. J. (2020). Impulsivity and Cognitive Flexibility as Neuropsychological Markers for Suicidality: A Multi-Modal Investigation Among Military Veterans with Alcohol Use Disorder and PTSD. *Arch Suicide Res*, *24* (3), 313-26.

[103] Wild, J., Smith, K. V., Thompson, E., Béar, F., Lommen, M. J. J. & Ehlers, A. (2016). A prospective study of pre-trauma risk

factors for post-traumatic stress disorder and depression. *Psychological Medicine*, *46* (12), 2571-82.

[104] American Psychiatric Association., American Psychiatric Association. DSM-5 Task Force. 2013. *Diagnostic and statistical manual of mental disorders: DSM-5*. 5th ed. Washington, D.C.: American Psychiatric Association; xliv, 947 p. p.

[105] Moulds, M. L., Bisby, M. A., Wild, J. & Bryant, R. A. (2020). Rumination in posttraumatic stress disorder: A systematic review. *Clinical Psychology Review*, *82*, 101910.

[106] Miller, B. R. & Hen, R. (2015). The current state of the neurogenic theory of depression and anxiety. *Current Opinion in Neurobiology*, *30*, 51-8.

[107] Schmaal, L., Han, L., Dinga, R., Thompson, P., Veltman, D. & Penninx, B. (2018). 44. Brain Aging in Major Depressive Disorder: Results From the ENIGMA MDD Consortium. *Biological psychiatry*, *83* (9), S18.

[108] Smith, M. E. (2005). Bilateral hippocampal volume reduction in adults with post-traumatic stress disorder: A meta-analysis of structural MRI studies. *Hippocampus*, *15* (6), 798-807.

[109] Boldrini, M., Santiago, A. N., Hen, R., Dwork, A. J., Rosoklija, G. B., Tamir, H., Arango, V. & John Mann, J. (2013). Hippocampal granule neuron number and dentate gyrus volume in antidepressant-treated and untreated major depression. *Neuropsychopharmacology*, *38* (6), 1068-77.

[110] Boldrini, M., Butt, T. H., Santiago, A. N., Tamir, H., Dwork, A. J., Rosoklija, G. B., Arango, V., Hen, R. & Mann, J. J. (2014). Benzodiazepines and the potential trophic effect of antidepressants on dentate gyrus cells in mood disorders. *The International Journal of Neuropsychopharmacology*, *17* (12), 1923-33.

[111] West, M. J., Coleman, P. D., Flood, D. G. & Troncoso, J. C. (1994). Differences in the pattern of hippocampal neuronal loss in normal ageing and Alzheimer's disease. *Lancet*, *344* (8925), 769-72.

[112] Lucassen, P. J., Stumpel, M. W., Wang, Q. & Aronica, E. (2010). Decreased numbers of progenitor cells but no response to antidepressant drugs in the hippocampus of elderly depressed patients. *Neuropharmacology*, *58* (6), 940-9.

[113] Wang, S. H. & Morris, R. G. (2010). Hippocampal-neocortical interactions in memory formation, consolidation, and reconsolidation. *Annual Review of Psychology*, *61*, 49-79, C1-4.

[114] Huang, Y., Coupland, N. J., Lebel, R. M., Carter, R., Seres, P., Wilman, A. H. & Malykhin, N. V. (2013). Structural Changes in Hippocampal Subfields in Major Depressive Disorder: A High-Field Magnetic Resonance Imaging Study. *Biological Psychiatry*, *74* (1), 62-8.

[115] Hill, A. S., Sahay, A. & Hen, R. (2015). Increasing Adult Hippocampal Neurogenesis is Sufficient to Reduce Anxiety and Depression-Like Behaviors. *Neuropsychopharmacology: official publication of the American College of Neuropsychopharmacology*, *40* (10), 2368-78.

[116] Mateus-Pinheiro, A., Pinto, L., Bessa, J. M., Morais, M., Alves, N. D., Monteiro, S., Patrício, P., Almeida, O. F. X. & Sousa, N. (2013). Sustained remission from depressive-like behavior depends on hippocampal neurogenesis. *Translational Psychiatry*, *3* (1), e210-e.

[117] Santarelli, L. (2003). Requirement of Hippocampal Neurogenesis for the Behavioral Effects of Antidepressants. *Science*, *301* (5634), 805-9.

[118] Perera, T. D., Coplan, J. D., Lisanby, S. H., Lipira, C. M., Arif, M., Carpio, C., Spitzer, G., Santarelli, L., Scharf, B., Hen, R., Rosoklija, G., Sackeim, H. A. & Dwork, A. J. (2007). Antidepressant-induced neurogenesis in the hippocampus of adult nonhuman primates. *The Journal of Neuroscience*, *27* (18), 4894-901.

[119] Jaako-Movits, K., Zharkovsky, T., Pedersen, M. & Zharkovsky, A. (2006). Decreased Hippocampal Neurogenesis Following

Olfactory Bulbectomy is Reversed by Repeated Citalopram Administration. *Cellular and Molecular Neurobiology*, *26* (7-8), 1557-68.

[120] Anacker, C., Zunszain, P. A., Cattaneo, A., Carvalho, L. A., Garabedian, M. J., Thuret, S., Price, J. & Pariante, C. M. (2011). Antidepressants increase human hippocampal neurogenesis by activating the glucocorticoid receptor. *Molecular psychiatry*, *16* (7), 738-50.

[121] Bauer, M., Severus, E., Möller, H. J. & Young, A. H. (2017). Pharmacological treatment of unipolar depressive disorders: summary of WFSBP guidelines. *International Journal of Psychiatry in Clinical Practice*, *21* (3), 166-76.

[122] Bandelow, B., Zohar, J., Hollander, E., Kasper, S., Möller, H.-J., Wfsbp Task Force On Treatment, G., Bandelow, B., Zohar, J., Hollander, E., Kasper, S., Möller, H. J. & Wfsbp Task Force On Treatment, G. (2008). World Federation of Societies of Biological Psychiatry (WFSBP) Guidelines for the Pharmacological Treatment of Anxiety, Obsessive-Compulsive and Post-Traumatic Stress Disorders – First Revision. *The World Journal of Biological Psychiatry*, *9* (4), 248-312.

[123] Arnone, D., McKie, S., Elliott, R., Juhasz, G., Thomas, E. J., Downey, D., Williams, S., Deakin, J. F. W. & Anderson, I. M. (2012). State-dependent changes in hippocampal grey matter in depression. *Molecular Psychiatry*, *18* (12), 1265-72.

[124] Boldrini, M., Underwood, M. D., Hen, R., Rosoklija, G. B., Dwork, A. J., John Mann, J. & Arango, V. (2009). Antidepressants increase neural progenitor cells in the human hippocampus. *Neuropsychopharmacology*, *34* (11), 2376-89.

[125] Boldrini, M., Hen, R., Underwood, M. D., Rosoklija, G. B., Dwork, A. J., Mann, J. J. & Arango, V. (2012). Hippocampal angiogenesis and progenitor cell proliferation are increased with antidepressant use in major depression. *Biological Psychiatry*, *72* (7), 562-71.

[126] Cuijpers, P., Berking, M., Andersson, G., Quigley, L., Kleiboer, A. & Dobson, K. S. (2013). A Meta-Analysis of Cognitive-Behavioural Therapy for Adult Depression, Alone and in Comparison with other Treatments. *The Canadian Journal of Psychiatry*, *58* (7), 376-85.

[127] Amick, H. R., Gartlehner, G., Gaynes, B. N., Forneris, C., Asher, G. N., Morgan, L. C., Coker-Schwimmer, E., Boland, E., Lux, L. J., Gaylord, S., Bann, C., Pierl, C. B. & Lohr, K. N. (2015). Comparative benefits and harms of second generation antidepressants and cognitive behavioral therapies in initial treatment of major depressive disorder: systematic review and meta-analysis. *BMJ*, *351*, h6019-h.

[128] Mavranezouli, I., Megnin-Viggars, O., Daly, C., Dias, S., Welton, N. J., Stockton, S., Bhutani, G., Grey, N., Leach, J., Greenberg, N., Katona, C., El-Leithy, S. & Pilling, S. (2020). Psychological treatments for post-traumatic stress disorder in adults: a network meta-analysis. *Psychological Medicine*, *50* (4), 542-55.

[129] Beck, A. T. (2008). The Evolution of the Cognitive Model of Depression and Its Neurobiological Correlates. *American Journal of Psychiatry*, *165* (8), 969-77.

[130] Early, B. P. & Grady, M. D. (2016). Embracing the Contribution of Both Behavioral and Cognitive Theories to Cognitive Behavioral Therapy: Maximizing the Richness. *Clinical Social Work Journal*, *45* (1), 39-48.

[131] Moustafa, A. A. (2013). Increased hippocampal volume and gene expression following cognitive behavioral therapy in PTSD. *Frontiers in Human Neuroscience*, *7*, 747.

[132] Smith, N. B., Doran, J. M., Sippel, L. M. & Harpaz-Rotem, I. (2017). Fear extinction and memory reconsolidation as critical components in behavioral treatment for posttraumatic stress disorder and potential augmentation of these processes. *Neuroscience Letters*, *649*, 170-5.

[133] van Praag, H., Kempermann, G. & Gage, F. H. (1999). Running increases cell proliferation and neurogenesis in the adult mouse dentate gyrus. *Nature Neuroscience*, *2* (3), 266-70.

[134] Gourgouvelis, J., Yielder, P., Clarke, S. T., Behbahani, H. & Murphy, B. A. (2018). Exercise Leads to Better Clinical Outcomes in Those Receiving Medication Plus Cognitive Behavioral Therapy for Major Depressive Disorder. *Frontiers in Psychiatry*, *9*, 37.

[135] Gelfo, F. (2019). Does experience enhance cognitive flexibility? An overview of the evidence provided by the environmental enrichment studies. *Frontiers in Behavioral Neuroscience*, *13*, 150.

[136] Bratman, G. N., Hamilton, J. P., Hahn, K. S., Daily, G. C. & Gross, J. J. (2015). Nature experience reduces rumination and subgenual prefrontal cortex activation. *Proceedings of the National Academy of Sciences of the United States of America*, *112* (28), 8567-72.

[137] Hanson, N. D., Owens, M. J. & Nemeroff, C. B. (2011). Depression, antidepressants, and neurogenesis: a critical reappraisal. *Neuropsychopharmacology: official publication of the American College of Neuropsychopharmacology*, *36* (13), 2589-602.

[138] Kobayashi, K., Ikeda, Y., Sakai, A., Yamasaki, N., Haneda, E., Miyakawa, T. & Suzuki, H. (2010). Reversal of hippocampal neuronal maturation by serotonergic antidepressants. *Proceedings of the National Academy of Sciences of the United States of America*, *107* (18), 8434-9.

[139] Bessa, J. M., Ferreira, D., Melo, I., Marques, F., Cerqueira, J. J., Palha, J. A., Almeida, O. F. X. & Sousa, N. (2008). The mood-improving actions of antidepressants do not depend on neurogenesis but are associated with neuronal remodeling. *Molecular Psychiatry*, *14* (8), 764-73.

[140] Yang, Z., Oathes, D. J., Linn, K. A., Bruce, S. E., Satterthwaite, T. D., Cook, P. A., Satchell, E. K., Shou, H. & Sheline, Y. I. (2018).

Cognitive Behavioral Therapy Is Associated With Enhanced Cognitive Control Network Activity in Major Depression and Posttraumatic Stress Disorder. *Biol Psychiatry Cogn Neurosci Neuroimaging*, *3* (4), 311-9.

[141] Yasinski, C., Hayes, A. M., Ready, C. B., Abel, A., Görg, N. & Kuyken, W. (2019). Processes of change in cognitive behavioral therapy for treatment-resistant depression: psychological flexibility, rumination, avoidance, and emotional processing. *Psychotherapy Research*, *30* (8), 983-97.

[142] Wang, Z., Neylan, T. C., Mueller, S. G., Lenoci, M., Truran, D., Marmar, C. R., Weiner, M. W. & Schuff, N. (2010). Magnetic resonance imaging of hippocampal subfields in posttraumatic stress disorder. *Archives of General Psychiatry*, *67* (3), 296-303.

In: The Dentate Gyrus
Editor: Feng-Ru Tang
ISBN: 978-1-68507-212-4

Chapter 9

Maturational Arrest of the Dentate Gyrus Granule Cell Layer in Schizophrenia

Ayda Tavitian and Hyman M. Schipper*
Department of Neurology and Neurosurgery, McGill University,
Montreal, QC, Canada

Abstract

The hippocampal dentate gyrus has been extensively implicated in the pathogenesis of schizophrenia. Here, we discuss evidence from human and animal research for arrested maturation of the dentate gyrus granule cell layer in this neuropsychiatric disorder. This perpetually immature dentate gyrus exhibits distinct dysmorphogenesis of the granule cell layer which could potentially serve as an anatomical biomarker for the diagnosis of schizophrenia. Although of probable neurodevelopmental origin, schizophrenia becomes clinically evident in late adolescence or early adulthood. The retention of immature properties of the dentate gyrus may explain cardinal features of the illness and the delay of symptom onset into early adulthood.

* Corresponding Author's Email: hyman.schipper@mcgill.ca.

Keywords: astrocyte, dentate gyrus, granule cell layer, heme oxygenase-1 (HO-1), hippocampus, maturation, morphology, neuroanatomy, neurodevelopmental disorder, schizophrenia, transgenic mouse

Introduction

Since Kraepelin delineated "dementia praecox" in 1899 [1] and Bleuler renamed it "schizophrenia" in 1911 [2], much has been uncovered about this enigmatic syndrome, yet much more remains a mystery. The chance discovery in 1952 of chlorpromazine as the first effective medication for schizophrenia [3] was a major advance and re-established the temporarily forgotten biological basis of the disorder [4]. Unfortunately, chlorpromazine and other antipsychotic medications, while ameliorating symptoms of schizophrenia, do not arrest the pathogenesis of the disease. In the absence of biomarkers, diagnosis of schizophrenia is currently based solely on clinical manifestations which include symptoms categorized into positive, negative and cognitive domains with typical onset in late-adolescence or early-adulthood [5]. The causes of schizophrenia are still not known, but both genetic and environmental factors have been implicated [6]. More than a century ago, the neuropathologist Southard recognized that the brains of individuals with schizophrenia had diffuse structural abnormalities that appeared to be maldevelopmental in nature [7]. He considered the disease to have a structural basis and surmised that "the potential victim of dementia praecox is probably born with the normal stock of brain cells, although their arrangement and development are at times early interfered with" [7, p.662]. Nevertheless, postmortem neuropathological studies by various researchers during the many decades that followed failed to identify a characteristic lesion in the schizophrenic brain, leading to a declining interest in the field [8]. With the advent of *in vivo* neuroimaging technology, interest was revived in the neuroanatomy of schizophrenia and alterations were revealed in the sizes of certain brain structures in living patients and corroborated to a certain extent by new postmortem investigations [9-17]. Still, the search for a characteristic neuropathological lesion in the schizophrenia-affected brain has remained elusive. In this chapter, we discuss our recently published position [18] that such a lesion may indeed be present within the schizophrenic dentate gyrus and correspond to a maturational arrest of the granule cell layer in this brain region.

THE HIPPOCAMPUS AND DENTATE GYRUS IN SCHIZOPHRENIA

Aberrations in the structure and function of the hippocampus have been documented in the brains of schizophrenic subjects. Structurally, the schizophrenia-affected hippocampus shows a reduction in its size and a deformation of its shape [12, 16, 19-24]. A bilateral reduction in hippocampal volume is already present when schizophrenia patients present with their first episode of psychosis [15, 17, 19]. This volume deficit may be the result of arrested growth rather than atrophy of the hippocampus, especially in light of imaging evidence that during late adolescence, contrary to a progressive increase in healthy controls, the volume of the hippocampus remains static in subjects at high-risk for schizophrenia [25]. The anomalous structure of the hippocampus in schizophrenia is accompanied by abnormal function characterised by high intrinsic activity and low evoked activation [26-34].

In addition to the whole hippocampus, the dentate gyrus/CA4 region of schizophrenia patients also displayed volume deficits in *in vivo* neuroimaging studies [35-40], as did the granule cell layer of the dentate gyrus [39, 41]. The latter finding has also been demonstrated in two separate postmortem investigations [22, 42]. Postmortem studies assessing the number of dentate gyrus granule cells in schizophrenia patients relative to controls have reported varying results, with the majority having found no significant difference between the two groups

[22, 42-46]. Further studies are needed to determine whether granule cell numbers are altered in this disorder. Morphological modifications in the schizophrenia-affected dentate gyrus include a significantly higher percentage of granule cells with basal dendrites compared to controls which may reflect the retention of an immature form of plasticity by these cells [45, 47].

At the molecular level, an immature profile characterised by elevated expression of calretinin and diminished expression of calbindin has been described in dentate gyrus granule cells of adult schizophrenia patients [43, 48]. The immature molecular profile of the schizophrenia-affected dentate gyrus extends to *N*-methyl-D-aspartate (NMDA) glutamatergic receptors with a low expression of the GluN1 (NR1, NMDAR1) subunit [49-51] and a high mossy fiber synaptic expression of the GluN2B subunit [49, 52]. This is accompanied by a diminished density of synapses between mossy fiber terminals and CA3 pyramidal neurons [53].

An immature molecular profile has also been detected in whole hippocampal preparations from the brains of schizophrenic patients in the form of increased flip:flop ratio in GluR2 subunit isoforms of the glutamatergic α-amino-3-hydroxy-5-methyl-4-isoxazolepropionic acid (AMPA) receptor [54].

Animal Models of Schizophrenia Research

The immature dentate gyrus molecular profile as a possible endophenotype of schizophrenia has been described in calcium calmodulin-dependent protein kinase II alpha heterozygous knockout (α-CaMKII–HKO) [55] and schnurri-2 knockout (Shn-2 KO) [56] mice that exhibit behavioural abnormalities relevant to schizophrenia, and confirmed in human brain tissue derived from schizophrenia patients [43, 48] attesting to its translational validity. In these mouse models, dentate gyrus granule cells also have morphological and electrophysiological properties similar to those of immature granule cells [48, 55-58]. The immature dentate gyrus profile becomes evident only in late adolescence in these models [56, 57].

Animal models currently in use for investigations into the etiopathogenesis of schizophrenia are conceptualized within the five major categories of pharmacologic, lesion, genetic, developmental and gene-environment interaction models. Each category has its inherent strengths and weaknesses and no single model can fully recapitulate the human illness, yet every model can provide an important piece of the final picture (for reviews see [18, 59-64]).

Conditional transgenic GFAP.HMOX1$^{0\text{-}12m}$ mice developed in our laboratory to overexpress the human stress protein heme oxygenase-1 (HO-1) in astrocytes exhibit many behavioural, neurochemical, molecular, neuroanatomical and craniofacial features relevant to schizophrenia, with several features emerging after adolescence [65-67, Tavitian and Schipper, unpublished results].

IMMATURE MORPHOLOGY OF THE DENTATE GYRUS GRANULE CELL LAYER IN GFAP.HMOX1$^{0\text{-}12M}$ MICE

The granule cell layer of the dentate gyrus has an unusually "stunted" appearance in adult GFAP.HMOX1$^{0\text{-}12m}$ mice compared to that of wild-type counterparts [65]. This morphology, which is abnormal in the adult animal, is qualitatively and quantitatively indistinguishable from that of the normal granule cell layer in adolescent wild-type mice, as well as adolescent GFAP.HMOX1$^{0\text{-}12m}$ mice [18, Tavitian and Schipper, unpublished results], strongly suggesting that it corresponds to a maturational arrest of the dentate gyrus granule cell layer at the adolescent stage (Figure 1).

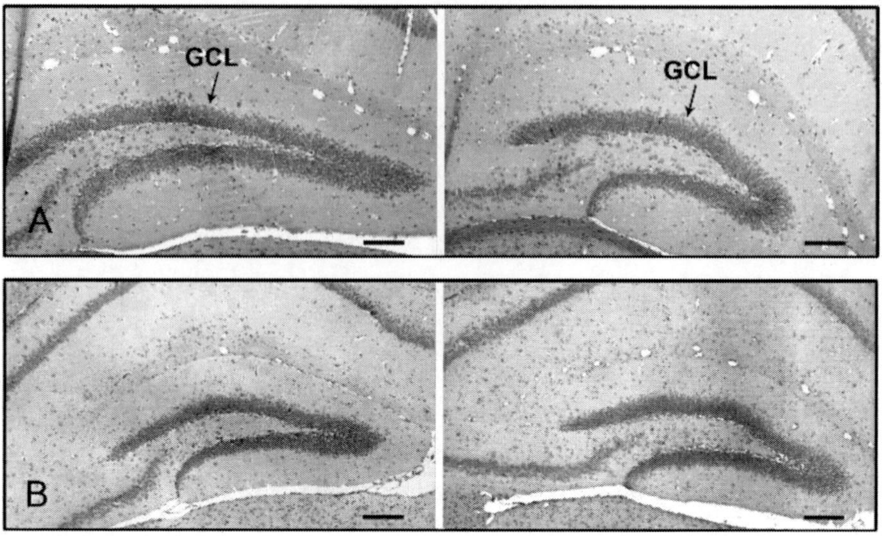

Figure 1. Morphology of the dentate gyrus granule cell layer in GFAP.HMOX1$^{0\text{-}12m}$ (right panels) and wild-type (left panels) mice. (A) adult age. (B) adolescent age. Scale bars, 100μm. GCL, granule cell layer. Reproduced with permission from Song et al. Schizophrenia-like features in transgenic mice overexpressing human HO-1 in the astrocytic compartment. J. Neurosci. (Volume 32, Issue 32) pp. 10841-10853 [65]. Copyright © 2012 (The Authors). DOI: 10.1523/JNEUROSCI.6469-11.2012 (A) and Tavitian A., Song W., Schipper H.M. Dentate gyrus immaturity in schizophrenia. The Neuroscientist (Volume 25, Issue 6) pp. 528–547 [18]. Copyright © 2019 (The Authors). DOI: 10.1177/1073858418824072 (B).

Immature Morphology of the Dentate Gyrus Granule Cell Layer in Other Rodent Models

Subsequent to our observations in GFAP.HMOX1$^{0\text{-}12m}$ mice, a survey of published photomicrographs of the adult hippocampus in other rodent models of schizophrenia disclosed similar, if not identical, abnormalities of dentate gyrus morphology. We identified this previously undetected "signature" morphology of the dentate gyrus granule cell layer in ten distinct models, underscoring the notion that this feature may be central to the disorder. Genetic models in which we saw this abnormality include α-CAMKII-HKO [55], STOP null [68], NR1 hypomorphic (NR1neo/neo) [69], 14-3-3 zeta deficient [70, 71], TLR-2 KO [72] and Disc1tr [73] mice. In the developmental category of preclinical schizophrenia models, we observed this neuroendophenotype in the MAM-E17 [74-76] and AraC [77] rat models, and the maternal immune activation models of PolyI:C treatment [78] and early IL-6 exposure [79]. For a compilation of photomicrographs depicting the abnormal morphology in these models, we refer the reader to figure 4 of our position paper on this subject [18], as well as to the original publications listed above. Future studies directed at systematic analyses of dentate gyrus granule cell layer morphology in animal models of schizophrenia, as we have performed in the GFAP.HMOX1$^{0\text{-}12m}$ model, may lead to the inculcation of the maturationally arrested dentate gyrus into a validation tool for animal models useful for schizophrenia research.

Morphology of the Human Dentate Gyrus Granule Cell Layer in Schizophrenia

To date, no systematic examination of dentate gyrus granule cell layer morphology has been done on human postmortem tissue in schizophrenia. As a result, there is no record of this morphology in comparison to the healthy control brain. However, in figure 2 of Benes, Sorensen and Bird (1991), relative to the control preparation, the dentate gyrus granule cell layer of the schizophrenia specimen [80] may represent a human correlate of the "signature" stunted morphology which we have identified in rodent brains and bears an interesting resemblance to the normal adolescent appearance of this structure [81]. For a compilation of the described photomicrographs, we refer the reader to figure 3 of our position paper on this subject [18] as well as to the original publications listed above. Empirical validation of our hypothesis warrants further studies. Our model of morphological immaturity of the dentate gyrus granule cell layer in schizophrenia is presented in Figure 2.

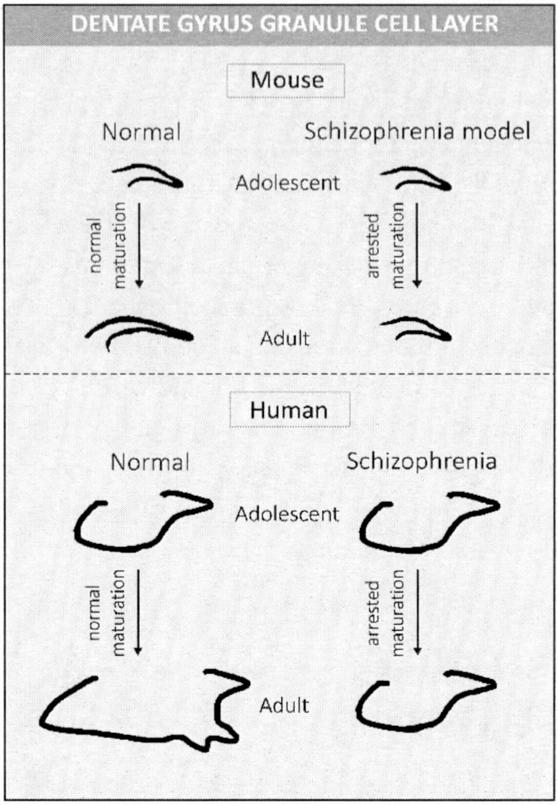

Figure 2. Morphological immaturity of the dentate gyrus granule cell layer in schizophrenia: a model. Reproduced with permission from Tavitian A., Song W., Schipper H.M. Dentate gyrus immaturity in schizophrenia. The Neuroscientist (Volume 25, Issue 6) pp. 528–547 [18]. Copyright © 2019 (The Authors). DOI: 10.1177/1073858418824072.

CONCLUSION

In this chapter, we have described a discrete morphological abnormality of the dentate gyrus granule cell layer in schizophrenia, which we propose represents arrested maturation of this brain region in this condition. Maturational arrest of the dentate gyrus granule cell layer may constitute the elusive neuropathological lesion long sought after in schizophrenia. Technological advances in magnetic resonance imaging now permit reliable high-resolution mapping of the human hippocampal dentate gyrus granule cell layer [82]. Once this technology is in wider use, the "stunted" dentate gyrus granule cell layer morphology - if empirically validated in the human schizophrenia-affected brain - may serve as an effective diagnostic biomarker of this disease.

ACKNOWLEDGMENT

We thank Adrienne Liberman for assembly of the figure plates.

REFERENCES

[1] Kraepelin, E. 1899. Psychiatrie: Ein lehrbuch für studierende und ärzte. Leipzig: J.A. Barth. p 2 vol. [Kraepelin, E. 1899. *Psychiatry: A textbook for students and physicians*. Vol. 2 vol. Leipzig: J.A. Barth].

[2] Bleuler, E. 1911. Dementia praecox, oder gruppe der schizophrenien. Handbuch der Psychiatrie. Leipzig: Deuticke. p xii, 420 p. [Bleuler, E. 1911. Dementia praecox, or the group of schizophrenias. Vol. xii, 420 p. *Manual of Psychiatry*. Leipzig: Deuticke].

[3] Delay, J., Deniker, P. 1955. Neuroleptic effects of chlorpromazine in therapeutics of neuropsychiatry. *J. Clin. Exp. Psychopathol.* 16, 104-12.

[4] Kandel, E. R. 1998. A new intellectual framework for psychiatry. *Am. J. Psychiatry* 155, 457-69.

[5] Tandon, R., Nasrallah, H. A., Keshavan, M. S. 2009. Schizophrenia, "just the facts" 4. Clinical features and conceptualization. *Schizophr. Res.* 110, 1-23.

[6] Tandon, R., Keshavan, M. S., Nasrallah, H. A. 2008. Schizophrenia, "just the facts": What we know in 2008: 2. Epidemiology and etiology. *Schizophr. Res.* 102, 1-18.

[7] Southard, E. B. 1915. On the topographical distribution of cortex lesions and anomalies in dementia praecox, with some account of their functional significance. *Am. J. Psychiatry* 71, 603-71-20.

[8] Harrison, P. J. 1999. The neuropathology of schizophrenia. A critical review of the data and their interpretation. *Brain* 122 (Pt 4), 593-624.

[9] Andreasen, N., Nasrallah, H. A., Dunn, V., Olson, S. C., Grove, W. M., Ehrhardt, J. C., Coffman, J. A., Crossett, J. H. W. 1986. Structural abnormalities in the frontal system in schizophrenia: A magnetic resonance imaging study. *Arch. Gen. Psychiatry* 43, 136-44.

[10] Bogerts, B., Meertz, E., Schönfeldt-Bausch, R. 1985. Basal ganglia and limbic system pathology in schizophrenia: A morphometric study of brain volume and shrinkage. *Arch. Gen. Psychiatry* 42, 784-91.

[11] Heckers, S., Heinsen, H., Heinsen, Y., Beckmann, H. 1991. Cortex, white matter, and basal ganglia in schizophrenia: A volumetric postmortem study. *Biol. Psychiatry* 29, 556-66.

[12] Okada, N., Fukunaga, M., Yamashita, F., Koshiyama, D., Yamamori, H., Ohi, K., Yasuda, Y., Fujimoto, M., Watanabe, Y., Yahata, N., Nemoto, K., Hibar, D. P., Van Erp, T. G. M., Fujino, H., Isobe, M., Isomura, S., Natsubori, T., Narita, H., Hashimoto, N., Miyata, J., Koike, S., Takahashi, T., Yamasue, H., Matsuo, K., Onitsuka, T., Iidaka, T., Kawasaki, Y., Yoshimura, R., Watanabe, Y., Suzuki, M., Turner, J.A., Takeda, M., Thompson, P. M., Ozaki, N., Kasai, K., Hashimoto, R. 2016. Abnormal asymmetries in subcortical brain volume in schizophrenia. *Mol. Psychiatry* 21, 1460.

[13] Pakkenberg, B. 1987. Post-mortem study of chronic schizophrenic brains. *Br. J. Psychiatry* 151, 744-52.

[14] Roeske, M. J., Konradi, C., Heckers, S., Lewis, A. S. 2020. Hippocampal volume and hippocampal neuron density, number and size in schizophrenia: A systematic review and meta-analysis of postmortem studies. *Mol. Psychiatry* Jul 28:10.1038/s41380-020-0853-y. Epub ahead of print.

[15] Steen, R. G., Mull, C., Mcclure, R., Hamer, R.M., Lieberman, J. A. 2006. Brain volume in first-episode schizophrenia: Systematic review and meta-analysis of magnetic resonance imaging studies. *Br. J. Psychiatry* 188, 510-8.

[16] Van Erp, T. G., Hibar, D. P., Rasmussen, J. M., Glahn, D. C., Pearlson, G. D., Andreassen, O. A., Agartz, I., Westlye, L. T., Haukvik, U. K., Dale, A. M., Melle, I., Hartberg, C. B., Gruber, O., Kraemer, B., Zilles, D., Donohoe, G., Kelly, S., Mcdonald, C., Morris, D. W., Cannon, D. M., Corvin, A., Machielsen, M. W., Koenders, L., De Haan, L., Veltman, D. J., Satterthwaite, T. D., Wolf, D. H., Gur, R. C., Gur, R. E., Potkin, S. G., Mathalon, D. H., Mueller, B. A., Preda, A., Macciardi, F., Ehrlich, S., Walton, E., Hass, J., Calhoun, V. D., Bockholt, H. J., Sponheim, S. R., Shoemaker, J. M., Van Haren, N. E., Hulshoff Pol, H. E., Ophoff, R. A., Kahn, R. S., Roiz-Santianez, R., Crespo-Facorro, B., Wang, L., Alpert, K. I., Jonsson, E. G., Dimitrova, R., Bois, C., Whalley, H. C., Mcintosh, A. M., Lawrie, S. M., Hashimoto, R., Thompson, P. M., Turner, J. A. 2016. Subcortical brain volume abnormalities in 2028 individuals with schizophrenia and 2540 healthy controls via the ENIGMA consortium. *Mol. Psychiatry* 21, 547-53.

[17] Vita, A., De Peri, L., Silenzi, C., Dieci, M. 2006. Brain morphology in first-episode schizophrenia: A meta-analysis of quantitative magnetic resonance imaging studies. *Schizophr. Res.* 82, 75-88.

[18] Tavitian, A., Song, W., Schipper, H. M. 2019. Dentate gyrus immaturity in schizophrenia. *Neuroscientist* 25, 528-47.

[19] Adriano, F., Caltagirone, C., Spalletta, G. 2012. Hippocampal volume reduction in first-episode and chronic schizophrenia: A review and meta-analysis. *Neuroscientist* 18, 180-200.

[20] Bogerts, B., Falkai, P., Haupts, M., Greve, B., Ernst, S., Tapernon-Franz, U., Heinzmann, U. 1990. Post-mortem volume measurements of limbic system and basal ganglia structures in chronic schizophrenics: Initial results from a new brain collection. *Schizophr. Res.* 3, 295-301.

[21] Csernansky, J. G., Wang, L., Jones, D., Rastogi-Cruz, D., Posener, J. A., Heydebrand, G., Miller, J. P., Miller, M. I. 2002. Hippocampal deformities in schizophrenia characterized by high dimensional brain mapping. *Am. J. Psychiatry* 159, 2000-6.

[22] Falkai, P., Bogerts, B. 1986. Cell loss in the hippocampus of schizophrenics. *Eur. Arch. Psychiatry Neurol. Sci.* 236, 154-61.

[23] Haijma, S. V., Van Haren, N., Cahn, W., Koolschijn, P. C., Hulshoff Pol, H. E., Kahn, R. S. 2013. Brain volumes in schizophrenia: A meta-analysis in over 18 000 subjects. *Schizophr. Bull.* 39, 1129-38.

[24] Harrison, P. 2004. The hippocampus in schizophrenia: A review of the neuropathological evidence and its pathophysiological implications. *Psychopharmacology* (Berl.) 174, 151-62.

[25] Bois, C., Levita, L., Ripp, I., Owens, D. C. G., Johnstone, E. C., Whalley, H. C., Lawrie, S. M. 2016. Longitudinal changes in hippocampal volume in the Edinburgh High Risk Study of Schizophrenia. *Schizophr. Res.* 173, 146-51.

[26] Heckers, S., Rauch, S. L., Goff, D., Savage, C. R., Schacter, D. L., Fischman, A. J., Alpert, N. M. 1998. Impaired recruitment of the hippocampus during conscious recollection in schizophrenia. *Nat. Neurosci.* 1, 318-23.

[27] Ledoux, A. A., Phillips, J. L., Labelle, A., Smith, A., Bohbot, V. D., Boyer, P. 2013. Decreased fMRI activity in the hippocampus of patients with schizophrenia compared to healthy control participants, tested on a wayfinding task in a virtual town. *Psychiatry Res.* 211, 47-56.

[28] Malaspina, D., Harkavy-Friedman, J., Corcoran, C., Mujica-Parodi, L., Printz, D., Gorman, J. M., Van Heertum, R. 2004. Resting

neural activity distinguishes subgroups of schizophrenia patients. *Biol. Psychiatry* 56, 931-7.

[29] Medoff, D. R., Holcomb, H. H., Lahti, A. C., Tamminga, C.A. 2001. Probing the human hippocampus using rCBF: Contrasts in schizophrenia. *Hippocampus* 11, 543-50.

[30] Molina, V., Sanz, J., Sarramea, F., Benito, C., Palomo, T. 2005. Prefrontal atrophy in first episodes of schizophrenia associated with limbic metabolic hyperactivity. *J. Psychiatr. Res.* 39, 117-27.

[31] Thoresen, C., Endestad, T., Sigvartsen, N. P., Server, A., Bolstad, I., Johansson, M., Andreassen, O. A., Jensen, J. 2014. Frontotemporal hypoactivity during a reality monitoring paradigm is associated with delusions in patients with schizophrenia spectrum disorders. *Cogn. Neuropsychiatry* 19, 97-115.

[32] Tregellas, J. R., Smucny, J., Harris, J. G., Olincy, A., Maharajh, K., Kronberg, E., Eichman, L. C., Lyons, E., Freedman, R. 2014. Intrinsic hippocampal activity as a biomarker for cognition and symptoms in schizophrenia. *Am. J. Psychiatry* 171, 549-56.

[33] Wiesel, F. A., Wik, G., Sjogren, I., Blomqvist, G., Greitz, T., Stone-Elander, S. 1987. Regional brain glucose metabolism in drug free schizophrenic patients and clinical correlates. *Acta Psychiatr. Scand.* 76, 628-41.

[34] Wölwer, W., Stroth, S., Brinkmeyer, J., Gaebel, W. 2012. Electrophysiological correlates of planning and monitoring in first episode schizophrenia. *Psychiatry Res. Neuroimaging* 203, 83-8.

[35] Haukvik, U. K., Westlye, L. T., Morch-Johnsen, L., Jorgensen, K. N., Lange, E. H., Dale, A. M., Melle, I., Andreassen, O. A., Agartz, I. 2015. In vivo hippocampal subfield volumes in schizophrenia and bipolar disorder. *Biol. Psychiatry* 77, 581-8.

[36] Kawano, M., Sawada, K., Shimodera, S., Ogawa, Y., Kariya, S., Lang, D. J., Inoue, S., Honer, W. G. 2015. Hippocampal subfield volumes in first episode and chronic schizophrenia. *PLoS One* 10, e0117785.

[37] Kraguljac, N. V., White, D. M., Reid, M. A., Lahti, A. C. 2013. Increased hippocampal glutamate and volumetric deficits in

unmedicated patients with *schizophrenia. JAMA Psychiatry* 70, 1294-302.

[38] Mathew, I., Gardin, T. M., Tandon, N., Eack, S., Francis, A. N., Seidman, L. J., Clementz, B., Pearlson, G. D., Sweeney, J. A., Tamminga, C.A., Keshavan, M.S. 2014. Medial temporal lobe structures and hippocampal subfields in psychotic disorders: Findings from the Bipolar-Schizophrenia Network on Intermediate Phenotypes (B-SNIP) study. *JAMA Psychiatry* 71, 769-77.

[39] Nakahara, S., Turner, J. A., Calhoun, V. D., Lim, K. O., Mueller, B., Bustillo, J. R., O'Leary, D. S., McEwen, S., Voyvodic, J., Belger, A., Mathalon, D. H., Ford, J. M., Macciardi, F., Matsumoto, M., Potkin, S. G., Van Erp, T. G. M. 2020. Dentate gyrus volume deficit in schizophrenia. *Psychol. Med.* 50, 1267-77.

[40] Ota, M., Sato, N., Hidese, S., Teraishi, T., Maikusa, N., Matsuda, H., Hattori, K., Kunugi, H. 2017. Structural differences in hippocampal subfields among schizophrenia patients, major depressive disorder patients, and healthy subjects. *Psychiatry Res. Neuroimaging* 259, 54-9.

[41] Ho, N. F., Iglesias, J. E., Sum, M. Y., Kuswanto, C. N., Sitoh, Y. Y., De Souza, J., Hong, Z., Fischl, B., Roffman, J. L., Zhou, J., Sim, K., Holt, D. J. 2017. Progression from selective to general involvement of hippocampal subfields in schizophrenia. *Mol. Psychiatry* 22, 142-52.

[42] Chen, F., Bertelsen, A. B., Holm, I. E., Nyengaard, J. R., Rosenberg, R., Dorph-Petersen, K.-A. 2020. Hippocampal volume and cell number in depression, schizophrenia, and suicide subjects. *Brain Res.* 1727, 146546.

[43] Altar, C. A., Jurata, L. W., Charles, V., Lemire, A., Liu, P., Bukhman, Y., Young, T. A., Bullard, J., Yokoe, H., Webster, M. J., Knable, M. B., Brockman, J. A. 2005. Deficient hippocampal neuron expression of proteasome, ubiquitin, and mitochondrial genes in multiple schizophrenia cohorts. *Biol. Psychiatry* 58, 85-96.

[44] Luts, A., Jonsson, S.A., Guldberg-Kjaer, N., Brun, A. 1998. Uniform abnormalities in the hippocampus of five chronic schizophrenic men compared with age-matched controls. *Acta Psychiatr. Scand.* 98, 60-4.

[45] Senitz, D., Beckmann, H. 2003. Granule cells of the dentate gyrus with basal and recurrent dendrites in schizophrenic patients and controls. A comparative Golgi study. *J. Neural Transm.* 110, 317-26.

[46] Walker, M. A., Highley, J. R., Esiri, M. M., Mcdonald, B., Roberts, H.C., Evans, S.P., Crow, T.J. 2002. Estimated neuronal populations and volumes of the hippocampus and its subfields in schizophrenia. *Am. J. Psychiatry* 159, 821-8.

[47] Lauer, M., Beckmann, H., Senitz, D. 2003. Increased frequency of dentate granule cells with basal dendrites in the hippocampal formation of schizophrenics. *Psychiatry Res. Neuroimaging* 122, 89-97.

[48] Walton, N. M., Zhou, Y., Kogan, J. H., Shin, R., Webster, M., Gross, A. K., Heusner, C. L., Chen, Q., Miyake, S., Tajinda, K., Tamura, K., Miyakawa, T., Matsumoto, M. 2012. Detection of an immature dentate gyrus feature in human schizophrenia/bipolar patients. *Transl. Psychiatry* 2, e135.

[49] Gao, X. M., Sakai, K., Roberts, R. C., Conley, R. R., Dean, B., Tamminga, C. A. 2000. Ionotropic glutamate receptors and expression of N-methyl-D-aspartate receptor subunits in subregions of human hippocampus: Effects of schizophrenia. *Am. J. Psychiatry* 157, 1141-9.

[50] Law, A. J., Deakin, J. F. 2001. Asymmetrical reductions of hippocampal NMDAR1 glutamate receptor mRNA in the psychoses. *Neuroreport* 12, 2971-4.

[51] Stan, A. D., Ghose, S., Zhao, C., Hulsey, K., Mihalakos, P., Yanagi, M., Morris, S. U., Bartko, J. J., Choi, C., Tamminga, C. A. 2015. Magnetic resonance spectroscopy and tissue protein concentrations together suggest lower glutamate signaling in dentate gyrus in schizophrenia. *Mol. Psychiatry* 20, 433-9.

[52] Li, W., Ghose, S., Gleason, K., Begovic, A., Perez, J., Bartko, J., Russo, S., Wagner, A. D., Selemon, L., Tamminga, C.A. 2015. Synaptic proteins in the hippocampus indicative of increased neuronal activity in CA3 in schizophrenia. *Am. J. Psychiatry* 172, 373-82.

[53] Kolomeets, N. S., Orlovskaya, D. D., Uranova, N. A. 2007. Decreased numerical density of CA3 hippocampal mossy fiber synapses in schizophrenia. *Synapse* 61, 615-21.

[54] Eastwood, S. L., Burnet, P. W. J., Harrison, P. J. 1997. GluR2 glutamate receptor subunit flip and flop isoforms are decreased in the hippocampal formation in schizophrenia: A reverse transcriptase-polymerase chain reaction (RT–PCR) study. *Brain Res. Mol. Brain Res.* 44, 92-8.

[55] Yamasaki, N., Maekawa, M., Kobayashi, K., Kajii, Y., Maeda, J., Soma, M., Takao, K., Tanda, K., Ohira, K., Toyama, K., Kanzaki, K., Fukunaga, K., Sudo, Y., Ichinose, H., Ikeda, M., Iwata, N., Ozaki, N., Suzuki, H., Higuchi, M., Suhara, T., Yuasa, S., Miyakawa, T. 2008. Alpha-CAMKII deficiency causes immature dentate gyrus, a novel candidate endophenotype of psychiatric disorders. *Mol. Brain* 1, 6.

[56] Takao, K., Kobayashi, K., Hagihara, H., Ohira, K., Shoji, H., Hattori, S., Koshimizu, H., Umemori, J., Toyama, K., Nakamura, H. K., Kuroiwa, M., Maeda, J., Atsuzawa, K., Esaki, K., Yamaguchi, S., Furuya, S., Takagi, T., Walton, N. M., Hayashi, N., Suzuki, H., Higuchi, M., Usuda, N., Suhara, T., Nishi, A., Matsumoto, M., Ishii, S., Miyakawa, T. 2013. Deficiency of schnurri-2, an MHC enhancer binding protein, induces mild chronic inflammation in the brain and confers molecular, neuronal, and behavioral phenotypes related to schizophrenia. *Neuropsychopharmacology* 38, 1409-25.

[57] de Koning, A., Walton, N. M., Shin, R., Chen, Q., Miyake, S., Tajinda, K., Gross, A. K., Kogan, J. H., Heusner, C. L., Tamura, K.,

Matsumoto, M. 2013. Derivation of neural stem cells from an animal model of psychiatric disease. *Transl. Psychiatry* 3, e323.

[58] Schmidt-Hieber, C., Jonas, P., Bischofberger, J. 2004. Enhanced synaptic plasticity in newly generated granule cells of the adult hippocampus. *Nature* 429, 184-7.

[59] Kannan, G., Sawa, A., Pletnikov, M.V. 2013. Mouse models of gene–environment interactions in schizophrenia. *Neurobiol. Dis.* 57, 5-11.

[60] Lazar, N. L., Neufeld, R. W. J., Cain, D. P. 2011. Contribution of nonprimate animal models in understanding the etiology of schizophrenia. *J. Psychiatry Neurosci.* 36, E5-E29.

[61] Lipska, B. K., Weinberger, D. R. 2000. To model a psychiatric disorder in animals: Schizophrenia as a reality test. *Neuropsychopharmacology* 23, 223-39.

[62] Marcotte, E. R., Pearson, D. M., Srivastava, L. K. 2001. Animal models of schizophrenia: A critical review. *J. Psychiatry Neurosci.* 26, 395-410.

[63] O'Tuathaigh, C. M., Waddington, J. L. 2015. Closing the translational gap between mutant mouse models and the clinical reality of psychotic illness. *Neurosci. Biobehav. Rev.* 58, 19-35.

[64] Young, J. W., Zhou, X., Geyer, M. A. 2010. Animal models of schizophrenia. In Behavioral neurobiology of schizophrenia and its treatment. *Current topics in behavioral neurosciences*, edited by Neal R. Swerdlow, 4: 391-433. Berlin, Heidelberg: Springer.

[65] Song, W., Zukor, H., Lin, S. H., Hascalovici, J., Liberman, A., Tavitian, A., Mui, J., Vali, H., Tong, X. K., Bhardwaj, S. K., Srivastava, L. K., Hamel, E., Schipper, H. M. 2012. Schizophrenia-like features in transgenic mice overexpressing human HO-1 in the astrocytic compartment. *J. Neurosci.* 32, 10841-53.

[66] Song, W., Tavitian, A., Cressatti, M., Galindez, C., Liberman, A., Schipper, H.M. 2017. Cysteine-rich whey protein isolate (Immunocal (R)) ameliorates deficits in the GFAP.HMOX1 mouse model of schizophrenia. *Free Radic. Biol. Med.* 110, 162-75.

[67] Tavitian, A., Cressatti, M., Song, W., Turk, A.Z., Galindez, C., Smart, A., Liberman, A., Schipper, H. M. 2020. Strategic timing of glial *HMOX1* expression results in either schizophrenia-like or parkinsonian behavior in mice. *Antioxid. Redox Signal.* 32, 1259-72.

[68] Powell, K.J., Hori, S.E., Leslie, R., Andrieux, A., Schellinck, H., Thorne, M., Robertson, G.S. 2007. Cognitive impairments in the STOP null mouse model of schizophrenia. *Behav. Neurosci.* 121, 826-35.

[69] Duncan, G. E., Inada, K., Koller, B. H., Moy, S. S. 2010. Increased sensitivity to kainic acid in a genetic model of reduced NMDA receptor function. *Brain Res.* 1307, 166-76.

[70] Cheah, P. S., Ramshaw, H. S., Thomas, P. Q., Toyo-Oka, K., Xu, X., Martin, S., Coyle, P., Guthridge, M. A., Stomski, F., Van Den Buuse, M., Wynshaw-Boris, A., Lopez, A. F., Schwarz, Q. P. 2012. Neurodevelopmental and neuropsychiatric behaviour defects arise from 14-3-3zeta deficiency. *Mol. Psychiatry* 17, 451-66.

[71] Xu, X., Jaehne, E. J., Greenberg, Z., Mccarthy, P., Saleh, E., Parish, C. L., Camera, D., Heng, J., Haas, M., Baune, B. T., Ratnayake, U., Buuse, M. V. D., Lopez, A.F., Ramshaw, H. S., Schwarz, Q. 2015. 14-3-3ζ deficient mice in the BALB/c background display behavioural and anatomical defects associated with neurodevelopmental disorders. *Sci. Rep.* 5, 12434.

[72] Park, S. J., Lee, J. Y., Kim, S. J., Choi, S. Y., Yune, T. Y., Ryu, J. H. 2015. Toll-like receptor-2 deficiency induces schizophrenia-like behaviors in mice. *Sci. Rep.* 5, 8502.

[73] Shen, S., Lang, B., Nakamoto, C., Zhang, F., Pu, J., Kuan, S.-L., Chatzi, C., He, S., Mackie, I., Brandon, N. J., Marquis, K. L., Day, M., Hurko, O., Mccaig, C. D., Riedel, G., St Clair, D. 2008. Schizophrenia-related neural and behavioral phenotypes in transgenic mice expressing truncated Disc1. *J. Neurosci.* 28, 10893-904.

[74] Le Pen, G., Gourevitch, R., Hazane, F., Hoareau, C., Jay, T. M., Krebs, M. O. 2006. Peri-pubertal maturation after developmental disturbance: A model for psychosis onset in the rat. *Neuroscience* 143, 395-405.

[75] Matricon, J., Bellon, A., Frieling, H., Kebir, O., Le Pen, G., Beuvon, F., Daumas-Duport, C., Jay, T. M., Krebs, M. O. 2010. Neuropathological and reelin deficiencies in the hippocampal formation of rats exposed to MAM; differences and similarities with schizophrenia. *PLoS One* 5, e10291.

[76] Moore, H., Jentsch, J. D., Ghajarnia, M., Geyer, M. A., Grace, A. A. 2006. A neurobehavioral systems analysis of adult rats exposed to methylazoxymethanol acetate on E17: Implications for the neuropathology of schizophrenia. *Biol. Psychiatry* 60, 253-64.

[77] Brown, P. L., Shepard, P. D., Elmer, G. I., Stockman, S., Mcfarland, R., Mayo, C. L., Cadet, J. L., Krasnova, I. N., Greenwald, M., Schoonover, C., Vogel, M.W. 2012. Altered spatial learning, cortical plasticity and hippocampal anatomy in a neurodevelopmental model of schizophrenia-related endophenotypes. *Eur. J. Neurosci.* 36, 2773-81.

[78] Nyffeler, M., Meyer, U., Yee, B. K., Feldon, J., Knuesel, I. 2006. Maternal immune activation during pregnancy increases limbic GABAA receptor immunoreactivity in the adult offspring: Implications for schizophrenia. *Neuroscience* 143, 51-62.

[79] Samuelsson, A. M., Jennische, E., Hansson, H. A., Holmang, A. 2006. Prenatal exposure to interleukin-6 results in inflammatory neurodegeneration in hippocampus with NMDA/GABA(A) dysregulation and impaired spatial learning. *Am. J. Physiol. Regul. Integr. Comp. Physiol.* 290, R1345-56.

[80] Benes, F. M., Sorensen, I., Bird, E. D. 1991. Reduced neuronal size in posterior hippocampus of schizophrenic patients. *Schizophr. Bull.* 17, 597-608.

[81] Green, R. C., Mesulam, M. M. 1988. Acetylcholinesterase fiber staining in the human hippocampus and parahippocampal gyrus. *J. Comp. Neurol.* 273, 488-99.

[82] Prudent, V., Kumar, A., Liu, S., Wiggins, G., Malaspina, D., Gonen, O. 2010. Human hippocampal subfields in young adults at 7.0 T: *Feasibility of imaging. Radiology* 254, 900-6.

Editor's Contact Information

Feng-Ru Tang
Radiation Physiology Laboratory, Singapore
Nuclear Research and Safety Initiative,
National University of Singapore, Singapore
Email: tangfr@gmail.com

INDEX

A

B

C

D

E

F

G

H

I

L

M

N

O

P

R

S

T

V

W

X